FREE Study Skills DVD Offer

Dear Customer,

Thank you for your purchase from Mometrix! We consider it an honor and a privilege that you have purchased our product and we want to ensure your satisfaction.

As a way of showing our appreciation and to help us better serve you, we have developed a Study Skills DVD that we would like to give you for <u>FREE</u>. This DVD covers our *best practices* for getting ready for your exam, from how to use our study materials to how to best prepare for the day of the test.

All that we ask is that you email us with feedback that would describe your experience so far with our product. Good, bad, or indifferent, we want to know what you think!

To get your FREE Study Skills DVD, email <u>freedvd@mometrix.com</u> with *FREE STUDY SKILLS DVD* in the subject line and the following information in the body of the email:

- The name of the product you purchased.
- Your product rating on a scale of 1-5, with 5 being the highest rating.
- Your feedback. It can be long, short, or anything in between. We just want to know your impressions and experience so far with our product. (Good feedback might include how our study material met your needs and ways we might be able to make it even better. You could highlight features that you found helpful or features that you think we should add.)
- Your full name and shipping address where you would like us to send your free DVD.

If you have any questions or concerns, please don't hesitate to contact me directly.

Thanks again!

Sincerely,

Jay Willis
Vice President
<u>jay.willis@mometrix.com</u>
1-800-673-8175

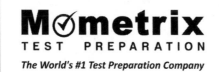

Paramedic
Exam
SECRETS

Study Guide
Your Key to Exam Success

Paramedic Test Review for the
NREMT Paramedic Exam

Published by
Mometrix Test Preparation
Mometrix Paramedic Certification Test Team

Written and edited by the Mometrix Paramedic Certification Test Team

Printed in the United States of America

This paper meets the requirements of ANSI/NISO Z39.48-1992 (Permanence of Paper).

Mometrix offers volume discount pricing to institutions. For more information or a price quote, please contact our sales department at sales@mometrix.com or 888-248-1219.

Mometrix Media LLC is not affiliated with or endorsed by any official testing organization. All organizational and test names are trademarks of their respective owners.

ISBN 13: 978-1-62733-888-2
ISBN 10: 1-62733-888-8

Dear Future Exam Success Story:

First of all, **THANK YOU** for purchasing Mometrix study materials!

Second, congratulations! You are one of the few determined test-takers who are committed to doing whatever it takes to excel on your exam. **You have come to the right place.** We developed these study materials with one goal in mind: to deliver you the information you need in a format that's concise and easy to use.

In addition to optimizing your guide for the content of the test, we've outlined our recommended steps for breaking down the preparation process into small, attainable goals so you can make sure you stay on track.

We've also analyzed the entire test-taking process, identifying the most common pitfalls and showing how you can overcome them and be ready for any curveball the test throws you.

Standardized testing is one of the biggest obstacles on your road to success, which only increases the importance of doing well in the high-pressure, high-stakes environment of test day. Your results on this test could have a significant impact on your future, and this guide provides the information and practical advice to help you achieve your full potential on test day.

Your success is our success

We would love to hear from you! If you would like to share the story of your exam success or if you have any questions or comments in regard to our products, please contact us at **800-673-8175** or **support@mometrix.com**.

Thanks again for your business and we wish you continued success!

Sincerely,
The Mometrix Test Preparation Team

Need more help? Check out our flashcards at: http://MometrixFlashcards.com/EMT

TABLE OF CONTENTS

INTRODUCTION 1

SECRET KEY #1 – PLAN BIG, STUDY SMALL 2
INFORMATION ORGANIZATION 2
TIME MANAGEMENT 2
STUDY ENVIRONMENT 2

SECRET KEY #2 – MAKE YOUR STUDYING COUNT 3
RETENTION 3
MODALITY 3

SECRET KEY #3 – PRACTICE THE RIGHT WAY 4
PRACTICE TEST STRATEGY 5

SECRET KEY #4 – PACE YOURSELF 6

SECRET KEY #5 – HAVE A PLAN FOR GUESSING 7
WHEN TO START THE GUESSING PROCESS 7
HOW TO NARROW DOWN THE CHOICES 8
WHICH ANSWER TO CHOOSE 9

TEST-TAKING STRATEGIES 10
QUESTION STRATEGIES 10
ANSWER CHOICE STRATEGIES 11
GENERAL STRATEGIES 12
FINAL NOTES 13

PREPARATORY 15

ANATOMY AND PHYSIOLOGY 42

LIFE SPAN DEVELOPMENT 44

PUBLIC HEALTH 45

PHARMACOLOGY 46

AIRWAY MANAGEMENT, RESPIRATIONS AND ARTIFICIAL VENTILATION 49

ASSESSMENT 63

MEDICINE 72

SHOCK AND RESUSCITATION 131

TRAUMA 137

SPECIAL PATIENT POPULATIONS 166

EMS OPERATIONS 180

PARAMEDIC PRACTICE TEST 197

ANSWER KEY AND EXPLANATIONS 219

HOW TO OVERCOME TEST ANXIETY 234
CAUSES OF TEST ANXIETY 234
ELEMENTS OF TEST ANXIETY 235
EFFECTS OF TEST ANXIETY 235

PHYSICAL STEPS FOR BEATING TEST ANXIETY 236
MENTAL STEPS FOR BEATING TEST ANXIETY 237
STUDY STRATEGY...238
TEST TIPS...240
IMPORTANT QUALIFICATION 241

THANK YOU..**242**

ADDITIONAL BONUS MATERIAL..**243**

Introduction

Thank you for purchasing this resource! You have made the choice to prepare yourself for a test that could have a huge impact on your future, and this guide is designed to help you be fully ready for test day. Obviously, it's important to have a solid understanding of the test material, but you also need to be prepared for the unique environment and stressors of the test, so that you can perform to the best of your abilities.

For this purpose, the first section that appears in this guide is the **Secret Keys**. We've devoted countless hours to meticulously researching what works and what doesn't, and we've boiled down our findings to the five most impactful steps you can take to improve your performance on the test. We start at the beginning with study planning and move through the preparation process, all the way to the testing strategies that will help you get the most out of what you know when you're finally sitting in front of the test.

We recommend that you start preparing for your test as far in advance as possible. However, if you've bought this guide as a last-minute study resource and only have a few days before your test, we recommend that you skip over the first two Secret Keys since they address a long-term study plan.

If you struggle with **test anxiety**, we strongly encourage you to check out our recommendations for how you can overcome it. Test anxiety is a formidable foe, but it can be beaten, and we want to make sure you have the tools you need to defeat it.

Secret Key #1 – Plan Big, Study Small

There's a lot riding on your performance. If you want to ace this test, you're going to need to keep your skills sharp and the material fresh in your mind. You need a plan that lets you review everything you need to know while still fitting in your schedule. We'll break this strategy down into three categories.

Information Organization

Start with the information you already have: the official test outline. From this, you can make a complete list of all the concepts you need to cover before the test. Organize these concepts into groups that can be studied together, and create a list of any related vocabulary you need to learn so you can brush up on any difficult terms. You'll want to keep this vocabulary list handy once you actually start studying since you may need to add to it along the way.

Time Management

Once you have your set of study concepts, decide how to spread them out over the time you have left before the test. Break your study plan into small, clear goals so you have a manageable task for each day and know exactly what you're doing. Then just focus on one small step at a time. When you manage your time this way, you don't need to spend hours at a time studying. Studying a small block of content for a short period each day helps you retain information better and avoid stressing over how much you have left to do. You can relax knowing that you have a plan to cover everything in time. In order for this strategy to be effective though, you have to start studying early and stick to your schedule. Avoid the exhaustion and futility that comes from last-minute cramming!

Study Environment

The environment you study in has a big impact on your learning. Studying in a coffee shop, while probably more enjoyable, is not likely to be as fruitful as studying in a quiet room. It's important to keep distractions to a minimum. You're only planning to study for a short block of time, so make the most of it. Don't pause to check your phone or get up to find a snack. It's also important to **avoid multitasking**. Research has consistently shown that multitasking will make your studying dramatically less effective. Your study area should also be comfortable and well-lit so you don't have the distraction of straining your eyes or sitting on an uncomfortable chair.

The time of day you study is also important. You want to be rested and alert. Don't wait until just before bedtime. Study when you'll be most likely to comprehend and remember. Even better, if you know what time of day your test will be, set that time aside for study. That way your brain will be used to working on that subject at that specific time and you'll have a better chance of recalling information.

Finally, it can be helpful to team up with others who are studying for the same test. Your actual studying should be done in as isolated an environment as possible, but the work of organizing the information and setting up the study plan can be divided up. In between study sessions, you can discuss with your teammates the concepts that you're all studying and quiz each other on the details. Just be sure that your teammates are as serious about the test as you are. If you find that your study time is being replaced with social time, you might need to find a new team.

Secret Key #2 – Make Your Studying Count

You're devoting a lot of time and effort to preparing for this test, so you want to be absolutely certain it will pay off. This means doing more than just reading the content and hoping you can remember it on test day. It's important to make every minute of study count. There are two main areas you can focus on to make your studying count:

Retention

It doesn't matter how much time you study if you can't remember the material. You need to make sure you are retaining the concepts. To check your retention of the information you're learning, try recalling it at later times with minimal prompting. Try carrying around flashcards and glance at one or two from time to time or ask a friend who's also studying for the test to quiz you.

To enhance your retention, look for ways to put the information into practice so that you can apply it rather than simply recalling it. If you're using the information in practical ways, it will be much easier to remember. Similarly, it helps to solidify a concept in your mind if you're not only reading it to yourself but also explaining it to someone else. Ask a friend to let you teach them about a concept you're a little shaky on (or speak aloud to an imaginary audience if necessary). As you try to summarize, define, give examples, and answer your friend's questions, you'll understand the concepts better and they will stay with you longer. Finally, step back for a big picture view and ask yourself how each piece of information fits with the whole subject. When you link the different concepts together and see them working together as a whole, it's easier to remember the individual components.

Finally, practice showing your work on any multi-step problems, even if you're just studying. Writing out each step you take to solve a problem will help solidify the process in your mind, and you'll be more likely to remember it during the test.

Modality

Modality simply refers to the means or method by which you study. Choosing a study modality that fits your own individual learning style is crucial. No two people learn best in exactly the same way, so it's important to know your strengths and use them to your advantage.

For example, if you learn best by visualization, focus on visualizing a concept in your mind and draw an image or a diagram. Try color-coding your notes, illustrating them, or creating symbols that will trigger your mind to recall a learned concept. If you learn best by hearing or discussing information, find a study partner who learns the same way or read aloud to yourself. Think about how to put the information in your own words. Imagine that you are giving a lecture on the topic and record yourself so you can listen to it later.

For any learning style, flashcards can be helpful. Organize the information so you can take advantage of spare moments to review. Underline key words or phrases. Use different colors for different categories. Mnemonic devices (such as creating a short list in which every item starts with the same letter) can also help with retention. Find what works best for you and use it to store the information in your mind most effectively and easily.

Secret Key #3 – Practice the Right Way

Your success on test day depends not only on how many hours you put into preparing, but also on whether you prepared the right way. It's good to check along the way to see if your studying is paying off. One of the most effective ways to do this is by taking practice tests to evaluate your progress. Practice tests are useful because they show exactly where you need to improve. Every time you take a practice test, pay special attention to these three groups of questions:

- The questions you got wrong
- The questions you had to guess on, even if you guessed right
- The questions you found difficult or slow to work through

This will show you exactly what your weak areas are, and where you need to devote more study time. Ask yourself why each of these questions gave you trouble. Was it because you didn't understand the material? Was it because you didn't remember the vocabulary? Do you need more repetitions on this type of question to build speed and confidence? Dig into those questions and figure out how you can strengthen your weak areas as you go back to review the material.

Additionally, many practice tests have a section explaining the answer choices. It can be tempting to read the explanation and think that you now have a good understanding of the concept. However, an explanation likely only covers part of the question's broader context. Even if the explanation makes sense, **go back and investigate** every concept related to the question until you're positive you have a thorough understanding.

As you go along, keep in mind that the practice test is just that: practice. Memorizing these questions and answers will not be very helpful on the actual test because it is unlikely to have any of the same exact questions. If you only know the right answers to the sample questions, you won't be prepared for the real thing. **Study the concepts** until you understand them fully, and then you'll be able to answer any question that shows up on the test.

It's important to wait on the practice tests until you're ready. If you take a test on your first day of study, you may be overwhelmed by the amount of material covered and how much you need to learn. Work up to it gradually.

On test day, you'll need to be prepared for answering questions, managing your time, and using the test-taking strategies you've learned. It's a lot to balance, like a mental marathon that will have a big impact on your future. Like training for a marathon, you'll need to start slowly and work your way up. When test day arrives, you'll be ready.

Start with the strategies you've read in the first two Secret Keys—plan your course and study in the way that works best for you. If you have time, consider using multiple study resources to get different approaches to the same concepts. It can be helpful to see difficult concepts from more than one angle. Then find a good source for practice tests. Many times, the test website will suggest potential study resources or provide sample tests.

Practice Test Strategy

When you're ready to start taking practice tests, follow this strategy:

Untimed and Open-Book Practice

Take the first test with no time constraints and with your notes and study guide handy. Take your time and focus on applying the strategies you've learned.

Timed and Open-Book Practice

Take the second practice test open-book as well, but set a timer and practice pacing yourself to finish in time.

Timed and Closed-Book Practice

Take any other practice tests as if it were test day. Set a timer and put away your study materials. Sit at a table or desk in a quiet room, imagine yourself at the testing center, and answer questions as quickly and accurately as possible.

Keep repeating timed and closed-book tests on a regular basis until you run out of practice tests or it's time for the actual test. Your mind will be ready for the schedule and stress of test day, and you'll be able to focus on recalling the material you've learned.

Secret Key #4 – Pace Yourself

Once you're fully prepared for the material on the test, your biggest challenge on test day will be managing your time. Just knowing that the clock is ticking can make you panic even if you have plenty of time left. Work on pacing yourself so you can build confidence against the time constraints of the exam. Pacing is a difficult skill to master, especially in a high-pressure environment, so **practice is vital**.

Set time expectations for your pace based on how much time is available. For example, if a section has 60 questions and the time limit is 30 minutes, you know you have to average 30 seconds or less per question in order to answer them all. Although 30 seconds is the hard limit, set 25 seconds per question as your goal, so you reserve extra time to spend on harder questions. When you budget extra time for the harder questions, you no longer have any reason to stress when those questions take longer to answer.

Don't let this time expectation distract you from working through the test at a calm, steady pace, but keep it in mind so you don't spend too much time on any one question. Recognize that taking extra time on one question you don't understand may keep you from answering two that you do understand later in the test. If your time limit for a question is up and you're still not sure of the answer, mark it and move on, and come back to it later if the time and the test format allow. If the testing format doesn't allow you to return to earlier questions, just make an educated guess; then put it out of your mind and move on.

On the easier questions, be careful not to rush. It may seem wise to hurry through them so you have more time for the challenging ones, but it's not worth missing one if you know the concept and just didn't take the time to read the question fully. Work efficiently but make sure you understand the question and have looked at all of the answer choices, since more than one may seem right at first.

Even if you're paying attention to the time, you may find yourself a little behind at some point. You should speed up to get back on track, but do so wisely. Don't panic; just take a few seconds less on each question until you're caught up. Don't guess without thinking, but do look through the answer choices and eliminate any you know are wrong. If you can get down to two choices, it is often worthwhile to guess from those. Once you've chosen an answer, move on and don't dwell on any that you skipped or had to hurry through. If a question was taking too long, chances are it was one of the harder ones, so you weren't as likely to get it right anyway.

On the other hand, if you find yourself getting ahead of schedule, it may be beneficial to slow down a little. The more quickly you work, the more likely you are to make a careless mistake that will affect your score. You've budgeted time for each question, so don't be afraid to spend that time. Practice an efficient but careful pace to get the most out of the time you have.

Secret Key #5 – Have a Plan for Guessing

When you're taking the test, you may find yourself stuck on a question. Some of the answer choices seem better than others, but you don't see the one answer choice that is obviously correct. What do you do?

The scenario described above is very common, yet most test takers have not effectively prepared for it. Developing and practicing a plan for guessing may be one of the single most effective uses of your time as you get ready for the exam.

In developing your plan for guessing, there are three questions to address:

- When should you start the guessing process?
- How should you narrow down the choices?
- Which answer should you choose?

When to Start the Guessing Process

Unless your plan for guessing is to select C every time (which, despite its merits, is not what we recommend), you need to leave yourself enough time to apply your answer elimination strategies. Since you have a limited amount of time for each question, that means that if you're going to give yourself the best shot at guessing correctly, you have to decide quickly whether or not you will guess.

Of course, the best-case scenario is that you don't have to guess at all, so first, see if you can answer the question based on your knowledge of the subject and basic reasoning skills. Focus on the key words in the question and try to jog your memory of related topics. Give yourself a chance to bring the knowledge to mind, but once you realize that you don't have (or you can't access) the knowledge you need to answer the question, it's time to start the guessing process.

It's almost always better to start the guessing process too early than too late. It only takes a few seconds to remember something and answer the question from knowledge. Carefully eliminating wrong answer choices takes longer. Plus, going through the process of eliminating answer choices can actually help jog your memory.

Summary: Start the guessing process as soon as you decide that you can't answer the question based on your knowledge.

How to Narrow Down the Choices

The next chapter in this book (**Test-Taking Strategies**) includes a wide range of strategies for how to approach questions and how to look for answer choices to eliminate. You will definitely want to read those carefully, practice them, and figure out which ones work best for you. Here though, we're going to address a mindset rather than a particular strategy.

Your chances of guessing an answer correctly depend on how many options you are choosing from.

How many choices you have	How likely you are to guess correctly
5	20%
4	25%
3	33%
2	50%
1	100%

You can see from this chart just how valuable it is to be able to eliminate incorrect answers and make an educated guess, but there are two things that many test takers do that cause them to miss out on the benefits of guessing:

- Accidentally eliminating the correct answer
- Selecting an answer based on an impression

We'll look at the first one here, and the second one in the next section.

To avoid accidentally eliminating the correct answer, we recommend a thought exercise called **the $5 challenge**. In this challenge, you only eliminate an answer choice from contention if you are willing to bet $5 on it being wrong. Why $5? Five dollars is a small but not insignificant amount of money. It's an amount you could afford to lose but wouldn't want to throw away. And while losing $5 once might not hurt too much, doing it twenty times will set you back $100. In the same way, each small decision you make—eliminating a choice here, guessing on a question there—won't by itself impact your score very much, but when you put them all together, they can make a big difference. By holding each answer choice elimination decision to a higher standard, you can reduce the risk of accidentally eliminating the correct answer.

The $5 challenge can also be applied in a positive sense: If you are willing to bet $5 that an answer choice *is* correct, go ahead and mark it as correct.

Summary: Only eliminate an answer choice if you are willing to bet $5 that it is wrong.

Which Answer to Choose

You're taking the test. You've run into a hard question and decided you'll have to guess. You've eliminated all the answer choices you're willing to bet $5 on. Now you have to pick an answer. Why do we even need to talk about this? Why can't you just pick whichever one you feel like when the time comes?

The answer to these questions is that if you don't come into the test with a plan, you'll rely on your impression to select an answer choice, and if you do that, you risk falling into a trap. The test writers know that everyone who takes their test will be guessing on some of the questions, so they intentionally write wrong answer choices to seem plausible. You still have to pick an answer though, and if the wrong answer choices are designed to look right, how can you ever be sure that you're not falling for their trap? The best solution we've found to this dilemma is to take the decision out of your hands entirely. Here is the process we recommend:

Once you've eliminated any choices that you are confident (willing to bet $5) are wrong, select the first remaining choice as your answer.

Whether you choose to select the first remaining choice, the second, or the last, the important thing is that you use some preselected standard. Using this approach guarantees that you will not be enticed into selecting an answer choice that looks right, because you are not basing your decision on how the answer choices look.

This is not meant to make you question your knowledge. Instead, it is to help you recognize the difference between your knowledge and your impressions. There's a huge difference between thinking an answer is right because of what you know, and thinking an answer is right because it looks or sounds like it should be right.

Summary: To ensure that your selection is appropriately random, make a predetermined selection from among all answer choices you have not eliminated.

Test-Taking Strategies

This section contains a list of test-taking strategies that you may find helpful as you work through the test. By taking what you know and applying logical thought, you can maximize your chances of answering any question correctly!

It is very important to realize that every question is different and every person is different: no single strategy will work on every question, and no single strategy will work for every person. That's why we've included all of them here, so you can try them out and determine which ones work best for different types of questions and which ones work best for you.

Question Strategies

Read Carefully

Read the question and answer choices carefully. Don't miss the question because you misread the terms. You have plenty of time to read each question thoroughly and make sure you understand what is being asked. Yet a happy medium must be attained, so don't waste too much time. You must read carefully, but efficiently.

Contextual Clues

Look for contextual clues. If the question includes a word you are not familiar with, look at the immediate context for some indication of what the word might mean. Contextual clues can often give you all the information you need to decipher the meaning of an unfamiliar word. Even if you can't determine the meaning, you may be able to narrow down the possibilities enough to make a solid guess at the answer to the question.

Prefixes

If you're having trouble with a word in the question or answer choices, try dissecting it. Take advantage of every clue that the word might include. Prefixes and suffixes can be a huge help. Usually they allow you to determine a basic meaning. Pre- means before, post- means after, pro - is positive, de- is negative. From prefixes and suffixes, you can get an idea of the general meaning of the word and try to put it into context.

Hedge Words

Watch out for critical hedge words, such as *likely, may, can, sometimes, often, almost, mostly, usually, generally, rarely,* and *sometimes.* Question writers insert these hedge phrases to cover every possibility. Often an answer choice will be wrong simply because it leaves no room for exception. Be on guard for answer choices that have definitive words such as *exactly* and *always.*

Switchback Words

Stay alert for *switchbacks.* These are the words and phrases frequently used to alert you to shifts in thought. The most common switchback words are *but, although,* and *however.* Others include *nevertheless, on the other hand, even though, while, in spite of, despite, regardless of.* Switchback words are important to catch because they can change the direction of the question or an answer choice.

Face Value

When in doubt, use common sense. Accept the situation in the problem at face value. Don't read too much into it. These problems will not require you to make wild assumptions. If you have to go beyond creativity and warp time or space in order to have an answer choice fit the question, then you should move on and consider the other answer choices. These are normal problems rooted in reality. The applicable relationship or explanation may not be readily apparent, but it is there for you to figure out. Use your common sense to interpret anything that isn't clear.

Answer Choice Strategies

Answer Selection

The most thorough way to pick an answer choice is to identify and eliminate wrong answers until only one is left, then confirm it is the correct answer. Sometimes an answer choice may immediately seem right, but be careful. The test writers will usually put more than one reasonable answer choice on each question, so take a second to read all of them and make sure that the other choices are not equally obvious. As long as you have time left, it is better to read every answer choice than to pick the first one that looks right without checking the others.

Answer Choice Families

An answer choice family consists of two (in rare cases, three) answer choices that are very similar in construction and cannot all be true at the same time. If you see two answer choices that are direct opposites or parallels, one of them is usually the correct answer. For instance, if one answer choice says that quantity x increases and another either says that quantity x decreases (opposite) or says that quantity y increases (parallel), then those answer choices would fall into the same family. An answer choice that doesn't match the construction of the answer choice family is more likely to be incorrect. Most questions will not have answer choice families, but when they do appear, you should be prepared to recognize them.

Eliminate Answers

Eliminate answer choices as soon as you realize they are wrong, but make sure you consider all possibilities. If you are eliminating answer choices and realize that the last one you are left with is also wrong, don't panic. Start over and consider each choice again. There may be something you missed the first time that you will realize on the second pass.

Avoid Fact Traps

Don't be distracted by an answer choice that is factually true but doesn't answer the question. You are looking for the choice that answers the question. Stay focused on what the question is asking for so you don't accidentally pick an answer that is true but incorrect. Always go back to the question and make sure the answer choice you've selected actually answers the question and is not merely a true statement.

Extreme Statements

In general, you should avoid answers that put forth extreme actions as standard practice or proclaim controversial ideas as established fact. An answer choice that states the "process should be used in certain situations, if..." is much more likely to be correct than one that states the "process should be discontinued completely." The first is a calm rational statement and doesn't even make a definitive, uncompromising stance, using a hedge word *if* to provide wiggle room, whereas the second choice is a radical idea and far more extreme.

Benchmark

As you read through the answer choices and you come across one that seems to answer the question well, mentally select that answer choice. This is not your final answer, but it's the one that will help you evaluate the other answer choices. The one that you selected is your benchmark or standard for judging each of the other answer choices. Every other answer choice must be compared to your benchmark. That choice is correct until proven otherwise by another answer choice beating it. If you find a better answer, then that one becomes your new benchmark. Once you've decided that no other choice answers the question as well as your benchmark, you have your final answer.

Predict the Answer

Before you even start looking at the answer choices, it is often best to try to predict the answer. When you come up with the answer on your own, it is easier to avoid distractions and traps because you will know exactly what to look for. The right answer choice is unlikely to be word-for-word what you came up with, but it should be a close match. Even if you are confident that you have the right answer, you should still take the time to read each option before moving on.

General Strategies

Tough Questions

If you are stumped on a problem or it appears too hard or too difficult, don't waste time. Move on! Remember though, if you can quickly check for obviously incorrect answer choices, your chances of guessing correctly are greatly improved. Before you completely give up, at least try to knock out a couple of possible answers. Eliminate what you can and then guess at the remaining answer choices before moving on.

Check Your Work

Since you will probably not know every term listed and the answer to every question, it is important that you get credit for the ones that you do know. Don't miss any questions through careless mistakes. If at all possible, try to take a second to look back over your answer selection and make sure you've selected the correct answer choice and haven't made a costly careless mistake (such as marking an answer choice that you didn't mean to mark). This quick double check should more than pay for itself in caught mistakes for the time it costs.

Pace Yourself

It's easy to be overwhelmed when you're looking at a page full of questions; your mind is confused and full of random thoughts, and the clock is ticking down faster than you would like. Calm down and maintain the pace that you have set for yourself. Especially as you get down to the last few minutes of the test, don't let the small numbers on the clock make you panic. As long as you are on track by monitoring your pace, you are guaranteed to have time for each question.

Don't Rush

It is very easy to make errors when you are in a hurry. Maintaining a fast pace in answering questions is pointless if it makes you miss questions that you would have gotten right otherwise. Test writers like to include distracting information and wrong answers that seem right. Taking a little extra time to avoid careless mistakes can make all the difference in your test score. Find a pace that allows you to be confident in the answers that you select.

Keep Moving

Panicking will not help you pass the test, so do your best to stay calm and keep moving. Taking deep breaths and going through the answer elimination steps you practiced can help to break through a stress barrier and keep your pace.

Final Notes

The combination of a solid foundation of content knowledge and the confidence that comes from practicing your plan for applying that knowledge is the key to maximizing your performance on test day. As your foundation of content knowledge is built up and strengthened, you'll find that the strategies included in this chapter become more and more effective in helping you quickly sift through the distractions and traps of the test to isolate the correct answer.

Now it's time to move on to the test content chapters of this book, but be sure to keep your goal in mind. As you read, think about how you will be able to apply this information on the test. If you've already seen sample questions for the test and you have an idea of the question format and style, try to come up with questions of your own that you can answer based on what you're reading. This will give you valuable practice applying your knowledge in the same ways you can expect to on test day.

Good luck and good studying!

Preparatory

EMS history

Historically, the first use of an ambulance was in the Siege of Málaga in Spain in 1487. Napoleon Bonaparte assigned battlefield vehicles and attendants in 1793, but the first use of medics and ambulances in the United States was in 1860, with the first ambulance service operating in 1869 in New York City. Hospital-based ambulance services increased in the 1900s, but many hospital ambulance services shut down during World War II, so fire and police departments filled the roles, but there were no laws regarding minimum training. Following World War II, the use of ambulance services increased, but the quality was often poor until basic training standards were developed in 1968 along with the 9-1-1 emergency system. The first paramedic program was developed in 1969, and the use of helicopters in rescues was explored in 1970. The EMS Systems Act was passed in 1973, the EMS for Children Act in 1983, and the Trauma Care Systems Planning and Development Act in 1990. In 1991, standards and benchmarks for ambulance services were established by the Commission on Accreditation of Ambulance Services.

EMS systems

The National Highway Traffic Safety Administration (NHTSA) is the lead agency for coordinating and promoting evidence-based emergency medical services (EMS) (fire based, third service, and hospital based) and the 9-1-1 system. The public safety answering point (PSAP) is the designated call-receiving site that directs calls to the appropriate emergency services. Each state defines the scope of practice, licensure, and credentialing for prehospital personnel and sets education standards based on national EMS standards. The paramedic is expected to maintain certification through the maintenance of skills and continuing education and should exhibit professional behavior, including working with integrity and empathy, being an effective member of a team, showing respect and tact, maintaining a professional appearance, communicating effectively, and advocating for patients. The paramedic must be alert to patient safety and recognize that most errors result from skills-based, rules-based, and knowledge-based failures. Error reduction requires the use of decision aids and protocols, asking for assistance when appropriate, questioning assumptions, and debriefing calls.

EMS service types and direct and indirect medical direction

EMS service types include the following:

- Fire based: EMS is provided by fire departments, but requirements vary. Some jurisdictions require all fire personnel to be EMTs or paramedics, whereas others may have varying requirements.
- Third service: EMS is a separate service from the fire and police departments, so personnel are not trained in fire suppression. EMS is sent out independently of other departments.
- Private: Profit and nonprofit companies/organizations manage EMS. EMS may vary widely in terms of training of personnel and equipment.
- Hospital based: They may be stationed at the hospital or at satellite areas, or they may be roving, depending on the area to be covered and available rigs.
- Hybrid: This is some combination of the above.

Medical direction types include the following:

- Online/Direct: The paramedic has voice contact via the phone or radio with an EMS physician who directs care and can assist in dealing with emergent problems.
- Offline/Indirect: The paramedic follows protocols established for care but does not have direct voice contact with an EMS physician.

Patient safety and high-risk situations

Up to 98,000 patients die each year because of medical errors. Patients are especially at risk of further injury or death in **high-risk situations and activities** such as the following:

- Hand-off: A standard procedure, such as SBAR, should be used, as follows:
  - (S) Situation: Overview of current situation and important issues.
  - (B) Background: Important history and issues leading to current situation.
  - Assessment: Summary of important facts and condition.
  - (R) Recommendation: Actions needed.
- Communications: Problems may result in delayed or inadequate care, wrong address, or wrong destination.
- Dropping: Patients can be easily dropped if the gurney isn't positioned properly or if too few personnel are involved in transport.
- Ambulance crashes: Unnecessary speeding and failing to stop at intersections are the most common causes of ambulance crashes.
- Inadequate spinal immobilization: If unsure, it's always best to immobilize.
- Medication errors: Administration of wrong medication, wrong mode of administration, and wrong dosage.

Continuous quality improvement (CQI)

Continuous Quality Improvement (CQI) emphasizes the organization and systems and processes within that organization rather than focusing on individuals. It recognizes internal customers (staff) and external customers (patients) and uses data to improve processes. CQI represents the concept that most processes can be improved. CQI uses the scientific method of experimentation to meet needs and improve services and uses various tools, such as brainstorming, multivoting, various charts and diagrams, storyboarding, and meetings. Core concepts include the following:

- Quality and success is meeting or exceeding internal and external customers' needs and expectations.
- Problems relate to processes, and variations in processes lead to variations in results.
- Change can be made in small steps.

Steps to CQI include the following:

- Forming a knowledgeable team.
- Identifying and defining measures used to determine success.
- Brainstorming strategies for change.
- Plan, collect, and use data as part of making decisions.
- Test changes and revise or refine as needed.

National EMS Education Agenda for the Future: A Systems Approach

The **National EMS Education Agenda for the Future: A Systems Approach** proposed an education system for EMS with five primary components, establishing the following goals for 2010 and 2020:

Core content: Core content to be developed by the EMS medical community, educators, and providers under the leadership of the National Highway Traffic Safety Administration (NHTSA) to ensure consistency of content and reciprocity of certification. The core content should be tied to licensure and accreditation.
Scope-of-practice model: National models to be used by states for all levels of EMS certification/licensure.
Education standards: Standards developed by EMS educators with input from the medical community and regulators and that are peer reviewed. Education program accreditation: A single national accreditation agency will develop standards and guidelines.
EMS certification: There are four levels of national certification with different educational requirements, standards, scopes of practice, and certification: (1) entry-level emergency medical responder (EMR), (2) next-level emergency medical technician (EMT), (3) advanced EMT (AEMT), and (4) paramedic.

Research

Research is especially important in identifying the need for change in procedures and protocols in order to improve patient outcomes. Research depends on the gathering of data. Data collection may include direct observations, surveys, interviews, and various other sources of information, such as documents and audiovisual materials. Literature research requires a comprehensive evaluation of current ($\leq$5 years) and/or historical information. Most literature research begins with an Internet search of databases, which provides listings of books, journals, and other materials on specific topics. Databases vary in content, and many contain only a reference listing with or without an abstract, so once the listing is obtained, the researcher must do a further search (publisher, library, etc.) to locate the material. Some databases require a subscription, but access is often available through educational or healthcare institutions. In order to search effectively, the researcher should begin by writing a brief explanation of the research to help identify possible keywords and synonyms to use as search words.

Qualitative and quantitative research

Qualitative and quantitative research methods are both used for research and analysis, but the focus is quite different.

- Qualitative: Data are described verbally or graphically, and the results are subjective, depending upon observers to provide information. Interviews and observations may be used as tools to gather information, and the researcher's interpretation of data is important. Gathering this type of data can be time intensive, and it usually cannot be generalized to a larger population. Analysis is done through summarizing and interpreting.
- Quantitative: Data are described in terms of numbers within a statistical format. This type of information gathering is done after the design of data collection is outlined, usually in later stages. Tools may include surveys, questionnaires, review of records, statistical analysis, and other methods of obtaining numerical data. The researcher's role is objective, and research may be experimental or nonexperimental.

Evidence-based decision making

Although traditional medical practice has been based on knowledge, intuition, and judgment, these practices have not always been supported by evidence. Outcomes-based research focuses on achieving positive outcomes. **Evidence-based decision making** results in best practices based on best evidence for procedures, medications, and treatments. Steps include the following:

- Formulating a question regarding treatment and/or procedures.
- Conducting a search of the appropriate medical literature (government sites, journal articles), often beginning with the search of an online database to find research that is related to the question.
- Determining the validity (measure of accuracy) and reliability (consistency) of the evidence. Evaluating the level of evidence (1a and 1b are the most valid, and 1c is required by state or federal regulations or is an industry standard).
- Assessing the data to determine if they apply to current needs.
- Drawing up a plan for change with input from all staff members.
- Implementing changes.
- Monitoring changes and outcomes.

Methods of data collection

When developing **data collection procedures** to determine needs, the following must be considered: the purpose of the data collection, the audience for which the data are intended, the types of questions to be answered, the scope of the research, and the resources available to carry out data collection.

Method	Issues regarding procedures
Direct observation	Observers must be selected and trained on how to observe and when and how to record observations.
Interviews	Interview questions must be developed and validated, and the interviewers must be given practice time.
Questionnaires	The type of questionnaire, the questions, and the Likert scale must be determined as well as the method of distribution (one-on-one, group, email, Internet).
Record review	A form or checklist should be developed to guide record review, and the records should be selected based on criteria established for the research.
Secondary analysis	The databases to be mined should be selected, and the criteria for the research should be established, including keywords, time frames, and populations.

Descriptive statistics and inferential statistics

Descriptive statistics organize raw data in a meaningful manner, such as through measures of central tendency (average, mean, median) and measures of spread (range, standard deviation, quartile, variance). These descriptive terms are referred to as parameters because they provide information about the entire population (group). Descriptive statistics may also be organized in various types of graphs, tables, and charts. **Inferential statistics** use sampling (a sample is a subset of a larger population) to arrive at conclusions about the population as a whole using data derived from the sample. So, the results from a sample of 1000 paramedics may be applied to all paramedics. However, if the sample does not accurately reflect the larger population, then a sampling error occurs. Sampling may be nonprobability (intentionally biased) or probability (nonbiased). Nonprobability sampling is not generalizable to an entire population, whereas probability sampling is generalizable to an entire population. Polling is an example of gathering inferential statistics.

PICOT

The **PICOT** format is one method of developing appropriate questions to use in searching quantitative research. This method helps clarify the question and necessary information and to identify keywords used in searching.

P	Patient/ Population	List important characteristics: 35-year-old male with low back pain.
I	Intervention/ Indicator	Explain the desired intervention under consideration: Acupuncture.
C	Comparison/ Control	List other possible interventions or alternatives: Surgery.
O	Outcome	Provide the desired measurable outcomes: Decreased pain levels (from 6–7 to 1–2) and increased mobility.
T	Time	Time frame (if appropriate).

This format is then used to formulate a question such as the following:

- In a 35-year-old male with low back pain, how does spinal immobilization compare to nonimmobilization regarding pain levels and mobility?

Based on this question, the search may be conducted with the following (including synonyms) phrasing: (back pain or sciatica) and (spinal immobilization or spinal nonimmobilization) and (pain management or pain free or pain control).

Human research subject protection

Protection of human subjects is covered in the Health and Human Services, Title 45 Code of Federal Regulations, part 46. This regulation provides guidance for institutional review boards (IRBs) for those involved in research and outlines requirements. Institutions engaged in nonexempt research must submit an assurance of compliance (document) to the Office for Human Research Protections (OHRP), agreeing to comply with all requirements for research projects. Subjects cannot be used solely as a means to an end, but research should hold the possibility of benefit to the subject. Risks should be minimal, and selection of subjects should be equitable. Some research populations are granted additional protections because of their vulnerability and susceptibility to coercion; these populations include children, prisoners, pregnant women, human fetuses and neonates, mentally disabled people, and people who are economically or educationally disadvantaged. When cooperative research projects are conducted involving more than one institution, then each must safeguard the rights of subjects, ensuring informed consent and privacy.

Informed consent

Patients or their families must provide **informed consent** for all treatments that they receive. This includes a thorough explanation of all procedures and treatment and the associated risks. Patients/families should be apprised of all options and allowed input on the type of treatments. Patients/families should be apprised of all reasonable risks and any complications that might be life threatening or increase morbidity.

The American Medical Association has established guidelines for informed consent as follows:

- Explanation of the diagnosis.
- Nature of and reason for the treatment or procedure.
- Risks and benefits.
- Alternative options (regardless of cost or insurance coverage).
- Risks and benefits of alternative options.
- Risks and benefits of not having a treatment or procedure.
- Providing informed consent is a requirement of all states.

The requirement for informed consent may be waived in life-threatening situations and if the paramedic cannot obtain informed consent because the patient cannot communicate and legal consent cannot be obtained.

Health Insurance Portability and Accountability Act of 1996 (HIPAA)

Sensitive information is classified under the **Health Insurance Portability and Accountability Act of 1996** (HIPAA) as protected health information (PHI) and it includes the following:

- Any information about an individual's past, present, or future health or condition (mental or physical).
- Provision of health care.
- Any identifying information related to payment for healthcare services.
- Identifying information: Name, address, Social Security number, birth date, and any document or material that contains the identifying information.

Personal information can be shared with a spouse, legal guardians, those with durable power of attorney for the patient, and those involved in the care of the patient, such as physicians, without a specific release. HIPAA mandates the following privacy and security rules to ensure that health information and individual privacy are protected:

- Privacy rule: Protected information includes any information included in the medical record (electronic or paper), conversations between the doctor and other healthcare providers, billing information, and any other form of health information.
- Security rule: Any electronic health information must be secure and protected against threats, hazards, or nonpermitted disclosure.

National EMS Research Agenda

The **National EMS Research Agenda** (2004) is a document published by the NHTSA and the Maternal and Child Health Bureau. The document stresses the need for EMS research to improve patient care and advance the profession, discusses a number of issues (such as the need for outcome measurement), and provides recommendations. The three domains of EMS research include the following:

- Clinical: Prehospital interventions.
- Systems: Components of the system, such as level of training and procedures for restocking supplies.
- Education: Suitability and adequacy of a curriculum.

Barriers to research include a lack of adequate funding. Funding sources include public, corporate, foundation, and state and federal grants. The document stresses the importance of changing the EMS culture to recognize the importance of research and the need for academic commitment to teaching research. Research must be carried out with informed consent and within the guidelines of human research subject protection.

Immunizations for EMS personnel

The Centers for Disease Control and Prevention (CDC) recommends the following **immunizations** for all healthcare workers, including EMS personnel:

- Hepatitis B: Three-dose series (now, in one month, and five months later) followed by an anti-HBs serologic test 30 to 60 days after the third immunization.
- Measles, mumps, rubella (MMR): Two-dose series with second immunization at least 28 days after the first for those born during or after 1957 and those born before 1957 without proof of immunity.
- Varicella (chickenpox): Two doses, four weeks apart. (A combined MMRV immunization is available.)
- Influenza: Annually.
- Tetanus, diphtheria, and pertussis (Tdap): One time with a tetanus (TD) booster every 10 years. The TD injection does not protect against pertussis (whooping cough).
- Meningococcal: One dose.

Screening for tuberculosis with a chest x-ray or skin test is also recommended.

CDC isolation guidelines

The **2007 CDC Guideline for Isolation Precautions** includes the standard precautions that apply to all patients and transmission-based precautions for those with known or suspected infections. **Standard precautions** should be used for all patients because all body fluids (sweat, urine, feces, blood, and sputum) and nonintact skin and mucous membranes may be infected.

Hand hygiene	Wash hands before and after each patient contact and after any contact with body fluids and contaminated items. Use soap and water for visible soiling.
Protective equipment	Use personal protective equipment (PPE), such as gloves, gowns, and masks, eye protection, and/or face shields, when anticipating contact with body fluids or contaminated skin.
Respiratory hygiene/ Cough etiquette	Use source-control measures, such as covering cough, disposing of tissues, using a surgical mask on the person coughing or on staff to prevent inhalation of droplets, and properly disposing of dressings and used equipment. Wash hands after contacting respiratory secretions. Maintain a distance of >3 feet from a coughing person when possible.
Sharps	Dispose of sharps, such as needles, carefully in sharps containers. Do not recap needles.

The **2007 CDC Guideline for Isolation Precautions** includes the standard precautions that apply to all patients and **transmission-based precautions** for those with known or suspected infections as well as those with excessive wound drainage, other discharge, or fecal incontinence. Transmission-based precautions include the following:

Contact	Use PPE, including gown and gloves, for all contacts with the patient or the patient's immediate environment.
Droplet	(Appropriate for influenza, streptococcus infection, pertussis, rhinovirus, and adenovirus and pathogens that remain viable and infectious for only short distances.) Use a mask while caring for the patient. Maintain patient >3 feet away from other patients (with a curtain separating them in an emergency department). Use a patient mask if transporting a patient.
Airborne	(Appropriate for measles, chickenpox, tuberculosis, and severe acute respiratory syndrome [SARS] because pathogens remain viable and infectious for long distances.) Use ≥N95 respirators (or masks) while caring for the patient. The patient should be placed in an airborne infection isolation room in an emergency department.

Hand hygiene and gloves

Hand hygiene should be done before eating, before and after direct contact with a patient's skin, after contact with any body fluids, after contact with inanimate objects in the patient's immediate vicinity, when moving hands from a dirty to a clean area, after removing gloves, and after using the restroom. Hand hygiene is carried out in the following two manners:

- Antiseptic soaps/detergents: For visible soiling, after exposure to diarrhea stool or a patient with diarrhea, before eating, and after using the restroom. Wet hands, apply product, rub hands together vigorously for 15 seconds covering all surfaces, rinse hands with water, and use a disposable towel to dry.
- Alcohol-based hand sanitizers (the most effective way to kill bacteria): For all other situations. Apply product and rub hands together, including between the fingers, for about 20 seconds until the skin surfaces are dry.

Gloves must be worn when touching any body fluids, nonintact skin, open wounds, or mucous membranes (eyes, mouth, nose); gloves should be changed when moving from a dirty area to a clean one or from one patient to another.

Personal protective equipment (PPE)

Personal protective equipment (PPE) should be readily available in the appropriate sizes for each EMS individual.

- Gowns: Should be worn for risk of splash or spray with body fluids (severe bleeding, childbirth) and should be fluid resistant.
- Eye protectors: Should be worn for risk of splash or spray with body fluids or contact with debris, such as at a worksite or in a collapsing building. Goggles should fit snugly and have antifog features. (Prescription eyeglasses do not take the place of goggles.)
- Face shields: Provide protection for the face, eyes, nose, and mouth. These are preferred to goggles when there is a risk of spray or splash of body fluids. They should wrap around and cover the forehead and extend to below the chin.
- Masks: Protect the nose and mouth from fluids and particles and should be fluid resistant, fit snugly, and have a flexible nosepiece.

- Respirators (such as N95, N99, and N100): Protect the nose, mouth, and airway passages exposed to hazardous or infectious aerosols, including bacteria (tuberculosis [TB], measles patients).

Procedures for exposure/contamination

Any **exposure/contamination** should be reported at hand-off and to the appropriate infection control person following protocols, and follow-up care should be sought if necessary. Decontamination procedures are as follows:

- Skin: Cleanse the area thoroughly with soap and water.
- Eyes: Flush with water for 20 minutes.
- Needlestick: Wash the area with soap and water and report immediately.
- Clothing: Remove the clothing as soon as possible, and wash visible soiling of skin with soap and water if a shower is not immediately available, but shower as soon as possible. Clothes should be washed separately in a washing machine at the workplace.
- Equipment/Vehicles: Clean thoroughly with disinfectant. Dispose of equipment if unable to adequately decontaminate it.

When reporting exposures/contamination, note the type of exposure, the date and time of exposure, circumstances, actions taken to decontaminate, and any other required information.

Dealing with stress

The paramedic must often deal with **stressful incidents**, such as dangerous situations (storm conditions, gunshots, falling debris); critically ill patients; unpleasant sights, sounds, and odors; multipatient incidents; and angry/upset patients, family members, and bystanders. The paramedic should not argue or become defensive but should remain calm and supportive, allowing the patient to express his or her feelings and trying to defuse the situation while administering medical care and cooperating with other first responders. If a patient has no pulse or respirations and does not have a valid do-not-resuscitate (DNR) order, the paramedic should attempt resuscitation unless doing so puts the paramedic at risk; the injuries are not compatible with life; or obvious signs of death are present, such as tissue decay, livor mortis, which is discoloration in the lowermost blood vessels from pooled blood shortly after death, or rigor mortis, which is stiffening of the joints that occurs within 2 to 6 hours of death (verified by checking two or more joints). After 24 to 48 hours of rigor mortis, the muscles become flaccid.

Warning signs of stress often begin with difficulty sleeping and nightmares about work, loss of appetite, and lack of interest in usual activities including work and intimacy. The individual may feel increasingly sad and depressed and may have difficulty concentrating, making decisions, and carrying out tasks. The individual may also begin to isolate from others and exhibit irritability with coworkers, family, and friends. Some individuals develop physical symptoms related to stress, such as stomach upset, headaches, nausea, and high blood pressure (BP), whereas others may experience panic attacks. Some individuals may try to self-medicate with alcohol or drugs. When experiencing the warning signs of stress, the individual should talk about the problems with someone trusted, such as a physician, coworker, supervisor, or family member, and he or she may need to seek assistance from a professional counselor. Lifestyle changes, such as decreasing the use of alcohol or drugs, exercising regularly, and practicing relaxation exercises, may help to relieve stress.

Stress reactions include:

- <u>Acute stress reaction:</u> This reaction usually occurs quickly (minutes to hours) in response to an event that is stressful (such as the death of a child or a multiple-casualty incident). The individual may experience physical symptoms (with the release of adrenaline), such as rapid pulse, nausea, chest tightness, headache, fast respirations, and increased perspiration. An acute stress reaction usually recedes quickly, but it may persist for weeks in some individuals.
- <u>Delayed stress reaction:</u> Although the individual may cope well with a stressful event initially, months later, the person may begin to have nightmares, anxiety, and other indications of post-traumatic stress.
- <u>Cumulative stress reaction:</u> This type of stress reaction occurs when the individual has repeated stressors (either in the workplace or in his or her personal life) that cause repeated acute stress reactions, resulting in various physical and psychological problems. This is especially common in EMS personnel.

End of life/death and dying

Grief is a normal response to the death or severe illness/abnormality of a patient. How a person deals with grief is very personal, and each will grieve differently. Elisabeth Kübler-Ross identified **five stages of grief**, which can apply to patients and family members. A person may not go through each stage, but he or she usually goes through two of the five stages.

Stage	Patient/Family	Appropriate paramedic response
Denial	Resistive to information, stunned, immobile, detached, unable to respond appropriately	Be patient and supportive and repeat information as needed.
Anger	Lashing out, overt hostility, self-blame, blaming others	Do not respond in anger or take statements personally. Remain calm and supportive, but be alert to risk of physical attack.
Bargaining	If–then thinking, demanding another opinion or expert, praying	Avoid making any judgmental statements.
Depression	Tearful, crying, withdrawn, sad, isolated	Encourage expression of feelings, remain supportive, and assure the individual that these feelings are normal.
Acceptance	Resolution	Listen patiently and remain supportive.

Prevention of response-related injuries

Prevention of response-related injuries includes the following:

- <u>Infectious diseases:</u> Use PPE and understand the spread of infectious diseases—air (coughing), direct contact (blood, vomitus, other body fluids), needlestick, contaminated food/equipment, and sexual transmission. Maintain current immunizations.
- <u>Personal habits:</u> Obtain adequate sleep, nutrition, and exercise. Avoid excessive alcohol and tobacco.
- <u>Environmental hazards:</u> Conduct a 360° assessment. Note traffic hazards, the vehicle's condition, fire, leaking fluids, downed power lines, hazardous materials (look for placards and warning symbols; avoid the area until it is cleared). Use PPE and respirators as indicated.

- **Violence:** Defuse situations, make a safe response (with the assistance of law enforcement), and use restraints if necessary for dangerous or violent individuals.
- **Collisions:** Drive safely; avoid speeding and driving through stop signs and red lights when possible. Wear seat belts and/or safety harnesses.

Signs and symbols

Sign/Symbol	Interpretation
	Flame: Includes flammable materials and gases and those that are self-heating or self-reactive.
	Corrosion: Includes substances that can cause skin burns, metal corrosion, and eye damage.
	Health hazard: Includes carcinogens, toxic substances, and respiratory irritants.
	Poison: Includes materials, gases, or substances that are extremely toxic and may result in death or severe illness.
	Irritant: Includes material, gases, or substances that are irritants to skin, eyes, and/or respiratory tract, are acutely toxic, or have a narcotic effect.
	Biohazard: Includes biological substances, such as body fluids, that pose a threat to humans. Appears on sharps containers that hold contaminated needles.

Body mechanics

Basic principles of body mechanics include the following:

- Avoid reaching for prolonged periods of time, overhead, or more than 20 inches away.
- Avoid pulling—push, roll, or slide instead.
- Avoid lifting—push, roll, or slide instead.
- Lift with the leg muscles, not with the back.
- Hold the weight close to your body rather than at arm's length.
- Flex at the hips and knees, not the waist.

- Carry patients head first upstairs and feet first downstairs.
- Maintain a straight back and avoid twisting.
- Assess weight and recognize limitations in lifting/carrying.
- Get help when necessary and communicate every step with your partner ("Lift on the count of three").
- Maintain a firm base of support with your feet apart (shoulder width) to stabilize your stance.
- Maintain the line of gravity (the imaginary line between your center of gravity and the ground) within the base of support.
- Position yourself close to an object that is to be lifted or carried.
- Lift patients from stable ground.

Techniques for moving and lifting patients

Techniques for moving patients include the following:

- Direct ground lift: Use only for lightweight individuals with no suspected spinal injuries. Three rescuers line up on one side of the patient, and each one kneels on the same knee. The paramedic at the head places one arm under the patient's neck and shoulder and the other arm under the patient's lower back. The middle paramedic places his or her arms above and below the patient's waist, and the paramedic at the patient's feet places his or her arms under the knees and lower legs. On the count of three, they roll the patient onto their knees and toward their chests. On the count of three, they stand and move the patient.
- Power lift: Place feet (shoulder width) apart and pointing slightly outward; tighten the back and abdominal muscles. Squat down as though sitting. Place hands 10 inches apart with the palms upward (power grip) while grasping the stretcher and lift with the upper body becoming vertical before the hips rise.
- Extremity lift: Requires two paramedics. One paramedic squats at the patient's head, and another is at one side by the patient's knees. The paramedic at the head folds the patient's arms across the chest and grasps the patient by wrapping both arms around the torso under the patient's arms and grasping the patient's wrists. The second paramedic slides his or her hands beneath the patient's knees and lower legs, and together they stand and lift the patient.
- Squat lift: Requires two paramedics. One paramedic squats with the back straight and the weak foot slightly forward at the head of patient, and the other paramedic is in the same position at the patient's feet. Grasp the patient's upper body as for the extremity lift and grasp the patient's feet. Both paramedics push up with the stronger foot and lift with the upper body becoming vertical before the hips rise.
- Logroll: Used to position carrying devices under the patient and for some transfers; it requires two paramedics positioned on the same side of the patient. Place the patient's arm on the side that he or she is being turned to above his or her head or over the chest. Place the patient's other arm across his or her chest. If on the ground, squat close to the patient. The paramedic at the patient's head reaches across the patient and grasps his or her shoulders and trunk while the second paramedic grasps his or her trunk and legs. On the count of three, they turn the patient in one smooth move.

- 26 -

- Draw-sheet transfer: Requires four paramedics with two positioned on one side of the patient and two positioned on the other side but on the opposite side of the bed or stretcher to which the patient will be transferred. The logroll technique is used to place a draw sheet under the patient. The paramedics on both sides roll the edges of the draw sheet until the edges are close to the patient. On the count of three, they lift the patient slightly and move the patient across to the bed.

Backboards and cervical collars

Backboards were originally designed to transfer patients. However, **backboards and cervical collars** have been routinely used for EMS rescues for many years without evidence-based studies supporting their use. The premise was that stabilizing the spine and neck would prevent further injury in case a spinal injury had occurred, but spinal injuries are relatively rare, and some studies indicate that these devices do not provide any protection and, in fact, may cause damage. Additionally, cervical collars restrict the airway by 20% or more and may worsen injuries if not properly sized for the patient. Because of these findings, some EMS no longer routinely use backboards but use a vacuum mattress in a scoop basket instead. The American Association of Neurological Surgeons/Congress of Neurological Surgeons (AANS/CNS) guidelines advise that spinal immobilization with a backboard be reserved for known or suspected spinal cord injury without penetrating injury, although the use of the cervical collar is still recommended until the cervical spine is assessed for injury. Short backboards may be used to support a patient's back in a sitting position.

Restraints

Restraints should be avoided if possible, although if a combative patient poses a risk to him- or herself or EMS personnel, restraints may be necessary to safely assess, treat, and transport the patient, keeping in mind that the altered state of consciousness may result from drug or alcohol use; traumatic injury; or from a mental or physical disorder, such as schizophrenia, dementia, or hypoglycemia (insulin reaction). Protocols for use of restraints must be followed, and restraints should be applied under medical direction. If possible, the police should be present and there should be one EMS personnel for each limb, staying beyond the limb's range of motion until ready to secure the limb, with one paramedic talking to the patient and explaining the procedure. The paramedic should avoid unnecessary force, which may result in increased combativeness and injury to the patient or others. Patients should not be restrained in the prone (face-down) position. Documentation must include the reason for restraining the patient, the time, and the method of restraint.

Common **types of physical restraints** include the following:

- Soft: Padded cuffs (often leather) that fasten about the wrists and ankles and are attached to a long board. These are the most commonly used restraints.
- Stretcher/Spinal board straps: These may be strapped across the chest (not too tight), abdomen, or legs to help restrict movement.
- Long board/Spinal board: The patient should be restrained to the long board and then placed on a wheeled stretcher and never tied to or fastened to the stretcher.
- Spit sock: A hood that fits over the patient's head to prevent him or her from biting or spitting.
- Cervical collar: This is used to protect the patient's cervical spine and to prevent him or her from biting.

The paramedic should not place the patient in handcuffs or hard plastic ties. If these were placed on a patient by a law enforcement officer and must stay in place, such as with a criminal or an extremely violent patient, then a law enforcement officer must stay with the patient at all times.

Emergency moves

Emergency moves may be needed if the patient and/or paramedic is in immediate danger from fire, explosives, or other hazards; if the patient requires life-saving treatment, such as cardiopulmonary resuscitation (CPR); or if the patient is in water, such as a pond or lake. Emergency moves include the following:

- Blanket drag: Logroll the patient onto a blanket, wrap the patient in the blanket, grasp the blanket near the patient's head while in a squatting position with your back straight, and drag. If there are two rescuers, the other one should be positioned at the patient's feet and should be pushing.
- Clothing drag: Squat down by the patient's head, securely grasp the clothing near the patient's neck or shoulders (avoid grasping by a T-shirt), and drag the patient.
- Arm drag: Squat down by the patient's head. Fold the patient's arms across his or her chest. Grasp the patient under the arms, wrapping your arms about the torso and grasping the patient's wrists to stabilize his or her arms. Drag the patient.
- Firefighter's drag: Tie the patient's wrists together with any available material. Straddle the patient and pull the patient's arms over your neck and then crawl forward, dragging him or her beneath you.
- Firefighter's carry: Grasp the patient's knees and pull them together and up. Stand on the patient's feet and reach out and grab one of the patient's arms with one hand. Pull the patient upright, and, as the patient elevates, place your other hand between the patient's legs. Place the patient's arm behind your neck and continue to pull the patient and lift until he or she is draped across your upper back with the arm hanging free. Then grasp the patient's arm that is hanging with the hand that is between the legs to secure the patient.

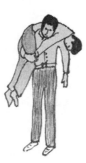

Urgent moves, such as with altered mental status, shock, or breathing difficulties, should also be done as quickly as possible.

Minimum data sets

Minimum data sets are the minimum data specifically required for EMS services. These consist of the following:

- Patient information: This derives from the assessment including the patient's primary complaint and the findings during the initial assessment, including the patient's name and address; vital signs (blood pressure [BP], pulse [P], respiration rate [R]); and descriptions of any wounds, injuries, pain, or other symptoms. The patient's demographics (age, gender, ethnic background) should be noted as well as any other identifying or essential information.
- Administrative information: This includes the time of the initial report, time the EMS unit was notified, time of arrival at the incident, time of leaving the scene, time of arrival at the destination (hospital, trauma center), and time of hand-off.
- Accurate/Synchronous clocks: All members of the EMS system should use accurate and synchronous clocks so that they all are set to the same time to ensure there is no disparity in time reporting.

Prehospital care report

The **prehospital care report** serves as a legal document to show that emergent care was provided. It describes the condition of the patient upon the paramedic's arrival at the scene, interventions provided, and changes in the patient's condition; it is essential to ensure continuity of care. The documenting paramedic may be called in to legal proceedings. The prehospital care report may also be used for educational purposes, such as through debriefing and case review. Additionally, the report is used administratively as the basis for billing as well as for the collection of data for research and evaluation of continuous quality improvement. Required elements of documentation include the time of events (receipt of call, arrival at incident, time of transport, arrival at destination), assessment findings (vital signs, injuries, bleeding, mental status), emergent care, changes in the patient's condition, response to the treatment provided, scene observations (specific place/area), hazards, and disposition of the patient (care refusal, transportation, hand-off). Documentation may be on paper or may be done electronically and may combine checkboxes and narrative reports. Run data are those data elements that are required for reporting of each run.

Patient refusal of medical care

According to the **Patient Self-Determination Act** (1990), competent patients have the right to refuse any medical treatment, and parents have the right to make this decision for minor children. If a patient refuses care, then the paramedic should try to persuade the patient to go to the hospital by giving the reasons and possible consequences of refusal. The patient should be asked to sign the refusal form, and a family member, police officer, or bystander should sign as a witness to the patient's signing or witness the patient's refusal to sign. The paramedic should complete documentation of any assessment carried out and any refusal of the patient to assessment. The paramedic should carefully document the conversation between the paramedic and patient regarding refusal of care and consequences and should document the proposed care as well as the information the paramedic gave the patient about alternate care (such as a visit to the patient's personal physician) and the willingness to return if the patient has a change of mind.

Special situations

Documentation errors: In handwritten documents, draw one line through the error, initial, and write the correct information beside the error. If information was omitted, add a note with the date and your initials. If documentation was electronic, follow the method prescribed for corrections.

Multiple-casualty incidents: Record information temporarily for later complete documentation, if necessary, following the procedures in place for such an incident.

Incident reports: Fill out forms as soon as possible, document any witnesses to the incident, and file forms according to protocol. Incident reports are often maintained separately from prehospital reports.

Special-situation reports: Used for events/incidents that must be reported to an outside authority or as a supplement to the prehospital report. Fill out the report as soon as possible, and include the names of all parties involved; use objective descriptions, and avoid stating conclusions. Maintain a personal copy.

Transfer reports: Ensure that they contain minimum data sets and provide a transfer signature. These are used during hand-off.

EMS system communication

With the paramedic's arrival at the scene of an incident, he or she should assess the situation and the need for added resources, such as additional EMS personnel or police, and contact the appropriate authorities to request assistance. When additional EMS personnel arrive or contact is made with medical control or the receiving facility, the paramedic should self-identify and provide a verbal report of the patient's current condition, including demographic information such as age and gender. The paramedic should report the patient's chief complaint and provide any history that is pertinent as well as the condition of the patient on arrival and any history of major illnesses. The paramedic should also report the results of the patient assessment, including the vital signs and any physical/psychological findings, as well as any treatment provided and the patient's response to the treatment. The paramedic should communicate with law enforcement officers and other responders, such as firefighters, especially regarding safety concerns.

Components of an EMS communication system include the base station of a two-way radio system, which is in a fixed location, such as a dispatch center. The base station facilitates communication among a number of handheld/mobile radios. There is often only one channel per base station, so additional base stations may be installed to add more channels. Radio transmitters/receivers may be vehicular mounted or mobile, although mobile transmitters/receivers may have a limited range because they tend to have lower power (1–5 watts) than do base stations (20–50 watts). Typically, the mobile device has a range of 10–15 miles over average terrain, but it is shorter in rugged terrain. The Federal Communications Commission (FCC) controls radio frequencies, and those used for EMS are in the public safety pool.

The paramedic may be in **communication with medical control** regarding a patient's condition and need for medication. Medical control may be at the receiving facility or at a separate site. Upon receiving an order by phone or radio, the paramedic should repeat back the order and dosage to ensure that the message was received correctly. When using the radio, the radio must be turned on and the press-to-talk (PTT) button must be pressed before beginning the transmission. The paramedic should address the medical control person by name and give the name of the paramedic's unit. Transmissions should be brief and to the point, avoiding unnecessary pleasantries, codes, agency-specific terms, profanity, and meaningless phrases, keeping in mind that the airways are public. The paramedic should give individual digits for long numbers, use "affirmative" and "negative" in place of "yes" and "no," and say "over" when the transmission is finished. Reports should be objective rather than opinion based and should avoid offering a diagnosis. The dispatcher must be notified when the unit leaves the scene.

Phone/cellular communication and interpersonal communication with patients

Phone/Cellular communication: This is similar to radio communication, but the paramedic should be familiar with important phone numbers (such as medical control, hospitals, trauma centers) or have the numbers prominently posted for access. The paramedic should also be aware of dead spots that may prevent communication and should have a backup plan (radio) for when cellular transmission fails. **Interpersonal communication:** Upon arrival at the scene of an incident, the paramedic should self-introduce, making eye contact, and he or she should communicate using language that the patient can understand, that is age-appropriate, and that avoids any medical jargon. The paramedic should be positioned at or below the level of the patient if possible to avoid intimidating the patient and should remain aware of body language. The paramedic should be honest and speak slowly and calmly, using the patient's first or last name, depending on the age of the patient and the circumstances. The paramedic may request interpreters if necessary.

Dynamics of the communication process

The **communication process**, which includes the sender-receiver feedback loop, is based on Claude Shannon's article, "A Mathematical Theory of Communication" (1948), in which he provided the basis for information theory and described three necessary steps of successful communication: encoding a message, transmitting it through a channel, and decoding it. The resultant communication process begins with the sender, who serves as the encoder and determines the content of the message. The medium is the form the message takes (digital, written, audiovisual), and the channel is the method of delivery (mail, radio, TV, phone, email, text message). The recipient (receiver), who acts as the decoder determines the meaning from the message. Feedback helps to determine whether or not the communication is successful and whether the message is understood as intended. This process is referred to as the sender-receiver feedback loop. Context is the environment (physical and psychological) in which the communication occurs, and interference is any factor that impacts the communication process. Interference may be external, (such as environmental noise) or internal (such as emotional distress or anxiety).

Effective communication and interviewing techniques

Effective communication begins with a self-introduction and an introduction of other team members to the patient and family and includes respecting the patient's privacy by shielding the patient from passersby if possible and avoiding loudly repeating any patient information. If possible, the paramedic should adjust lighting and limit outside distractions, such as noise. When interviewing the patient, the paramedic should ask open-ended questions (such as "Can you describe your pain?") and avoid questions that can be answered with "yes" or "no." The paramedic should ask direct questions, such as "When did the pain start?" Questions should be asked one at a time while allowing the patient/family time to respond. It's especially important to observe the patient's body language (posture, eye contact, gestures, and tone of voice) to determine if it matches his or her words and to avoid medical/professional jargon. The paramedic should avoid giving false reassurances or advice, and he or she should avoid leading/biased questions, being too talkative, interrupting the patient, and asking "why" questions, such as "Why did you take an overdose of medication?"

Special interview situations

Interviewing **hostile patients** requires a calm response, avoiding negative responses and using reflective statements, such as "I can understand your feelings." The paramedic should maintain eye contact (50%–60% of the time) and try to defuse the situation, but he or she should avoid staring or standing too close and having crossed arms because this may be misinterpreted as threatening behavior. If patients are **sexually aggressive**, it's important to tell them that the behavior is inappropriate and to ask them to stop. When interviewing patients under the **influence of drugs or alcohol,** try to ask essential questions, such as the type and amount of drug/alcohol ingested. Obtain information from family or friends if necessary. When patients are **hearing impaired**, the paramedic should face the person directly, speak slowly and distinctly (but avoid shouting), provide information in writing if possible, use pantomime, and try to reduce environmental noise. Knowledge of the alphabet in sign language can be very useful to communicate with the deaf, especially if a sign-language translator is unavailable. When **interviewing elderly patients**, the paramedic should be alert to possible cognitive, hearing, or vision impairments, especially if the patient appears confused upon questioning or his or her answers are inappropriate. The paramedic should ask if the patient has eyeglasses or a hearing aid and should obtain them if possible. The patient's family may be able to assist with the interview. If the patient's speech is unclear, he or she may need to put in dentures. When communicating with a **pediatric patient**, the paramedic should have the parent or caregiver comfort the child and answer questions, especially if the child is an infant or is very young. The paramedic should use simple sentences and age-appropriate language and explain to the child what he or she is doing to help alleviate the child's fear. Adolescents should be addressed directly even if a parent or caregiver is providing some information, and, in some cases, the adolescent will provide more information if the parent/caregiver is not present.

Cultural considerations

Hmong	• The eldest male in the family makes the decisions for the family and is deferred to by other family members, so the paramedic should ask who should receive information about the patient. • Communication should be polite and respectful, avoiding direct eye contact, which is considered rude. • Disagreeing is considered rude, so "yes" may mean "I hear you" and NOT "I agree with you."
Mexican	• Mexican culture perceives time with more flexibility than does American culture, so if patients/family need to be present at a particular time, the paramedic should specify the exact time ("be here at 1:30 PM") and explain the reason rather than saying something that is more vague, such as "be here after lunch." • People may appear to be unassertive or unable to make decisions when they are simply showing respect to the paramedic by being deferent. • In traditional families, the males make decisions, so a woman may wait for the husband or other males in the family to make decisions about her treatment or care.

Middle Eastern	• In Middle Eastern countries, males make the decisions, so issues for discussion or decision should be directed to males, such as the patient's spouse or son, and males may be direct in stating what they want, sometimes appearing demanding.
	• Middle Easterners often require less personal space and may stand very close.
	• If a male paramedic must care for a female patient, then the family should be advised that *only* medical treatments, not personal care, will be done by the male paramedic.
Asian	• Asian families may expect the paramedic to remain authoritative and to give directions and may not question the paramedic's authority.
	• Disagreeing is considered impolite. "Yes" may only mean that the person is heard, not that they agree with the person. When asked if they understand, they may indicate that they do even when they clearly do not so as not to offend the paramedic.
	• Asians may avoid eye contact as an indication of respect.

Cultural competence

There are a number of issues related to cultural competence in communicating with others.

- **Eye contact:** Many cultures use eye contact differently than what is common in the United States. Some patients and families, such as Asians, Native Americans, and Arabs, may avoid direct eye contact, considering it rude, or they may look away to signal disapproval, or they may look down to signal respect. Careful observation of the way family members use eye contact can help to determine what will be most comfortable for the patient/family.
- **Distance**: Some cultures stand close to others (<4 feet) when speaking (Middle Easterners, Hispanics), and others stand at a greater distance (>4 feet) (Northern Europeans, many Americans). There is a considerable difference relating to concepts of personal space among cultures. Allowing the family to approach or observing whether they tend to move closer, lean forward, or move back can help to determine a comfortable distance for communication.
- **Time**: Americans tend to be time oriented, and they expect people to be on time, but time is viewed more flexibly in many other cultures.

Therapeutic communication

Therapeutic communication begins with respect for the individual/family and the assumption that all communication, verbal and nonverbal, has meaning. Listening must be done empathetically. Techniques that facilitate communication include the following:

| Introduction | Make a personal introduction and use the individual's name: "Mrs. Brown, I am Toby Williams, your paramedic." |

Encouragement	Use an open-ended opening question: "Is there anything you'd like to discuss?" Acknowledge comments: Say "Yes" and "I understand." Allow silence and observe nonverbal behavior rather than trying to force a conversation. Ask for clarification if the patient's statements are unclear. Reflect the patient's statements back (use sparingly): <ul><li>Individual: "I hate this hospital."</li><li>Paramedic: "You hate this hospital?"</li></ul>
Empathy	Make observations: "You are shaking," and "You seem worried." Recognize feelings: <ul><li>Individual: "I want to get well."</li><li>Paramedic: "It must be hard for you to deal with this illness."</li></ul>Provide information as honestly and completely as possible about the patient's condition, treatment, and procedures and respond to the individual's questions and concerns.
Exploration	Verbally express implied messages: <ul><li>Individual: "This treatment is too much trouble."</li><li>Paramedic: "Do you think the treatment isn't helping you?"</li></ul>Explore a topic but allow the individual to terminate the discussion without further probing: "I'd like to hear how you feel about that."
Orientation	Indicate reality: <ul><li>Individual: "Someone is screaming."</li><li>Paramedic: "That sound was a police siren."</li></ul>Comment on distortions without directly agreeing or disagreeing: Individual: "That policeman promised I could go to St. John's Hospital." Paramedic: "Really? That's surprising because this ambulance is based at County Hospital."
Collaboration	Work together to achieve better results: "Maybe if we talk about this, we can figure out a way to make the treatment easier for you."
Validation	Seek validation: "Do you feel better now?" or "Did the medication help you breathe better?"

Nontherapeutic communication

Although using therapeutic communication is important, it is equally important to avoid interjecting **nontherapeutic communication**, which can effectively block effective communication. **Avoid the following:**

Stating meaningless clichés	"Don't worry. Everything will be fine." "Isn't it a nice day?"
Providing advice	"You should…" or "The best thing to do is…." It's better when individuals ask for advice to provide facts and encourage individuals to make their own decisions.
Providing inappropriate approval	This can prevent the individual from expressing true feelings or concerns. Individual: "I shouldn't cry about this." Paramedic: "That's right. You're an adult."

Asking for explanations of behavior not directly related to individual care	Asking for explanations such as "Why are you upset?" may require analysis and an explanation of feelings on the individual's part.
Agreeing rather than accepting and responding	Agreeing with individual's statements "I agree with you" or "You are right" can make it difficult for the individual to change his/her statement or opinion later.
Making negative judgments	"You should stop arguing with the paramedics."
Devaluing an individual's feelings	"Everyone gets upset at times."
Disagreeing directly	"That can't be true" or "I think you are wrong."
Defending against criticism	"The doctor was not being rude; he's just very busy today."
Changing the subject	This avoids dealing with uncomfortable subjects: • Individual: "I'm never going to get well." • Paramedic: "We'll contact your family in a few minutes."
Making inappropriate literal responses	Even as a joke, this is not appropriate, especially if the individual is confused or having difficulty expressing ideas: • Individual: "There are bugs crawling under my skin." • Paramedic: "I'll get some bug spray."
Challenging to establish reality	This often increases confusion and frustration: • Individual: "I'm dying!" • Paramedic: If you were dying, you wouldn't be able to yell and kick."
Filling silence with words	Some cultures, such as Native Americans, allow more silent time in communication.

Assessing mental status

Assessing mental status during an interview begins with observing how the patient is behaving and responding as well as the patient's general appearance (neat, unkempt, sniffing, scratching, tremors), facial movements, and reactive movements (twitches, repetitive motions). The paramedic should ask questions that determine whether the patient is oriented to person, place, time, and event (oriented × 4) and observe speech patterns for clarity. An inability to concentrate, comprehend, or follow simple directions may indicate cognitive impairment. The patient's affect may be inappropriate (out of step with the situation), apathetic (indifferent), or flat (void of emotion). Questioning may help determine if a patient has remote, recent, and immediate memories because short-term memory loss is common with dementia. Mood disturbances may result from general medical conditions, prescription medications, drug abuse, and exposure to toxins. Patients may appear exceptionally depressed, irritable, or elated and "high." Mood disturbances are common with drug intoxication and withdrawal.

Interviewing a patient who does not speak English or who speaks limited English

The paramedic should begin an interview first in English. If a patient does not respond verbally and appears confused and/or frightened when questioned, and the paramedic suspects that the patient doesn't speak English, the paramedic should ask directly if he or she can understand English. When a patient is a **non-English speaking or a limited English speaker**, the important thing is to communicate. So although children, friends, bystanders, and family are not usually used as translators, in emergent or life-threatening situations, an exception is made. The paramedic may use signs, gestures, and pantomime to communicate and use simple words or phrases, such as "Pain?" and "OK?" because even non-English speakers may understand a few words. The paramedic may use a language line if available and the situation permits, and he or she should alert the receiving hospital of the need for a translator as well as providing information about the patient's language. The paramedic should point to a body part before touching it.

Conditions for consent

The **conditions for consent** for care and decision-making capacity include the following:

- 18 years or older: Patients who are younger may have the right to give consent for all or some medical treatment in some states. State laws vary; for example, the age of consent for medical treatment in Alabama is 14.
- Mentally competent to make decisions: The patient may be impaired by mental disability, injury, illness, or substance abuse (intoxication).
- Court-emancipated minor.
- Military service.
- Marriage.

Consent may be expressed if the patient is able to give informed consent, or it may be implied, such as when care is provided in an emergent situation in which the patient is unable to give consent. Parents or caregivers give consent for minors younger than the age of 18 unless they have been emancipated. If parents or caregivers are unavailable to give consent, life-saving emergent care, general medical assessment, and medical care to prevent further injury or harm can be provided without consent (*in loco parentis*).

Advance directives, durable power of attorney, and do-not-resuscitate (DNR) order

In accordance with federal and state laws, individuals have the right to self-determination in health care, including decisions about end-of-life care through **advance directives** such as living wills and the right to assign a surrogate person to make decisions through a **durable power of attorney**. Patients should routinely be questioned about an advanced directive because they may present at a healthcare organization without the document. Patients who have indicated that they desire a **do-not-resuscitate (DNR) order** should not receive resuscitative treatments for terminal illness or conditions in which meaningful recovery cannot occur. Patients and families of those with terminal illnesses should be questioned as to whether the patients are hospice patients. For those with DNR requests or those withdrawing life support, staff should provide the patient palliative rather than curative measures, such as pain control and/or oxygen, and emotional support to the patient and family. Religious traditions and beliefs about death should be treated with respect.

Civil and criminal offenses related to patient care

The four necessary elements of **negligence** (failure to follow the standards of care) are as follows:

1. <u>Duty of care:</u> The defendant (healthcare provider) had a duty to provide adequate care and/or protect the plaintiff's (patient's) safety.
2. <u>Breach of duty:</u> The defendant failed to carry out the duty to care, resulting in danger, injury, or harm to the plaintiff.

3. <u>Damages:</u> The plaintiff experienced illness or injury as a result of the breach of duty.
4. <u>Causation:</u> The plaintiff's illness or injury is directly caused by the defendant's negligent breach of duty.

Abandonment occurs if the paramedic withdraws from providing care contrary to a patient's desire or knowledge and fails to arrange for appropriate care by others, resulting in harm to the patient. Assault occurs if a paramedic threatens a patient in such a way that the patient becomes fearful of harm, whereas **battery** occurs when the paramedic intentionally injures a patient, such as by hitting or shoving the person. **Kidnapping** is forcefully transporting a patient, and **false imprisonment** is preventing a patient from leaving.

Types of negligence

Negligence indicates that *proper care* has not been provided, based on established standards. State regulations regarding negligence may vary, but they all have some statutes of limitation, governmental immunity, and Good Samaritan laws that may provide a defense. Types of negligence include the following:

- <u>Negligent conduct:</u> An individual failed to provide reasonable care or to protect/assist another, based on standards and expertise.
- <u>Gross negligence:</u> Willfully providing inadequate care while disregarding the safety and security of another person.
- <u>Contributory negligence:</u> The injured party contributes to his/her own harm.
- <u>Comparative negligence:</u> The percentage of negligence attributed to each individual involved.

If the charge of negligence is supported, the patient may collect physical (lost earnings due to injury), psychological (pain and suffering), and punitive damages. The principle of *res ipsa loquitur* (the thing speaks for itself) is often used to claim that an accident or injury itself suggests negligence even without direct evidence of harm. Under the borrowed servant doctrine, the paramedic who accepts assistance from other EMS personnel is responsible for their actions and any errors they commit.

Statutory responsibilities

The paramedic must practice within the **scope of responsibility**, which is outlined by each state's medical practice act. The paramedic must be certified by the National Registry of Emergency Medical Technicians (NREMT) (nongovernmental) and must be licensed according to state (government) requirements and meet appropriate educational standards, including completion of mandatory training and demonstration of skill competency. The medical director (physician) is responsible for assuring that the paramedic is competent and knowledgeable and is responsible for online direct supervision and offline protocols with standing orders. The paramedic has a duty to the patients, the medical director, and the public and functions under government and medical oversight. The paramedic must respect patients' civil and human rights and maintain confidentiality. Sharing information about a patient with unauthorized individuals and/or without written consent is considered to be an invasion of privacy and may result in charges of libel or slander.

Mandatory reporting

Although laws about **mandatory reporting** vary from state to state, healthcare providers, including EMS personnel, are considered mandatory reporters in all states and must report suspected cases of child and elder abuse and neglect. The paramedic must follow state guidelines for reporting because simply notifying the receiving facility of suspected child abuse is not adequate. The paramedic should be familiar with the signs of abuse and neglect (certain types of fractures; unexplained or multiple bruises; suspicious bruise patterns; burns; hair loss; and inadequate food, clothing, and shelter). Additionally, in most states, certain types of injuries or assaults must be reported to law enforcement, including stab wounds, gunshot wounds, and sexual assaults. Each state has lists of specific communicable diseases (such as TB and measles) that must be reported—some required by the CDC but others specific to the state or local area. Those classified as urgent (such as Ebola) must be reported immediately, whereas others may be reported within one to seven working days. Reporting procedures vary.

Evidence preservation

When an incident may involve **court cases**, such as with gunshot wounds, knife wounds, and rape, the paramedic should take steps to preserve evidence, although providing emergent medical care takes priority. The paramedic should try to avoid disturbing items at the scene of the incident and should assess the environment and document any unusual findings, remembering that the environment and the patient are both considered to be part of the crime scene. The paramedic should collaborate with law enforcement officers at the scene. If the patient has had a gunshot wound or a knife wound, the paramedic should not cut through the holes in the clothing but should cut along the seams or away from the injuries. Any clothing or belongings removed during treatment should be secured separately in a paper bag (or plastic if paper is not available) and delivered with the patient to the receiving facility or to law enforcement officers. When the patient is describing the event, the paramedic should document using quotations rather than summarizing.

Ethical principles and moral obligations

Ethics is a branch of philosophy that studies morality—concepts of right and wrong. Applied ethics is the use of ethical principles, such as autonomy (right to self-determination), beneficence (acting to benefit another), nonmaleficence (doing no harm), verity (being truthful), and justice (equally distributing resources/care). Ethical conflicts may occur because of differences in cultural and ethical values, but they may also result from decisions that must be made regarding care, such as whether to provide CPR in a wilderness situation when the treatment is likely futile, situations involving triage in which some patients are given priority over others, situations that involve professional misconduct (such as EMS personnel being abusive toward patients), and incidents of patient dumping because the patient has inadequate insurance or an inability to pay. EMS personnel have a moral obligation to make decisions about care in good faith and in the patient's best interest.

Decision-making models

Do no harm   This model is based on nonmaleficence, the requirement that a treatment provided do no harm; however, by their nature, some treatments can and often do harm patients, so the underlying intent and goal of treatment must be considered when making decisions. For example, CPR may be carried out to save a patient's life and may be done with correct technique but still may result in rib fractures.

In good faith	The motive for a decision should be honest and fair, and decisions should be made with a sincere intention to do good even though the outcome may be negative. For example, EMS personnel may provide a treatment for a patient in good faith although the treatment proves to be ineffective for that particular patient.
Patient's best interest	Making a decision in the patient's best interest includes considering the patient's or parents' (in the case of children) wishes, the best clinical judgment, the best choice of various options, the chances for improvement/decline, and religious/cultural preferences.

Emergency Medical Treatment and Active Labor Act (EMTALA) regulations

The **Emergency Medical Treatment and Active Labor Act** (EMTALA) of 1986 is designed to prevent patient "dumping" from emergency departments (EDs) and is an issue of concern for risk management, requiring staff training for compliance.

- Transfers from the ED may be intrahospital or to another facility.
- Stabilization of the patient with an emergent condition or active labor must be done in the ED prior to transfer, and an initial screening must be given prior to inquiring about insurance or ability to pay.
- Stabilization requires treatment for emergency conditions and a reasonable belief that, although the emergent condition may not be completely resolved, the patient's condition will not deteriorate during transfer (not applicable to older adults).
- Women in the ED in active labor should deliver the child and the placenta before transfer.
- The receiving department or facility should be capable of treating the patient and dealing with complications that might occur.
- Transfer to another facility is indicated if the patient requires specialized services not available intrahospital, such as to a burn center.

Americans with Disabilities Act

The 1990 **Americans with Disabilities Act** is civil rights legislation that provides the disabled, including those with mental impairment, access to employment and the community. Although employers must make reasonable accommodations for the disabled, the provisions related to the community apply more directly to older Americans. The ADA covers not only obvious disabilities but also disorders such as arthritis, seizure disorders, and cardiovascular and respiratory disorders. Communities must provide transportation services for the disabled, including accommodation for wheelchairs. Public facilities (schools, museums, physician offices, post offices, and restaurants) must be accessible with ramps and elevators as needed. Telecommunications must also be accessible through devices or accommodations for the deaf and blind. Compliance is not yet complete because older buildings are required to provide access that is possible without "undue hardship," but newer construction of public facilities must meet ADA regulations.

Employment law

The **Equal Employment Opportunity Commission (EEOC)** enforces federal laws against discrimination in employment for employers with ≥15 employers or ≥20 employers in age-discrimination cases. The EEOC investigates, provides guidance, and enforces a number of laws such as the following:

- <u>Civil Rights Act (1964), Title VII, including the Pregnancy Discrimination Act (1978)</u>: Employers cannot discriminate based on race, color, gender, pregnancy, religion, and national origin.
- <u>Civil Rights Act (1991), Sections 102 and 103:</u> Amends previous laws to allow for jury trials and punitive and compensatory damages.
- <u>Equal Pay Act (1963):</u> Males and females must receive equal pay for equal work.
- <u>Age Discrimination in Employment Act (ADEA) (1967):</u> This law provides protection against age discrimination for those ≥40.
- <u>Americans with Disabilities Act (ADA) (1990):</u> This law prevents discrimination in the private sector and at the state and local levels against qualified individuals with disabilities, and it requires reasonable accommodations to be provided.
- <u>Rehabilitation Act (1973), Sections 501 and 505</u>: This law is similar to the ADA, but it applies to discrimination against those with disabilities in the federal government.
- <u>Genetic Information Nondiscrimination Act (GINA) (2008):</u> Employers cannot discriminate based on genetic information.

Family and Medical Leave Act and the Ryan White CARE Act

The **Family and Medical Leave Act** (FMLA) (1993) requires that employers with 50 or more employees offer up to 12 weeks of unpaid leave each year for maternity or other medical needs. To qualify, the individual must have worked at least one full year or a total of 1250 hours or more within the previous 12 months. Employers have discretion as to whether or not the leave is paid. Individuals may take leave because of the birth or adoption of a child, sickness, or the need to care for a family member with a serious illness.

The **Ryan White Comprehensive AIDS Resources Emergency Act** (Ryan White CARE Act) (1994) provides funding for human immunodeficiency virus (HIV) services but contains notification provisions requiring that emergency response employees (including paramedics, other EMS personnel, firefighters, and police) be notified if they are exposed to a communicable disease, such as HIV/acquired immune deficiency syndrome (AIDS) and measles. A designated infection control officer receives notification and in turn notifies the exposed employee.

End-of-life issues

Medical Orders for Life-Sustaining Treatment (MOLST) and **Physician's Orders for Life-Sustaining Treatment (POLST)** are forms, usually brightly colored, that are filled out with the patient or healthcare surrogate/proxy (next of kin if patient is unable to sign or the individual with power of attorney) and signed by the physician indicating the patient's/surrogate's wishes regarding end-of-life care and resuscitation, including do-not-resuscitate (DNR) orders. MOLST/POLST forms are generally intended for those who live in long-term-care facilities or require long-term care, who do not want life-sustaining treatment, or who are expected to die within a year. The form should be posted in a prominent place within the patient's home or other place of habitation. Some states suggest placing the form on the refrigerator in the kitchen. If the paramedic works in a state that authorizes use of the MOLST/POLST, the paramedic should ask about the form and look for it on arrival because the orders may determine the type of emergent care provided.

Limited resuscitation occurs when a patient's advance directive indicates that only some aspects of resuscitation may be carried out while others are to be avoided. If a patient or surrogate wants limited resuscitation rather than a full do-not-resuscitate order, the order should specify whether or not to use the following:

- Cardiac compression.
- Defibrillation.
- Intubation.
- Ventilation, assisted.
- Pediatric advanced life support (PALS) drugs/Advanced cardiac life support (ACLS) drugs.

Resuscitation is withheld if obvious signs of death (tissue decay, livor mortis, rigor mortis) are present, and resuscitation is terminated according to established protocols. Protocols for termination usually include unwitnessed cardiac arrest, no rescue shock, and no return of pulse. If a patient has an **organ donor** card or indicates the desire to donate on a driver's license, CPR should be continued until the patient is handed off at the receiving facility, even though the patient's death has been established, because CPR is necessary to maintain viability of his or her organs.

Anatomy and Physiology

Body planes and anatomic terms

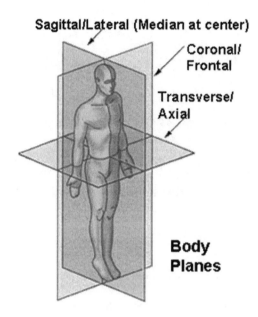

Sagittal/Lateral (Median at center)

Coronal/Frontal

Transverse/Axial

Body Planes

Body planes include the following:

- <u>Sagittal/Lateral:</u> Vertical plane separating right from left.
- <u>Median/Midsagittal:</u> Sagittal plane at the midline (middle) separating the body into equal halves.
- <u>Coronal/Frontal:</u> Vertical plane separating anterior (front) from posterior (back).
- <u>Axial/Transverse:</u> Horizontal plane that separates the body into superior (upper) and inferior (lower) parts.
- A <u>cross section</u> is an axial/transverse (horizontal) cut through a tissue specimen or body structure, whereas a <u>longitudinal section</u> is a sagittal or coronal (vertical) cut.
- <u>Medial</u> is toward the midline, whereas <u>lateral</u> is away from the midline and to the side. <u>Distal</u> is the farthest point from the point of reference, and <u>proximal</u> is the closest point. When describing an area of the patient's body, the description should be patient oriented, using phrases such as "patient's left" and "patient's right" to ensure accurate interpretation.

Abdominal regions of the body

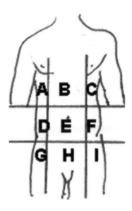

Abdominal regions include the following:

  A = Right hypochondriac
  B = Epigastric (epi = on, above)
  C = Left hypochondriac
  D = Right lumbar
  E = Umbilical
  F = Left lumbar
  G = Right iliac
  H = Hypogastric (hypo = below, beneath, less than normal)
   I = Left iliac

The abdomen may also be divided into four quadrants (sections) with the umbilicus (navel) at the center: right upper quadrant (RUQ), right lower quadrant (RLQ), left upper quadrant (LUQ) and left lower quadrant (LLQ).

Life Span Development

Normal vital signs from neonate to late adulthood

Age	Heart rate	Respirations	BP (mm Hg)
Neonate (newborn)	100–220 (average 140–160) begins to slow after 3 months	40–60 for a few minutes, then 30–40	Systolic 70–90
Toddler (12–36 mos.)	80–130	20–30	Systolic 70–100
Preschool (3 to 5)	80–120	20–30	Systolic 80–110
School age (6–12)	70–110	20–30	80–120/60–80
Adolescence (13–18)	55–100	12–20	110–131/64–84
Early adulthood (19–40)	60–100 (average 80)	12–20	100–119/60–79 to 140/90 (high)
Middle adulthood (41–60)	60–100 (average 80)	12–20	100–119/60–79 to 140/90 (high)
Late adulthood (61+)	60–100 (average 70)	12–20	100–119/60–79 to 140/90 (high)

Levels of disease prevention

Levels of disease prevention include the following:

- Primary: The goal is to prevent the initial occurrence of a health problem, such as a disease or injury, through activities such as immunizations, smoking cessation, fluoride supplementation of water, promotion of seat belt and helmet use, and use of child car seat restraints. Interventions are often aimed at the general public or large groups of people.
- Secondary: The goal is to identify diseases or conditions quickly and provide prompt intervention to provide treatment and prevent further disability through activities such as BP screenings, breast and testicular self-examinations, hearing and vision screenings, mammography, and pregnancy testing.
- Tertiary: The goal is to assist those who already have disease or disability to prevent further progress of the disease and to allow people to achieve the maximum quality of life through activities such as support groups, counseling, diet and exercise, stress management, and supportive services.

Public Health

Public health system

EMS are part of the **public health system**, a network of private, nonprofit, and government agencies and healthcare providers providing public health services in a wide range of areas. The primary services provided by the public health system include the following:

- Monitoring community health
- Identifying hazards to health in the environment/community.
- Educating people about health issues.
- Mobilizing various agencies and individuals to take action.
- Enforcing public safety laws/regulations.
- Ensuring that healthcare providers are qualified, licensed, and certified as required.
- Ensuring that health care is available.
- Assessing the effectiveness of health care.
- Researching health problems and finding solutions.

Public health laws/regulations may be federal, state, or tribal and cover issues such as immunization requirements, drinking water/sewage system standards, air quality, water fluoridation, restrictions on tobacco use (age and place), restrictions on drinking (age, driving), speed limits, prenatal care, abuse (child, older adult, sexual, and domestic), safety equipment, and safe lifting. Healthy People 2020, of the US. Department of Health and Human Services, provides goals and objectives for health-related public policies.

Pharmacology

Administration of medications

The paramedic may assist patients to self-administer medications or administer them directly depending on the scope of practice and protocols. Medical direction may be offline, which means that standing orders are available to treat specific conditions or written protocols have been established that must be followed. Online medical direction requires verbal contact with a medical director. When receiving an online medication order, the paramedic should use the echo technique (repeating back the orders to ensure that they were understood correctly) and clarify any orders that are confusing or unclear.

The **five rights of medication administration** include the following:

- Right patient: The medication should be prescribed specifically for that patient.
- Right medication: Correct choice for the patient's condition, and it matches the prescription.
- Right route: Appropriate for the patient's condition, enteral or parenteral.
- Right dose: As prescribed and appropriate for the patient's age, weight, and condition.
- Right time: The medication is not expired, and it is administered at the time ordered, such as "stat" (immediately) or "every 5 minutes × 3."

Drug dose calculations

Desired dose and volume/concentration on hand	Milligrams (mg) needed/mg available in dose × volume per dose = current dose.	If an infant is to receive 65 mg of acetaminophen elixir that contains 80 mg per 5 milliliters (mL): 65 mg/80 mg = 0.8125 ×5 = 4.06 = 4 mL.
Convert pounds (lb) to kilograms (kg)	No. of lb/2.2 kg.	Infant weight 16 lb.: 16/2.2 = 7.3 kg, rounded to 7 kg.
IV flow rate in drops per minute	Volume (mL)/time (minutes) × drop factor = flow rate. Note: The standard drop factor is 15 drops/mL, but microdrip infusion sets (used with pediatrics or small volumes) have 60 drops/mL.	If a patient is to receive 1200 mL of 5% dextrose in water (D5W) in 5 hours (300 minutes) and the drop factor of the infusion set is 15 drops per mL: 1000/300 × 15 = 49.9 = 50 drops/min.

Medication legislation

Act/Agency	Purpose
Pure Food and Drug Act (1906)	Consumer protection act intended to prevent the manufacture, sale, and transportation of adulterated foods, drugs, and alcoholic beverages.
Federal Food, Drug, and Cosmetic Act (1938)	Provides authority to the FDA to oversee food, drug, and cosmetic safety.

Harrison Narcotics Tax Act (1914)	Provides authority for regulation and taxation of the production, importation, and distribution of coca/opium products, such as narcotics.
Controlled Substances Act (1970)	Establishes U.S. drug policy and five schedules under which drugs are classified, implemented by the DEA and the FDA.
Food and Drug Administration (FDA)	Consumer protection agency that protects public health through the control and supervision of drugs, vaccines, blood transfusions, medical devices, cosmetics, foods, tobacco, and dietary supplements.
Drug Enforcement Agency (DEA)	Law enforcement agency, part of the Department of Justice, enforces the Controlled Substances Act and combats drug smuggling/use.

Commonly administered and assisted medications

Medication	Dose/Route/Use	Side effects/Interactions
Aspirin	Orally, 325 mg chew and swallow for fast action when having a heart attack.	Avoid with signs of stroke or gastrointestinal (GI) bleeding. Decreases clotting time and may increase the risk of bleeding.
Glucose	Orally for hypoglycemia. May be in liquid or tablet form, or a glass of orange juice may be given.	Minimal unless hyperglycemic.
Oxygen	Inhaled, usually 2–6 L, but it varies according to protocol.	Minimal, although oxygen toxicity can occur with high doses for prolonged periods of time.
Bronchodilators (albuterol, levalbuterol)	Inhaled, usually two puffs of a handheld inhaler. Dosage varies according to the medication. For bronchospasm, wheezing.	Adverse effects: tachycardia, dizziness, nervousness, tremor, headache, rhinitis, increased cough.
Epinephrine (EpiPen)	Autoinjector, 0.3 mg 1:1000 for ≥66 lb. 0.15 mg 1:2000 for 33–66 lb. for severe allergic reaction/anaphylaxis	Avoid using with antihistamines, thyroid hormones, and alpha blockers. Adverse effects: drowsiness, headache, palpitations, nervousness, tremors.
Nitroglycerin	Sublingually for angina (chest pain), 0.3–0.6 mg, repeated every 5 minutes up to three times.	Avoid with myocardial infarction. Adverse effects: headache, flushing, dizziness, orthostatic hypotension, palpitations. Interactions: avoid with erectile dysfunction drugs (sildenafil, tadalafil, vardenafil).

Principles of pharmacology

Pharmacodynamics relates to biological effects (therapeutic or adverse) of drug administration. Responses may be continuous, such as BP variations, or dichotomous, in which an event either occurs or does not occur (such as death). Information from pharmacodynamics provides feedback to modify medication dosage (pharmacokinetics). **Pharmacokinetics** relates to the route of administration, the absorption, the dosage, the frequency of administration, the distribution, and the serum levels achieved over time. Most drugs are cleared through the kidneys. Elimination half-time is the time needed to reduce plasma concentrations to 50% during elimination. Age and weight may impact the absorption and elimination of drugs. Drugs have a generic/scientific/nonproprietary name (acetaminophen) and a brand/trade/proprietary name (Tylenol). Emergency medications include solids (pills, capsules, powders), liquids (enteral [ingested] or parenteral [injected]), and gases (inhaled). Enteral medications may be given orally (glucose) or sublingually (nitroglycerin). Parenteral drugs are inhaled (oxygen, albuterol) or injected (epinephrine).

Airway Management, Respirations and Artificial Ventilation

Upper respiratory system

Air enters the **upper respiratory system** through the <u>nasal cavity</u> and/or mouth, where it is warmed and moistened by <u>nasal and oral mucosa</u>. The four pairs of <u>paranasal sinuses</u> aid in warming and moistening the air. The air passes through the <u>pharynx</u>: <u>nasopharynx, oropharynx,</u> and <u>laryngopharynx/hypopharynx</u> (below and behind the larynx and epiglottis). Air passes behind or past the <u>soft palate</u> (the soft tissue at the back of the mouth) and the <u>uvula</u>, which hangs from the soft palate and into the lower respiratory system. The <u>hyoid bone</u> is above the Adam's apple and helps support the larynx. The vallecula ("spit trap") is at the root of the tongue. The <u>adenoids</u> (pharyngeal tonsils) are located on the posterior wall of the nasopharynx, and the <u>palatine tonsils</u> are on the back of the mouth on either side of the tongue. The adenoids and tonsils may become infected and swollen, obstructing the airway. The jawbones include the maxilla (upper) and mandible (lower). The jugular notch is the visible depression between the neck and clavicles (collarbones).

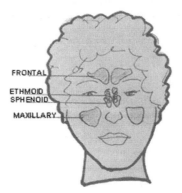

Lower respiratory system

Air passes from the upper respiratory system and the pharynx to the **lower respiratory system** and the <u>larynx</u> (voice box) into the <u>trachea</u> (windpipe). The <u>epiglottis</u> is a cartilage flap attached to the <u>thyroid cartilage</u> (above the cricoid cartilage), and it closes over the larynx and <u>glottis</u> (vocal cords) when swallowing so food enters the esophagus. The trachea branches into two (right and left) <u>bronchi</u> that carry the air into the <u>lungs</u>. Each bronchus branches into smaller <u>bronchioles</u> and <u>alveoli</u> (small air sacs), which are connected to the ends of the bronchioles. The alveoli are covered with webs of tiny venous capillaries that deliver carbon dioxide and arterial capillaries that pick up oxygen. Muscles of respiration are the <u>diaphragm</u>, which is enervated by the <u>phrenic nerve</u>, and the <u>intercostal muscles</u>, but <u>accessory muscles</u> in the neck and collarbone area may help during respiratory distress.

Breathing and pulmonary volumes

The **lungs**, located in the thoracic cavity and surrounded by pleural membranes, facilitate breathing through changes in pressure. When inhaling, the lungs and thoracic cavity expand, decreasing air pressure inside and forcing air from outside to enter. When exhaling, the pressure increases as the lungs and thoracic cavity contract, forcing air out of the lungs. The phrenic and intercostal nerves cause the diaphragm and intercostal muscles to contract and relax. <u>External respiration</u> occurs with gas exchange (oxygen for carbon dioxide) at the alveoli. The respiratory center in the brain (medulla oblongata) controls the breathing rate in response to chemoreceptors in the arteries that monitor levels of oxygen and carbon dioxide. Internal respiration occurs with gas exchange in the tissue cells. Physiologic dead spaces are those areas of the lung (including impaired alveoli) where gas exchange does not occur.

Pulmonary volumes are as follows:

- Tidal volume: The normal exchange of air between inhaling and exhaling is 500 mL.
- Minute respiratory volume: The volume of air inhaled or exhaled in one minute (tidal volume × respiratory rate).
- Vital capacity: The greatest volume of air exhaled after the greatest forced inhalation.

Acid/base balance

Respiratory acidosis: Hypoventilation (decreased breathing or inadequate mechanical ventilation) retains carbon dioxide and increases acid, which decreases the pH (acidity) to less than 7.35 (more acidic). The kidneys retain bicarbonate to compensate. Causes: COPD, pneumonia, muscle weakness, sedative/barbiturate overdose, obesity, muscle weakness (Guillain-Barré syndrome). Symptoms: Drowsiness, dizziness, headache, confusion, seizures, flushing, and low BP, tachypnea (tachy = rapid; pnea = breathing), tachycardia, and ventricular fibrillation. Treatment: Improved ventilation and bronchodilators.

Respiratory alkalosis: Hyperventilation (increased breathing) exhales more carbon dioxide and decreases acid, which increases the pH to greater than 7.45 (more alkalotic). The kidneys excrete increased bicarbonate to compensate. Causes: Hypoxia (low oxygen), brain injury, acetylsalicylic acid (ASA, i.e., aspirin) overdose, pulmonary embolism (clot), and septicemia. Symptoms: Confusion, lethargy, tachycardia, arrhythmia (irregular pulse), epigastric pain, nausea, and vomiting. Treatment: Identify and treat the underlying cause, and provide oxygen.

Metabolic acidosis: The kidneys excrete less bicarbonate, so pH decreases. Hyperventilation occurs in order to exhale additional carbon dioxide and acid to compensate. Causes: Diarrhea (it causes an excess loss of sodium bicarbonate), starvation, kidney disease, liver failure, excessive alcohol, shock, severe dehydration, and diabetic ketoacidosis (it causes acidic ketone bodies to build up). Symptoms: Headache, confusion, abnormal pulse, nausea, vomiting diarrhea, and low BP. Treatment: Identify and treat the underlying cause. Bicarbonate is rarely administered, but it may be indicated in severe cases.

Metabolic alkalosis: Kidneys excrete more bicarbonate, so pH increases, and hypoventilation occurs to retain carbon dioxide and acid. Causes: Excessive prolonged vomiting, low potassium level, advanced kidney failure. Symptoms: Confusion, anxiety, tremors, muscle cramping, seizures, tachycardia (rapid pulse), nausea, and vomiting. Treatment: Patient may respond to 0.9% IV saline (50 to 100 mL/hr.), but the underlying cause must be identified and treated. Some patients may require hemodialysis.

Life support chain

Critical to the **life support chain** are oxygenation and perfusion. Oxygenation involves gas exchange of carbon dioxide for oxygen at the alveolar/capillary level and at the cell/capillary level. Perfusion involves the transport of blood, which carries oxygen, glucose, and other nutrients as well as waste products throughout the body. Oxygen and glucose are essential for cell functioning. Glucose is produced by the digestion of carbohydrates (starches); it is the primary energy source for the body; and its use is controlled by insulin, which is produced by the pancreas. Excess glucose is stored in the liver as glycogen for later use or is converted to fat. These fundamental elements are affected by the composition of ambient air (usually 21% oxygen), airway patency, ventilation, regulation of respiration, blood volume and transport, heart action, and blood vessel size.

Differences in the respiratory system associated with pediatric patients and older adults

Pediatrics: Infants are obligate nasal breathers for their first two to four months of life, and they usually only breathe through the nose, although they can generally breathe through the mouth if necessary. However, if nasal passages are blocked, they may quickly develop respiratory distress. Chest wall compliance is greater in infants and small children, so they must work harder than an adult to move the same amount of air. In addition, proportionally, the airway is smaller, the tongue is larger, and the cartilage is softer, increasing the risk of obstruction.

Older adults: Breathing capacity tends to decline after age 40 because the number of alveoli decreases and the size of alveoli increases, resulting in less surface for and less efficient gas exchange. Lung elasticity also decreases, resulting in decreased vital capacity. The chest muscles tend to weaken and stiffen with age, and older adults have a lowered ability to clear the airways.

Airway assessment and manual measures to clear the airway

Indications of an adequate airway include a normal voice and speaking ability and audible and visible air exchange. Indications of inadequate airway include unusual breathing sounds (wheezing, stridor), hoarse voice/inability to speak, and no audible or visible air exchange. Airway obstruction may result from the tongue falling back, food, a foreign body, vomit, blood, teeth, and edema (swelling). Maneuvers include the following:

- Head tilt/chin lift: Hyperextend the neck by tilting the patient's head back with one hand on his or her forehead to straighten the airway and lift the tongue. Then lift the chin and pull forward with the fingers of the other hand under the chin with the thumb on top. The chin lift pulls the mandible (jaw) forward. This prevents the tongue from blocking the pharynx. Contraindications to the head tilt/chin lift include suspected cervical spine and neck injuries.
- Jaw thrust: This technique is used with a suspected spinal cord or neck injury in which extending the neck must be avoided. From behind, place the fingers behind the angles of the patient's lower jaw and place your thumbs on the chin; move the jaw upward until it is extended while using the thumbs to slightly open the patient's mouth. Contraindications include severe facial injuries.
- Modified chin lift/jaw thrust: This technique is used with a suspected spinal cord/neck injury with an unstable cervical spine. From the head of the patient, place your thumbs on his or her cheekbones and place your fingers under the patient's mandible, and then pull the mandible upward with the fingers while applying pressure with the thumbs. If using a mask for ventilation, place the mask in position and secure it with your thumbs while your fingers thrust the patient's jaw forward.

Oropharyngeal airway (OPA)

The **oropharyngeal airway (OPA)**, a blind-insertion airway device, may be inserted to provide better ventilation, but the OPA requires the head tilt/chin lift or modified jaw thrust as well because the device alone does not ensure a patent airway. The OPA is indicated for unconscious patients, patients with no gag reflex, and patients who are apneic (not breathing) and require ventilatory aid.

The OPA is often inserted if a patient stops breathing, such as with a cardiac arrest. The OPA is contraindicated in conscious patients and those with a gag reflex. To insert the OPA, perform the following steps:

- Estimate the OPA length by measuring the patient from the angle of the jaw or the tip of the earlobe to the corner of the mouth.
- Select the correct size.
- Open the patient's mouth using the cross-finger technique. Suction any secretions.
- Tilt the head back (if possible). Insert the device with the tip of the OPA pointing upward for adults and downward for children.
- Rotate the OPA into position for adults.
- Ensure that the phalanges of the mouthpiece are securely against the patient's mouth.
- Check to make sure that the OPA is patent (open).

Upper airway suctioning

- **Suctioning** devices may be vehicle mounted or portable and should be checked to ensure that the tubing is intact and the canister has an airtight seal. Patients at risk for aspiration include those with an altered level of consciousness, those having difficulty swallowing or breathing, trauma patients, obese patients, and those with recurrent vomiting. Oral suctioning is used to remove secretions, vomitus, and blood. Suctioning may be done with a rigid-tip catheter (Yankauer) or a soft-tip catheter. Techniques include the following: Don a mask and gloves.
- Measure the catheter from the tip of the ear to the corner of the mouth to determine how far to insert the catheter.
- Turn on the suction.
- Use the cross-finger technique to open the mouth.
- Insert the tube and apply suction. The rigid catheter has a finger control to start and stop suction.
- Move the catheter around the gum line and over the tongue to the back of the mouth, but avoid stimulating the gag reflex.
- Suction for no longer than 15 seconds at a time.
- Note: Clear a small infant's airway by suctioning nasal passages with a bulb syringe.

Tracheobronchial suctioning

Tracheobronchial suctioning may be done after intubating a patient so that secretions will not be forced into the lungs during artificial ventilation. A flexible "whistle-tip" catheter is used for suctioning. The patient should be on a cardiac monitor because hypoxia may produce cardiac arrhythmias (abnormal pulse). A pulse oximeter should be in place to monitor oxygen saturation.

The procedure is as follows:

- Preoxygenate the patient for at least 5 minutes with 100% oxygen to prevent suction-related hypoxia.
- Lubricate the catheter with a water-soluble lubricant.
- Detach the ventilation equipment and inject 3–5 mL sterile water/saline into the endotracheal tube (ETT) to loosen up any secretions.
- Gently insert the catheter into the ETT until resistance (the carina) is met.

- Then, apply suction while slowly withdrawing and rotating the catheter. Suction for no more than 15 seconds.
- If arrhythmias occur or if the oxygen saturation falls, discontinue suctioning immediately.
- Reattach the ventilation equipment.
- Preoxygenate again for at least 30 seconds if suctioning must be repeated.

Portable oxygen cylinders

Two commonly used sizes of **portable oxygen cylinders** are D tanks (M15; 350 L) and E tanks (M24; 625 L). The paramedic should use protective equipment (goggles, gloves). The cylinder should be placed upright. A label over the holes on the top of the cylinder indicates that the cylinder is full. Remove the label, leaving the washers in place unless the washers are built into the regulator. Face the opening of the tank away, and use the key to crack the cylinder by letting out a small amount of oxygen. Apply the regulator and slide it into place. Tighten and then open the cylinder to check for pressure (there should be at least 200 psi). Close the cylinder, attach the oxygen tubing to the regulator, set the oxygen flow to the correct amount of liters, and then open the cylinder and administer oxygen to the patient. When discontinuing use of the cylinder, turn off the cylinder, remove the oxygen tubing, turn the oxygen flow setting up to bleed air from the regular, and remove the regulator.

Assessment of respirations and supplemental oxygen administration

When **assessing respirations**, the paramedic should note the gag reflex by touching the back of the throat or tongue and should observe for partial or complete obstruction, such as from pharyngeal or laryngeal edema or foreign bodies. The paramedic should note the rate of respirations (normal for the patient's age or too fast, too slow, or absent). Patients who have difficulty breathing and speaking may have laryngospasm (spasms of the vocal cords causing them to close and shut off the air). The paramedic should assess any penetrating injuries, such as from knife wounds or gunshot wounds. The paramedic should also evaluate the rise and fall of the chest and any abnormal movements (such as sternal retraction, nasal flaring) noisy breathing (gurgling, wheezing, stridor), the use of accessory muscles, or the tripod position (sitting, leaning forward, and supporting the body with the hands). The paramedic should anticipate a difficult airway if the patient has trauma, bleeding, vomiting, obstructions, or facial hair. If breathing is abnormal or the pulse oximetry is less than 95%, the paramedic should take precautions against bloodstream infection (BSI) and administer **supplemental oxygen** with a nonrebreather mask with the oxygen level set at 12–15 L. The reservoir bag of the mask must be completely filled with oxygen before applying the mask to the patient; secure it with an elastic band around his or her head. Air is exhaled through a one-way valve that prevents rebreathing. The nonrebreather mask at 12–15 L/min is used for trauma patients, patients in respiratory distress, and those suffering from smoke inhalation and carbon monoxide inhalation, although it is not appropriate for those with facial or mouth injuries. If the patient cannot tolerate the nonrebreather mask or he or she is claustrophobic, then a nasal cannula may be used with the oxygen flow set at 4–6 L, the prongs inserted into the nostrils, and the tubing being secured by looping it over the ears and tightening under the chin, but the oxygen concentration will be lower.

Assessment of oxygenation

Assessment of oxygenation includes the following:

- <u>Evaluate respirations:</u> Note the signs of respiratory distress—rapid breathing, slow breathing, use of accessory muscles, nasal flaring, and sternal retraction—because they may indicate inadequate oxygenation.
- <u>Assess mental status:</u> Confusion may be associated with hypo-oxygenation (low oxygen), but it's important to determine a baseline mental status if possible because the patient may have dementia or may be confused because of medications.
- <u>Assess skin:</u> Note cyanosis (a blue tinge) especially around the mouth, fingertips, and oral mucous membranes because this indicates a lack of oxygen. Another sign is pallor. Mottling of the skin, purplish or reddish discoloration especially on the knees and feet, indicates hypo-oxygenation and is a common indication that death is near.
- <u>Monitor pulse oximetry:</u> It should be 95%–100%. If a patient has mild respiratory disease, the pulse oximetry level may be as low as 90% and still be within the normal range for the patient. Readings less than 90%–92% indicate hypoxemia (low oxygen in the blood).

Pulse oximetry

Pulse oximetry uses an external oximeter that attaches to the patient's finger or earlobe to measure the arterial oxygen saturation (SPO_2), the percentage of hemoglobin that is saturated with oxygen. The oximeter uses light waves to determine the SPO_2. Oxygen saturation should be maintained at $\geq 95\%$, although some patients with chronic respiratory disorders, such as COPD, may have lower SPO_2 readings. Results may be compromised by impaired circulation, excessive light, poor positioning, and nail polish. If the SPO_2 reading falls, the oximeter should be repositioned because incorrect positioning is a common cause of inaccurate readings. Oximetry is used for monitoring when patients are on oxygen or mechanical ventilation. Oximeters do not provide information about carbon dioxide levels, so they cannot monitor carbon dioxide retention. Oximeters also cannot differentiate between different forms of hemoglobin, so if the hemoglobin has picked up carbon monoxide, the oximeter will not recognize that.

Bag-valve mask (BVM) ventilation

Bag-valve mask (BVM) ventilation equipment used for positive-pressure ventilation includes a mask, a ventilator bag, an oxygen reservoir bag, and an attachment for oxygen delivery. The correct mask size is important: The mask should not cover the chin. BVM is contraindicated if the airway is not patent, but it is used for abnormal breathing and for respiratory distress/failure. BVM requires two EMS personnel—one to control the mask and the other to control the bag. Steps are as follows:

- Position yourself behind the patient's head, place the mask over the patient's nose and mouth, and make a tight seal by holding it in place with your thumbs and index fingers while your other fingers slide under the patient's jaw to lift the chin.
- Squeeze the bag with inhalations initially for 5 to 10 breaths, and then adjust the rate to at least 12 breaths per minute, slowly adjusting the rate and tidal volume delivered.

Assessment of lung compliance (the ability to expand and contract) includes observation of chest movement, rate of respirations, and the feel of the BVM. Difficult ventilation suggests impaired compliance. Note: The BVM can be used with or without oxygen.

Oxygen delivery devices

Oxygen delivery devices provide oxygen-enriched air. Ambient air is about 21% oxygen, so the fraction of inspired air (FIO_2) is 21%.

Oxygen delivery devices

Nasal cannula (prongs)	FIO_2 of 24%–40% with flows of ≤6 liters per minute (LPM). Humidification should be used for prolonged flow rates of >4 LPM.
Partial rebreather face mask	This mask covers the nose and mouth, delivering FIO_2 of 30%–60%, but the flow of oxygen should be maintained between 6 and 12 LPM to decrease the risk of rebreathing. Because of the higher flow rate, humidification should be used.
Venturi mask	Oxygen entrainment masks come with different-sized color-coded nozzles to more accurately control FIO_2, with different sizes providing different FIO_2 levels, usually ranging from 24% to 50%, although an FIO_2 reading of >35% is not always reliable. The flow rate is 12–15 LPM. Humidifiers may be used.
Nonrebreather mask	This mask covers the mouth and nose with a reservoir bag of oxygen. A one-way valve prevents the patient from rebreathing exhaled air. FIO_2 is about 60%–80% or greater at a flow rate of 15 LPM.

Sellick's maneuver (cricoid pressure)

Sellick's maneuver (cricoid pressure) may be used with PPV to prevent air from flowing down the esophagus and into the stomach rather than down the trachea and into the lungs because stomach distension increases the risk of vomiting. This maneuver may also be used with intubation to prevent regurgitation of stomach contents and aspiration. Sellick's maneuver may be used on unconscious patients receiving a mask or BVM. The procedure consists of applying pressure downward to the cricoid cartilage of the neck (which is at the bottom of the larynx and blocks the upper esophagus) with the thumb and index finger. Pressure is usually applied at 30 to 40 newtons but no greater than 40 newtons because too great of force may block the airway. The maneuver may also cause nausea and vomiting and, with severe pressure, may result in rupture of the esophagus. Vomiting is a contraindication.

Laryngeal-mask airway (LMA)

The laryngeal-mask airway (LMA), a blind-insertion airway device, is an intermediate airway allowing ventilation but not complete respiratory control. The LMA consists of an inflatable cuff (mask) with a connecting tube. It may be used when tracheal intubation can't be done or as a conduit for later blind insertion of an endotracheal tube. The head and neck must be in a neutral position for insertion. If the patient has a gag reflex, then conscious sedation or topical anesthesia (deep oropharyngeal) is required. The LMA is inserted by sliding the airway along the hard palate, using the finger as a guide, into the pharynx, and the ring is inflated to create a seal around the opening to the larynx, allowing ventilation with mild positive pressure. The LMA ProSeal has a modified cuff that extends onto the back of the mask to improve the seal. The CobraPLA (perilaryngeal airway) has a larger pharyngeal cuff and provides a better seal. The LMA is contraindicated in morbid obesity, with obstructions or abnormalities of the oropharynx, and in nonfasting patients because some aspiration is still possible.

Recovery position

The **recovery position** is used for patients who are unconscious but breathing, such as those with a drug overdose or after a seizure, and who have no life-threatening injuries. This position helps to maintain a patent airway and reduces the risk of aspiration from vomitus.

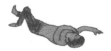

1. Kneeling beside the patient, lift his or her chin to ensure that the airway is open and place his or her closest arm at a right angle to the body with the hand up.
2. Place the patient's farthest arm around his or her neck with the hand touching the opposite cheek.
3. Flex the patient's knee to 90° until the foot is flat on the floor/surface.

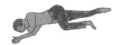

Using the patient's knee as a fulcrum and supporting the farthest arm and shoulder, roll the patient onto his or her side by pulling on the farthest knee.

Make sure that the top knee contacts the floor/surface to support the patient's body and that the top hand is under his or her head to keep the neck in a neutral position.

Normal negative-pressure breathing and positive-pressure breathing

Negative-pressure breathing (normal)

- The movement downward of the diaphragm (triggered by the phrenic nerves) creates a negative pressure in the lungs, drawing air into them.
- Blood flows from the lungs to the heart and back and to the body at a steady rate in normal breathing.
- The epiglottis closes the esophagus during inhalation, preventing air from entering the stomach.

Positive-pressure breathing

- Ventilation forces air into the lungs, and this can result in dysfunction of the diaphragm because it is responding to a change in pressure rather than stimulation by the phrenic nerve.
- Blood flow from the lungs is reduced, resulting in decreased cardiac (heart) output.
- The epiglottis may stay open during ventilation, allowing air into the stomach and increasing the risk of vomiting.

Esophageal tracheal Combitube (ETC)

The **esophageal tracheal Combitube** (ETC) is a blind-insertion airway device and an intermediate airway that contains two lumens (channels). It can be inserted into either the trachea or the esophagus (≤91%). The twin-lumen tube has a proximal cuff providing a seal for the oropharynx and a distal cuff providing a seal around the distal tube. Prior to insertion, the Combitube cuffs should be checked for leaks (with 15 mL of air into the distal cuff and 85 mL of air into the proximal cuff). The patient should be nonresponsive and with no gag reflex with his or her head in a neutral position. The tube is passed along the tongue and into the pharynx, using markings on the tube (black guidelines) to determine the depth by aligning the ETC with the upper incisors or the alveolar ridge. Once in place, the distal cuff is inflated (10–15 mL) and then placement in the trachea or esophagus should be determined so the proper lumen for ventilation can be used. The proximal cuff is inflated (usually to 50–75 mL), and ventilation is started. A capnogram should be used to confirm ventilation.

Nasopharyngeal airway (NPA)

The **nasopharyngeal airway (NPA),** a blind-insertion airway device, is indicated for unconscious or semiconscious patients who still have a gag reflex or those who cannot tolerate an oropharyngeal airway (OPA), but it should be avoided with severe head injury, risk of basal skull fracture, nasal bleeding, and a history of deviated septum or nasal fracture. It's important to use the appropriate size. To insert the NPA, perform the following steps: Choose a size that is slightly smaller in diameter than the patient's nostril. Measure from the tip of the earlobe to the tip of the nose. Lubricate the NPA with water-soluble lubricant and insert it in the larger and most patent (open) nostril. If inserting into the right nostril, insert with the bevel (tip) angled toward the nasal septum (the bony cartilage division between the nostrils). If inserting it into the left nostril, invert the NPA to angle the bevel toward the septum. When the NPA reaches the throat, rotate it 180° into the proper position.

Pocket-mask ventilation

Pocket-mask ventilation is used when administering cardiopulmonary resuscitation (CPR) to a patient who is in cardiac arrest and apneic (not breathing). If two EMS personnel are available, one should be positioned at the patient's head to administer pocket-mask ventilation while the other does compressions. If there is only one EMS personnel, then that person should be positioned at the patient's side. Administration is as follows:

- Remove the mask from the container and push the flattened mask to open it.
- Wipe the patient's face clean with an alcohol swab if necessary to remove secretions or vomitus.
- Do a chin tilt or jaw thrust and place the mask over the patient's nose and mouth, holding it in place with both hands to seal it tightly.
- Take a deep breath and blow in through the one-way valve, watching the chest rise to ensure that ventilation has occurred.
- Continue to ventilate the patient at a rate of 30 compressions to 2 ventilations for CPR.
- Attach supplemental oxygen if available to improve oxygenation.
- Upon patient recovery or completion of CPR, remove the mask, discard the valve, and disinfect the mask.

Confirmation of placement of an endotracheal tube (ETT) during intubation

There are several methods to **confirm correct placement of an endotracheal tube (ETT)** during intubation. Clinical assessment with auscultation alone is not adequate.

- Capnometry uses an end-tidal CO_2 (ETCO) detector that measures the concentration of CO_2 in expired air, usually through pH-sensitive paper that changes color (commonly purple to yellow). The capnometer is attached to the ETT, and a BVM ventilator is attached. The patient is provided six ventilations, and then the CO_2 concentration is checked.
- Capnography is attached to the ETT and provides a waveform graph, showing the varying concentrations of CO_2 in real time throughout each ventilation (with increased CO_2 on expiration); it can indicate changes in the patient's respiratory status.
- Esophageal detection devices fit over the end of the ETT so a large syringe can be used to attempt to aspirate. If the ETT is in the esophagus, the walls collapse on aspiration and resistance occurs, whereas the syringe fills with air if the ETT is in the trachea. A self-inflating bulb (the Ellick device) may also be used.

Airway management

A **fiber-optic laryngoscope** facilitates endotracheal intubation for difficult airways or for instability of the cervical spine. Fiber-optic intubation may be done nasally or orally and while the patient is awake or unconscious. However, fiber-optic intubation takes more time than standard procedures, so if an immediate airway is needed, it is contraindicated. There must be space around the scope for visualization, so tissue edema or mass (a tumor or hematoma) may preclude the use of fiber-optics. For awake intubation, a local anesthetic spray is applied to the back of the throat (Cetacaine aerosol and 3%–4% lidocaine spray), and the nose (both nares) should be sprayed with phenylephrine (Neo-Synephrine) to prevent bleeding for nasal intubation. Intubation is done by feeding the fiber-optic laryngoscope through the tip of the endotracheal tube and then inserting the tube into the airway. Fiber-optics may be more difficult to use in an unconscious patient because of relaxation of the soft tissue.

The **Shikani Optical Stylet** (SOS), a semimalleable, high-resolution fiber-optic endoscope (stainless steel), sometimes used as a stylet, allows visualization during intubation.

Lighted stylets have a malleable stylet and a lighted tip to provide light-guided intubation. Lighted stylets can be inserted without moving the head, so they are useful in patients with limited mobility, instability of the cervical spine, inadequate interincisor space, poor dentition, and facial trauma. One disadvantage is that insertion requires dim lighting. Contraindications include morbid obesity, foreign body obstruction, neck mass, and epiglottitis. The procedure for use is as follows:

- Lubricate the endotracheal tube (ETT) and lighted stylet.
- Insert the stylet into the ETT until the light is near the tip.
- Engage the locking piece and secure it.
- Bend the ETT and stylet at a right angle proximal to the cuff.
- Turn on the light.
- Insert the tube using the bend as a fulcrum and enter the glottic opening, at which time a pronounced glow will appear below the laryngeal prominence if the tube is in the trachea. If the light becomes diffuse, the tube is further away from the surface in the esophagus.
- Unlock the ETT connector and retract the stylet while advancing the ETT.
- Inflate the cuff.

Removing a foreign body from the airway

If the Heimlich maneuver is not successful in **removing a foreign body** from the airway, the paramedic may need to use a laryngoscope and Magill forceps to attempt to locate and remove the foreign body. The procedure for use is as follows:

- Select the correct size laryngoscope and blade; assemble it and check the light. Use a curved laryngoscope for the removal of foreign bodies.
- Place the patient in the sniffing position (chin up, neck extended, and cervical spine flexed to straighten the airway).
- Hold the laryngoscope in the left hand and insert it into the right side of the patient's mouth, displacing the tongue to the left.
- Visualize and grasp the foreign body with the Magill forceps.
- Remove the foreign body, using care to avoid dropping it and causing further obstruction.
- Remove the laryngoscope and check the ventilation.
- Ventilate if necessary.

Intubation with direction laryngoscopy (visualized)

Intubation with direct laryngoscopy is used when the upper airway is compromised, such as with burns, anaphylaxis, severe edema, trauma, and apnea. Prior to intubation, the patient's mouth should be suctioned to clear secretions and the patient should be oxygenated if possible. Estimate the correct size of the laryngoscope and endotracheal tube (ETT). ETTs are sized according to internal diameter. A large size increases airflow but can cause more trauma than smaller sizes. Adult ETTs usually have an inflatable cuff to effect a tracheal seal, which allows positive-pressure ventilation and prevents aspiration. Pediatric ETTs are usually uncuffed. The procedure for use is as follows:

- Extend the patient's neck if possible before intubation and position him or her in the sniffing position.
- Open the patient's mouth with the cross-finger technique.
- Examine the interior of the mouth.
- Insert the laryngoscope to the vallecula (base of the tongue) to raise the epiglottis and visualize the vocal cords.
- Insert the endotracheal tube into the right side of laryngoscope and through the vocal cords.
- Confirm the correct placement.
- Inflate the cuff or secure the ETT and attach ventilation equipment.

Assessing the difficulty of intubation and use of the Mallampati classification

The **Mallampati classification** is a 1 to 4 (good to bad) scale used to rate the difficulty of intubation based on visualization of the interior of the mouth. Classes 3 and 4 are especially difficult.

- Class I: The tonsils, hard and soft palate, and uvula are all visible.
- Class II: The hard and soft palate and upper part of the tonsils and uvula are visible.
- Class III: The hard and soft palate and base of the uvula are visible.
- Class IV: The hard palate and soft tissues only are visible.

Other indications of possible difficulty intubating include long upper incisors, overbite, inter-incisor distance of less than 3 cm, a narrow palate, a high arched palate, a short and/or thick neck, an inability to extend or fully flex the neck, and a thyromental distance (from the tip of the chin to the thyroid cartilage with the neck extended) of equal to or less than 6 cm.

Tracheostomy care

A **tracheostomy** is a surgical opening (stoma) into the trachea to form an airway in cases of upper respiratory obstruction or long-term mechanical ventilation. Tubes are inserted into the opening to provide a conduit and to maintain the opening. Tracheostomy tubes are usually metal or plastic— most are now lacking an inner cannula because they are nonadherent—and secured with ties around the neck. Tracheostomy tubes are changed using clean technique. For tracheostomy care, place the patient in the semi-Fowler's position and don PPE. Unlock and remove the inner cannula if present, clean with a 3% hydrogen peroxide, and rinse with sterile water. Wipe the area around the stoma with sterile water. If changing the outer cannula, remove the tube and clean it, then reinsert it at a 45° angle to the throat. If suctioning, preoxygenate, set the pressure to 120 to 150 mm Hg, and use sterile technique, inserting the catheter 0.5 cm longer than the length of the tracheostomy tube. Suction only on withdrawal for no more than 10 seconds. If repeating, oxygenate for three to four breaths between.

Percutaneous cricothyrotomy

Percutaneous cricothyrotomy provides an emergency airway when the paramedic is unable to effectively ventilate (to maintain oxygen saturation >90%) or intubate the patient. Needle cricothyrotomy is recommended for children ages 5 to 12 rather than surgical cricothyrotomy, but it is avoided in smaller children because the airway is narrower and softer, increasing the risk of bleeding or airway misplacement. The procedure for use is as follows:

- Position the patient supine with the neck in the neutral position and cleanse the skin.
- If possible, inject the site with 2–3 mL of 1% lidocaine with epinephrine.
- Stabilize the site with the thumb and middle finger, and use the index finger to palpate the area between the cricoid cartilage and thyroid membrane.
- Needle: Insert an over-the-needle catheter with a 10 mL syringe containing 5 mL water at a 45° angle and aspirate until bubbles appear. Change the angle to 20°, advance the catheter, and remove the needle. Connect the adapter and attach the BVM.
- Surgical/Open: Stab the site with a #10 scalpel, insert a hemostat or tracheal hook to enlarge the opening, insert a gum-elastic bougie until reaching resistance, and then insert the ETT over the bougie and secure.

Nasotracheal intubation

Nasotracheal intubation (nonvisualized) can be used with patients 12 years or older, but it is contraindicated with head (frontal) or midfacial trauma. The procedure for use is as follows:

- Spray 4% atomized lidocaine into both nares.
- Apply 4% lidocaine gel to the nasopharyngeal airway (NPA) (to dilate the nares).
- Preoxygenate the patient.
- Remove the NPA and insert a lubricated nasotracheal tube at a 90° angle, maintaining the bevel toward the septum.
- Advance the tube, listening for air sounds, which get louder at the larynx.
- At the glottic opening, continue to advance the tube with inhalations to reduce trauma to the vocal cords.
- As the tube enters the trachea, the patient may cough or gag, so observe for vomiting.
- Auscultate both lungs for air sounds, and observe the chest for symmetric movement.
- Inflate the cuff with 5–10 mL air.
- Confirm tube placement and secure the tube.
- Ventilate 8–10 times per minute.

Digital intubation

Digital intubation uses only the hand and an endotracheal tube (ETT) for intubation. It may be used for comatose or paralyzed patients and a trauma patient with cervical spine injuries, difficult airways, or a large amount of secretions or blood in the airway that prevents identification of landmarks.

The procedure for use is as follows:

- Apply BSI protective gear.
- Check the tube and cuff.
- Place the head in the sniffing position or do a jaw thrust.

- Open the mouth with the finger-scissor method and insert the index and middle finger of the dominant hand in the mouth to the glottis, depress the tongue, lift the epiglottis off of the back of the pharynx and creating a channel for the ETT to be inserted between fingers.
- Insert the tube down and through the glottis until the cuff passes the glottis.
- Secure the tube against the teeth, and attach the syringe to inflate the cuff.
- Detach the syringe and attach the BVM for ventilation.
- Confirm placement with capnography and auscultation, listing for bilateral air sounds and the absence of epigastric sounds.
- Secure the tube with ties.

Arterial blood gases

Arterial blood gases are monitored to assess the effectiveness of oxygenation, ventilation, and acid-base status and to determine oxygen flow rates. The partial pressure of a gas is the pressure that is exerted by each gas in a mixture of gases, proportional to its concentration, based on total atmospheric pressure of 760 mm Hg at sea level. Normal values include the following:

- Acidity/alkalinity (pH): 7.35–7.45.
- Partial pressure of carbon dioxide ($PaCO_2$): 35–45 mm Hg.
- Partial pressure of oxygen (PaO_2): ≥80 mg Hg.
- Bicarbonate concentration (HCO_3): 22–26 mEq/L. A lower level is a base deficit, and a higher level is a base excess.
- Oxygen saturation (SaO_2): ≥95%.

The relationship between these elements, particularly the $PaCO_2$ and the PaO_2, indicates the respiratory status. For example, $PaCO_2$ >55 and PaO_2 <60 in a patient previously in good health indicates respiratory failure. There are many issues to consider. Ventilator management may require a higher $PaCO_2$ to prevent barotrauma and a lower PaO_2 to reduce oxygen toxicity.

Positive airway pressure (PAP) devices

All **positive airway pressure (PAP) devices**, such as <u>continuous PAP</u> (CPAP), have an air blower that delivers pressurized room air to an interface/mask. The pressure can be increased or decreased by adjusting the speed or the amount of airflow, with most machines generating from 2 to 20 cm of water pressure. Carbon dioxide is expelled through a vent or a nonrebreather valve on expiration. <u>Bilevel PAP (BiPAP, BPAP)</u> devices deliver two levels of pressure, which can be preset. Inspiratory PAP (IPAP) is set at a higher level (10 cm H_2O) than expiratory PAP (EPAP) (5 cm H_2O) to allow the higher pressure needed to open the airway during inspiration but to reduce the pressure to facilitate expiration. PAP is indicated for pulmonary edema, CHF, COPD, asthma, and near drowning. The procedure includes the following:

- Fill the humidifier with distilled water.
- Program the settings.
- Fit the mask and headgear/straps.
- Begin with the pressure at the lowest setting, usually 5 cm H_2O (CPAP), and increase it slowly at 1 cm H_2O every few minutes until the optimal level is reached.
- Monitor the oxygen saturation and respirations.

Positive end-expiratory pressure (PEEP)

Positive end-expiratory pressure (PEEP) is a setting in mechanical ventilation, that is, the airway pressure at the end of an exhalation. The primary purpose of PEEP is to improve oxygenation by preventing airway collapse. The usual settings are 5 to 25 cm H_2O. PEEP is indicated for respiratory distress syndrome/acute lung injury, pulmonary edema, atelectasis, and severe pneumonia resulting in hypoxemia. PEEP may improve gas exchange and lung compliance and prevent alveolar collapse, but it may also decrease gas exchange and cardiac output and cause hypotension and hypoperfusion of internal organs as well as barotrauma and increased intracranial pressure. PEEP is contraindicated with increased intracranial pressure, low cardiac output, pneumothorax (without pleural catheter), and hypovolemia.

The procedure is as follows:

- Start the setting at 5 cm H_2O, and increase it by 2–3 cm H_2O (not to exceed 15) every 30 to 60 minutes to achieve oxygen saturation of greater than 88% or PaO_2 of greater than 55 mm Hg.

Assessment

Primary assessment on arrival at the scene

After surveying the environment for safety issues, the paramedic should quickly conduct a **primary assessment** to identify conditions that are life threatening, as follows:

- Level of consciousness: Alert, responsive to verbal stimuli, responsive to painful stimuli, nonresponsive.
- Breathing status: Normal, abnormal, rate abnormalities (>24 or <8), apnea, choking, normal or abnormal chest movement, chest rise and fall, noisy respirations, use of accessory muscles, tripod position, nasal flaring.
- Circulatory status: Radial and carotid pulse, pulse abnormalities, major bleeding, skin color—pink, blue, pale—skin temperature, skin moisture, capillary refill, signs of shock.

Life-threatening conditions must be treated immediately, as follows:

- If there is no radial pulse but there is a carotid pulse, lie the patient flat and elevate his or her feet 8–12 inches.
- No pulse: Begin CPR.
- Shock: Lay the patient flat, elevate his or her feet 8–12 inches, and administer oxygen at 15 L/min.
- Bleeding: Apply pressure to control any bleeding.
- Abnormal breathing: Provide oxygen with a nonrebreather mask. If the patient is unresponsive, cyanotic, or in respiratory distress, use a BVM with supplemental oxygen.
- Unresponsive: Ensure a patent airway.

Based on the assessment, the patient is classified as stable, potentially unstable, or unstable.

History taking

History taking should include the following:

- <u>Chief complaint:</u> If the patient is unable to explain, information may be gathered from his or her family, friends, or others who are present. Look for a medical alert bracelet or other such jewelry.
- <u>Nature of the illness or mechanism of injury:</u> Reason for calling EMS, cause of the injury, type of illness. Look for environmental clues (fire, drug paraphernalia, motor vehicle accident).
- <u>Signs and symptoms observed or reported by the patient:</u> Skin temperature, open wounds, BP abnormalities, pain, or difficulty breathing.
- <u>Precipitating events:</u> Falls, accidents, violence, eating, exercising, walking, driving.
- <u>Pediatric considerations:</u> Check capillary refill to assess blood flow in infants and children younger than 6 years of age. Assess the pulse at the brachial artery (inside of the upper arm) for infants up to 1 year of age and the carotid artery in the neck for children older than 1 year. The paramedic may need to use distraction to gain the child's trust and alleviate fears. Encourage the parents/caregivers to hold the child if possible and assist in calming the child.
- <u>Geriatric (older adult) considerations:</u> Determine if the patient needs assistive devices, such as hearing aids, eyeglasses, cane, walker, or dentures.

OPQRST method of history taking

O	Onset	The time that the symptoms associated with this event started.
P	Provocative; palliative. Positioning	That which makes it better; that which makes it worse. The position that the patient is in on arrival and the need to remain in this position or to move him or her.
Q	Quality of discomfort	Burning, stabbing, nagging, crushing, sharp, or dull.
R	Radiation of pain	Area to which pain moves from the original site.
S	Severity of pain	Based on a 1-to-10 or other appropriate scale.
T	Time	Historical onset, such as earlier, similar events.

SAMPLE method of history taking

S	Signs and symptoms	Pain, bleeding, shortness of breath, injuries, fever, rash.
A	Allergies	Medications, environmental (foods, insects, plants, animals).
M	Medications	Prescribed, over-the-counter (OTC) vitamins/minerals, birth control, erectile dysfunction medications, herbal preparations, recreational drugs, other people's medications.
P	Past pertinent history	Especially related to the current event.
L	Last oral intake	Foods, fluids, other substances.
E	Events (precipitating)	Occurrence just prior to the event.

Taking a history of sensitive topics

When asking a patient about **sensitive topics,** the paramedic should try to provide as much privacy as possible in an emergent situation in order to maintain confidentiality and protect the patient from reprisals. The paramedic should ask questions directly in a straightforward and nonjudgmental manner, stressing the need for information in order to help the patient, especially if the patient is reluctant to answer. Sensitive topics include the following:

- Sexual history: People who engage in unusual or unhealthy sexual practices, such as sadomasochism, autoerotic asphyxiation, swinging, and prostitution, are often reluctant to admit to those practices. Adolescents may be especially reluctant to admit that they are pregnant or have engaged in sexual activity or have had an abortion. Males (especially those older than age 40) should be asked about the use of erectile dysfunction drugs (such as Viagra) because they are a contraindication to some medical treatments.
- Physical/Sexual abuse and/or violence: Victims often lie about abuse to defend the abuser or out of shame or fear of further violence.
- Alcohol/Drug use and abuse: Patients often underreport the extent of their drinking or drug taking or deny it altogether. Patients may be concerned about legal actions, especially if they have been driving impaired and got into an accident.

Special history-taking challenges

Special history-taking challenges include the following:

- Silent patient: Be patient, sensitive, and alert for nonverbal clues.
- Talkative patient: Allow the patient to speak freely for a few minutes and then periodically summarize.
- Anxious patient: Be patient, provide reassurance, and explain all procedures.
- Patient with multiple complaints: Ask the patient to help prioritize his or her issues.
- Hostile/angry patient: Remain calm; respond as appropriate.
- Intoxicated patient: Avoid cornering, belittling, or challenging the patient or asking the patient to lower his or her voice or stop swearing. Remain calm and treat the patient with respect.
- Depressed, crying patient: Question the severity of the patient's depression; listen and remain supportive and nonjudgmental.
- Patient with a language barrier: Use a translator if possible. Use hand gestures. Show the equipment before using it; point to the part of the body where the equipment will be used.
- Patient with a visual impairment: Announce your presence and explain all procedures verbally. Tell the patient before touching him or her.
- Patient with a hearing impairment: Determine if the patient has a hearing aid, and obtain it if possible. Speak slowly and clearly, facing the patient for any hearing deficit. If the patient has no hearing, use writing, hand gestures, and demonstrations to communicate.

Instrumental Activities of Daily Living (IADL) assessment tool

Instrumental Activities of Daily Living (IADL) assessment tool measures eight activities necessary for an adult to function independently. This tool helps to determine the need for supportive services. Scores are assigned as 0 (cannot do independently) or 1 (minimal or adequate degree of ability), so the total score ranges from 0 to 8, with a higher score indicating more independence in care. Abilities that are measured include the following:

1. Telephone use (ability to look up numbers and/or call numbers).
2. Shopping for food, clothes, or needed items.
3. Food preparation (plans diet and prepares food).
4. Housekeeping (ability to perform all or part of household duties).
5. Laundry (can wash all or some of personal clothes and linen).
6. Transportation availability (ability to drive or use public transportation).
7. Medication (ability to be responsible for managing prescriptions and taking medications).
8. Financial responsibility (ability to keep track of finances, pay bills, and budget correctly).

Assessment of functional abilities

Functional abilities should ideally be assessed in an active manner, with the person demonstrating the ability to sit; stand; get on and off of the toilet; walk; bend down; remove shoes, shirt, or jacket and then put them on again; listen; read; and answer questions. However, in an emergent situation, this type of assessment is often not possible. Careful questioning about the home environment can help with approximating the type of activities required and physical limitations that the patient experiences. A careful history of functional ability can pinpoint when and if changes occurred. Again, specific questioning guides patients: "When did you begin to use a cane?" "How old were you when you stopped using the tub?" "What is the biggest problem with caring for yourself?" or "When did you have a hip replacement, and how has that changed your life?"

Secondary assessment

Following completion of the primary assessment and after attending to any life-threatening problems that are identified, carry out **a secondary assessment** as follows:

- Measure vital signs: Pulse (radial to carotid for adults and brachial for infants and small children), respiration rate, and BP. Using the correct BP cuff size is essential for accuracy. The length of the bladder in the cuff should be equal to 80% of the arm's circumference, and the lower edge of the cuff when positioned should end about 1 inch above the antecubital fossa (inner elbow). Inflate the cuff to 160 to 180 initially, and increase the pressure if pulse sounds are heard at that level.
- Ask further questions as indicated: This may focus on the primary complaint or other complaints, depending on the situation.
- Conduct a physical examination: Examine the body; palpate for areas of tenderness or swelling; auscultate heart, lung, and abdominal sounds; and note any injuries. Do a brief head-to-toe assessment, and compare one side of the body with the other, noting any asymmetry.
- Treat any life-threatening injuries or conditions noted immediately.

Assessing the patient's level of consciousness

The **AVPU** is a quick assessment done to determine the patient's level of consciousness. This may be one of the first assessments done when initially attending to a patient.

Alert, voice, pain, unresponsive (AVPU)

A	Alert and awake; aware of person, place, time, and condition. Follows commands. Pediatric: Active and responds to external stimuli and to caregiver.	Yes	No
V	Responds to verbal stimuli, but the eyes do not open spontaneously. Pediatric: Responds only when the caregiver calls the child's name.	Yes	No
P	Responds to painful stimuli, such as pinching the skin/earlobe, but not to verbal stimuli. Pediatric: Responds only to painful stimuli, such as pinching the nailbed.	Yes	No
U	Unresponsive; does not respond to painful or verbal stimuli. Pediatric: Unresponsive.	Yes	No

Assessment of lung sounds

The lungs should be auscultated for normal and abnormal **breath sounds.**

Vesicular	Normal low-pitched sound over lung bases and most lung fields.
Bronchovesicular	Medium-pitched sound heard over the main bronchi. Duration is the same in expiration and inspiration.
Bronchial	Normal high-pitched loud sound heard over the trachea. The expiratory sound is as long or longer than the inspiratory sound. It is abnormal if it is heard over the lung bases.
Rales (crackles)	High-pitched crackles usually heard at the end of expiration in the lung bases, indicating fluid in the alveoli. May be fine or coarse.
Rhonchi	Deep rumbling sound may be high-pitched and sibilant (whistling) or low-pitched and sonorous (snoring) caused by constricted airways or large amounts of secretions in the airways. It is more pronounced on expiration.
Wheezes	High- or low-pitched whistling or musical sounds most pronounced on expiration. They often indicate asthma or foreign-body obstruction.
Stridor	Crowing sound caused by inflammation and swelling of the larynx and trachea. Common finding in croup (associated with cough).
Grunts	Indicates respiratory distress in a newborn.
Friction rub	Grating sound heard over the area of the lungs where the pleura are inflamed.

Assessment of a patient's mental status

When **assessing a patient's mental status**, make note of the following:

- Level of consciousness: AVPU assessment.
- Posture and behavior: Abnormal findings include restlessness, agitation, bizarre posturing, catatonia (immobility), and tics or other abnormal movements.
- Dress, grooming, and hygiene: Kempt or unkempt, clean or dirty.
- Facial expressions: May vary widely (anxious, depressed, angry, sad, elated, or fearful). Note whether the patient's expressions seem appropriate to the situation/words.
- Speech/Language: Quantity, rate, fluency, appropriate/inappropriate. Note aphasia (inability to speak and/or understand words), dysphonia (abnormal voice/difficulty speaking), or dysarthria (difficulty speaking words).
- Mood: Nature and duration of the patient's current mood. Note suicidal ideation.
- Thoughts/Perceptions: Note logic, relevance, and organization of thoughts and abnormal findings, such as thought blocking (sudden period of silence in the middle of a sentence while speaking), flight of ideas (racing thoughts), incoherence, confabulation (producing distorted memories), loose association (responses not connected to questions or one sentence not connected to the next), or transference (redirecting emotions to a substitute). Note homicidal or suicidal thoughts, obsessions, compulsions, delusions, illusions, and hallucinations.
- Judgment: Note the patient's insight, ability to make decisions, and ability to plan.

Assessment of memory and attention

Techniques for the **assessment of memory and attention** include the following:

- Orientation: Ask patient questions to determine if he or she knows person (their name), place (where they are), time (date and hour), and event (what's happening). If a patient knows all of that information, then he or she is oriented × 4.
- Digit span test: Tell or show the patient a sequence of six or seven numbers and ask him or her to recall and repeat them.
- Word recall: Name three unrelated items and ask the patient to remember them. Wait a few minutes, and then ask the patient to name the items.
- Serial 7s test: Ask the patient to count backward from 100 by 7s (100, 93, 86. . .).
- Spell backward test: Ask the patient to spell "world" backward (D-L-R-O-W).
- Remote memory: Ask the patient to tell his/her birthdate or that of a close family member.
- Recent memory: Ask the patient to describe events earlier in the day.
- Current memory: Ask the patient to recall your name or the name of someone else present and to whom the patient was recently introduced.

Blood glucose monitoring

Blood glucose monitoring is done with a glucometer. Testing is indicated with a decreased level of consciousness or confusion in a diabetic patient or a decreased level of consciousness with the cause being unknown. The glucometer must be calibrated and tested regularly. Test results from capillary blood tend to be lower than test results on venous blood. The testing procedure is as follows:

- Wipe the site with an alcohol swab. The alcohol must be thoroughly dried before puncture, or it may interfere with the test results.
- Prick the side of the finger pad with a lancet or lancing device rather than the fingertip because the fingertip is more sensitive.
- Express a drop of blood onto the test strip.
- Insert the test strip into the glucometer according to the manufacturer's recommendations.
- Read the test results.
- Dispose of the lancet in a sharps container.

Warming the hand or lowering it may help to ensure adequate blood for the test. Hypoglycemia (low blood sugar/insulin reaction) is a reading of ≤70 mg/dL. Hyperglycemia (high blood sugar) is a reading of ≥160 mg/dL.

Cardiac electrical conduction system and the electrocardiogram (ECG)

The **electrocardiogram (ECG)** records and shows a graphic display of the electrical activity of the heart through a number of different waveforms, complexes, and intervals as follows:

- P wave: Start of the electrical impulse in the sinus node and spreading through the atria, muscle depolarization.
- QRS complex: Ventricular muscle depolarization and atrial repolarization.
- T wave: Ventricular muscle repolarization (resting state) as cells regain a negative charge.
- U wave: Repolarization of the Purkinje fibers.

A modified lead II ECG is often used to monitor basic heart rhythms and dysrhythmias. Typical placement of leads for a two-lead ECG is 3 to 5 cm inferior to the right clavicle and left lower rib cage. Typical placement for a three-lead ECG is the right arm (RA) near the shoulder, the V₅ position over the fifth intercostal space (LA), and the left upper leg (LL) near the groin.

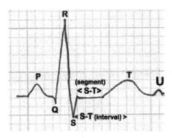

12-lead electrocardiography

The most common electrocardiography setup is the **12-lead ECG,** which assesses 12 different views of the heart. The 12-lead ECG actually comprises 10 electrodes and 12 sources of measurement as follows:

- Four limb electrodes: right and left arm and right and left leg (RA, LA, RL, LL). Put in place, avoiding heavily muscled areas.
- Six precordial (in front of the heart/pericardium) electrodes:

V1—Right sternum, fourth intercostal space.

V2—Left sternum, fourth intercostal space.

V3—Halfway between V2 and V4.

V4—Midclavicular line, fifth intercostal space.

V5—In line with V4 at the anterior axillary line.

V6—In line with V4 and V5 at the midaxillary line.

The patient should be placed in the flat supine position for the ECG, although he or she can sit in the semi-Fowler's position if unable to tolerate a flat position. The skin should be dry and the hair clipped or shaved to improve the electrode contact, and conductive gel is applied to the electrode. The skin can be wiped with an alcohol pad to remove oils or other residue before applying the electrodes. Electrodes should not be placed directly over a bone.

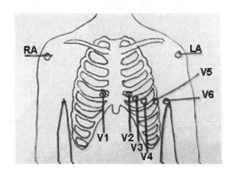

i-STAT CHEM 8+

There are many point-of-care testing devices available; the one most commonly used for comprehensive blood analysis is the i-STAT CHEM 8+, which includes the following tests plus hemoglobin and hematocrit:

Basic metabolic panel (i-STAT CHEM 8+)

Test	Normal	Purpose
Blood urea nitrogen (BUN)	7–20 mg/dL	Kidney function. It increases with kidney disease.
Carbon dioxide (CO_2)	20–29 mmol/L	Acid/base balance. It measures bicarbonate.
Anion gap	8–16 mEq/L	Sodium (chloride + bicarbonate). It helps identify metabolic acidosis.
Creatinine	0.8–1.4 mg/dL	Kidney function. It increases with kidney disease.
Glucose	70–128 mg/dL	Blood sugar level. An increase can indicate diabetic ketoacidosis, whereas a decrease can indicate an insulin reaction.
Serum chloride	101–111 mmol/L	Electrolyte level. An increase can indicate metabolic acidosis and respiratory alkalosis, whereas a decrease can indicate respiratory acidosis and metabolic alkalosis.
Serum sodium	136–144 mEq/L.	Electrolyte level. An increase can indicate excess sweating, diarrhea, burns, or the use of diuretics. A decrease can indicate dehydration, vomiting, and diarrhea.
Calcium (ionized)	4.4–5.4 mg/dL (1.1–1.35 mmol/L)	Electrolyte level. Critical values: <2 mg/dl (<0.5 mmol/L) may result in tetany and >7 mg/dL (>1.75 mmol/L) may result in coma.

Cardiac biomarkers

When the heart is damaged, it releases **cardiac biomarkers**, substances that aid in diagnosis. Biomarkers include the following:

- Creatine kinase (CK) and isoenzyme (MB): CK-MB is specific to the heart muscle, and the level increases within 4–8 hours of a heart attack; it peaks at about 24 hours (earlier with thrombolytic therapy), and it remains elevated for 72 hours.
- Myoglobin (heme protein that transports oxygen) is found in skeletal and cardiac muscles. The level increases 1–3 hours after a heart attack and peaks within 12 hours. Although an increase is not specific to a heart attack, a failure to increase can be used to rule out an MI.
- Troponin I is found only in the heart muscle. Levels increase 3–6 hours after a heart attack, peak in 14–20 hours, and return to normal within 5–7 days.
- Troponin T is found in heart and skeletal muscle. Levels increase 3–6 hours after a heart attack, peak in 12–24 hours, and return to normal in 10–15 days.
- Brain natriuretic peptide (BNP) is secreted by the ventricular muscle with increased volume and pressure. An increased level indicates heart failure.

Reassessment

Reassessment involves ongoing monitoring of the patient at regular intervals to determine changes in his or her condition or trends such as decreasing BP or increasing agitation.

- 70 -

Reassessment is done after a secondary assessment. Unstable patients should be reassessed at least every 5 minutes and stable patients every 15 minutes. Reassessment should include reviewing the primary assessment, taking vital signs, repeating the physical examination (including evaluation of mental status), and monitoring the chief complaint and response to interventions. Reassessment findings should be compared to baseline findings. The patient's airway, ventilation, and circulation should be reassessed as well as the patient's degree of pain—stable, better, or worse. Each intervention should be reassessed for effectiveness and the need for modifications of treatment or if new interventions should be determined. If the patient is receiving oxygen, the tank and all of the equipment should be checked to ensure that they are functioning properly.

Medicine

Neurological (nervous) system

The **neurological (nervous) system** consists of the central nervous system ([CNS] brain, spinal cord, and nerves) and the peripheral nervous system ([PNS] sensory neurons, ganglia [nerve clusters], and nerves connecting to the CNS). The brain consists of the cerebrum (frontal, temporal, parietal, and occipital lobes); the cerebellum; and the brain stem, which is continuous with the spinal cord. The PNS is divided into the autonomic nervous system (ANS) and the somatic nervous system (SoNS). The autonomic nervous system controls the body's organs and maintains homeostasis (balance). Functions of the ANS include control of the heart rate and function, respiration, digestion, sexual arousal, and other systems. The SoNS comprises cranial and spinal nerves that connect the CNS to the skeletal muscles and skin. The SoNS is the voluntarily controlled component of the PNS, and it receives and responds to external sensory stimuli from the skin and sensory organs.

Hemorrhagic and ischemic strokes

Strokes result from interruption of blood flow to an area of the brain. Ischemic strokes (80%) are caused by blockage of an artery supplying the brain, usually from a thrombus (blood clot) or embolus (traveling clot). Hemorrhagic strokes (20%) result from a ruptured cerebral artery, causing not only a lack of oxygen and nutrients but also edema (swelling) that causes widespread pressure and damage. With both types, patients may experience weakness, paralysis, and loss of sensation in one or more extremities; difficulty speaking or loss of speech; vision impairment; difficulty swallowing; headache; an altered state of consciousness (confusion, disorientation); or coma. Transient ischemic attacks (TIAs) from small clots cause similar but short-lived (minutes to hours) symptoms. Emergent treatment includes placing the patient in the semi-Fowlers or Fowler's position and administering oxygen. The patient may require oral suctioning if the secretions pool. The patient's airway, breathing, and circulation should be assessed, and an IV access line should be placed. Patients should be transported immediately to the receiving facility because thrombolytic therapy to dissolve blood clots should be administered within 1 to 3 hours.

Cincinnati Prehospital Stroke Scale

The **Cincinnati Prehospital Stroke Scale** should be administered to any patient who is suspected of having a stroke. The patient may be experiencing a stroke if testing positive for any of the three signs and should be transported to the receiving facility as soon as possible.

Cincinnati Prehospital Stroke Scale

Signs	Directions to patient	Abnormal results
Facial drooping	Smile. Show your teeth.	One side of the face is weak or paralyzed and doesn't move as well as the other.
Arm drifting	Close your eyes and hold your arms out straight and hold them there for 10 seconds.	One arm doesn't move at all or drifts downward.
Speaking abnormality	Repeat after me: "Don't count your chickens before they are hatched."	Patient slurs words, uses inappropriate words, or is unable to respond.

- 72 -

Los Angeles Prehospital Stroke Screen

The **Los Angeles Prehospital Stroke Screen** is used to assess patients in a prehospital setting who have symptoms that suggest a stroke (such as altered state of consciousness, difficulty speaking, one-sided weakness, or paralysis). The results are positive for stroke if all criteria are met or are unable to be measured and the physical exam shows an unequal response. Note: A patient may still be having a stroke even if all the criteria are not met.

General criteria	Yes	No	Unknown
Age >45	X		
No history of epilepsy or seizures	X		
Onset of symptoms <24 hours	X		
Patient was able to walk before the onset of symptoms	X		
Blood glucose between 60 and 400 mg/dL	X		

Physical criteria	Equal	Right	Left
Facial smile	Normal	Droop	Droop
Grip strength	Normal	Weak or no grip	Weak or no grip
Arm strength	Normal	Drifts or falls down	Drifts or falls down

Types of headaches

Type of headache	Characteristics	Prehospital
Tension	Steady, constant pressure-like pain usually starting in the forehead, temples, or the back of the neck.	May vary depending on the cause and severity. Manage the patient's airway/ventilation/oxygen supplementation as needed, dim the lights, place the patient in a position of comfort (usually semi-Fowler's or Fowler's), and apply a cold compress.
Cluster	Unilateral, occurring one to eight times daily, often for several weeks and associated with severe pain in the eye and orbit and radiating to the face and temporal area.	
Migraine	Severe recurring headaches often characterized by prodrome phase, aura phase, headache phase, and recovery phase.	
Head/Neck trauma related.	Vary but may start at neck or shoulders and radiate to the top of the head.	

Bleeding/Stroke related	Epidural: Sudden severe, intense. Subdural: Progressive headache worsening over time. Subarachnoid: "Thunderclap" severe headache with abrupt onset; it may be worse at the back of the head. Stroke: Tension-type headache with the site of pain relating to the area of injury. Often associated with alterations in mental status and other symptoms, such as weakness, paralysis, nausea and vomiting, and photophobia.	May vary depending on the cause and severity. Manage the patient's airway/ventilation/oxygen supplementation as needed, dim the lights, place the patient in a position of comfort (usually semi-Fowler's or Fowler's), and apply a cold compress.

Generalized seizures

Seizures are sudden, involuntary, abnormal electrical disturbances in the brain that can manifest as alterations of consciousness, spastic tonic and clonic movements, convulsions, and loss of consciousness.

- Tonic-clonic (grand mal): Occurs without warning.
- Tonic period (10–30 seconds): The eyes roll upward with loss of consciousness, the arms flex, and the body stiffens in symmetric contractions with cyanosis and salivating.
- Clonic period (usually 30 seconds or longer): Violent rhythmic jerking with contraction and relaxation and sometimes incontinence of urine and feces.

During the seizure, the patient's head and body should be protected from injury, but no attempt should be made to insert anything into the mouth or restrain the patient. If possible, the patient should be screened from spectators and turned onto his or her side (the recovery position) to prevent aspiration. Following seizures, there may be confusion, disorientation, and impairment of motor activity and speech and vision for several hours. Headache, nausea, and vomiting may occur. Prehospital: Monitor the airway, breathing, and circulation and suction and administer oxygen as needed. Insert a nasopharyngeal airway for assisted ventilation if the patient is cyanotic.

Partial seizures

Partial seizures are caused by an electrical discharge to a localized area of the cerebral cortex, such as the frontal, temporal, or parietal lobes with seizure characteristics related to the area of involvement. They may begin in a focal area and become generalized, often preceded by an aura.

- Simple partial: Unilateral motor symptoms including somatosensory, psychic, and autonomic.
- Aversive: The eyes and head are turned away from the focal side.
- Sylvan (usually during sleep): Tonic-clonic movements of the face, salivation, and arrested speech.
- Special sensory: Various sensations (numbness, tingling, prickling, or pain) spreading from one area. May include visual sensations, posturing, or hypertonia. These are rare in patients <8 years.

- **Complex (psychomotor):** There is no loss of consciousness, but there may be altered levels of consciousness, and patients may be nonresponsive with amnesia. May involve complex sensorium with bad tastes, auditory or visual hallucinations, and a feeling of déjà vu or strong fear. Patients may carry out repetitive activities, such as walking, running, smacking lips, chewing, or drawling. Patients are rarely aggressive. The seizure is usually followed by prolonged drowsiness and confusion. Occurs from age 3 through adolescence. Prehospital: Provide supportive care.

Status epilepticus

Status epilepticus (SE) is usually generalized tonic-clonic seizures that are characterized by a series of seizures with the intervening time being too short for the regaining of consciousness. The constant seizures and periods of apnea can lead to exhaustion, respiratory failure with hypoxemia and hypercapnia, hyperthermia, cardiac failure, and death. SE may result from uncontrolled epilepsy, noncompliance with anticonvulsive treatment, stroke, encephalopathy, drug toxicity, brain trauma, brain tumors (neoplasms), and metabolic disorders. SE is life threatening, so treatment should begin as soon as possible.

Prehospital care includes the following:

- Place an intravenous (IV) line.
- If opioid drug intoxication is the suspected cause, administer naloxone.
- Administer midazolam (intramuscular [IM]) (5 to 10 mg), lorazepam (IV), or diazepam (IV) to control seizures.
- Intubate and ventilate if the patient is in respiratory distress.
- Provide supportive care for seizures to prevent injury.
- Control hyperthermia with room-temperature water to the skin and an IV normal saline (NS) bolus of 500 mL.

AEIOU TIPS mnemonic to outline the potential causes for altered mental status

Many different conditions can lead to altered mental status, and the paramedic should consider all possibilities because emergent treatment may vary depending on the cause. Always check for medical alert jewelry. The following **AEIOU TIPS mnemonic** is a helpful guide to recalling potential causes:

A	Alcohol/ Acidosis	Note the smell of alcohol, empty alcohol containers.
E	Endocrine/Epilepsy	Consider electrolyte imbalance, encephalopathy; note oral trauma, urinary incontinence.
I	Infection	Consider urinary infection in older adults, meningitis, encephalitis, sepsis.
O	Opiates/ Overdose	Note if the pupils are constricted, drug paraphernalia, history of drug taking, empty medicine containers.
U	Uremia/ Underdose	Note generalized edema, history of kidney failure, failure to take prescribed medicines.
T	Trauma	Consider head injury, excessive bleeding, assault.
I	Insulin	Check refrigerator/medicine cabinet for diabetes medications; check the blood glucose level.
P	Poisoning/Psychosis	Note any history of psychiatric illness; observe the environment for poisons.

| S | Stroke/ Seizures | Note one-sided weakness, incontinence, difficulty speaking, somnolence. |

Glasgow Coma Scale (GCS)

The **Glasgow Coma Scale (GCS)** measures the depth and duration of coma or impaired levels of consciousness; it is used for postoperative assessment. The GCS measures three parameters: best eye response, best verbal response, and best motor response, with a total possible score that ranges from 3 to 15. The same scale is used with slight modifications for infants.

Eye opening	4: Spontaneous. 3: To verbal stimuli. 2: To pain (not of face). 1: No response.
Verbal	5: Oriented (Infant: Smiles, exhibits appropriate interactions). 4: Conversation is confused, but he or she can answer questions (Infant: Crying but consolable). 3: Uses inappropriate words (Infant: Moaning, sometimes inconsolable). 2: Speech incomprehensible (Infant: Inconsolable, agitated). 1: No response.
Motor	6: Moves on command (Infant: Moves spontaneously or with purpose). 5: Moves purposefully to respond to pain. 4: Withdraws in response to pain. 3: Decorticate posturing (flexion) in response to pain. 2: Decerebrate posturing (extension) in response to pain. 1: No response.

Injuries/conditions are classified according to the total score as follows: 3–8, coma; $\leq$ 8, severe head injury; 9–12, moderate head injury; 13–15, mild head injury.

Hydrocephalus

The brain's ventricular system produces and circulates cerebrospinal fluid (CSF). **Hydrocephalus** occurs with an imbalance between the production and absorption of cerebrospinal fluid in the ventricles, resulting from impaired absorption (communicating) or obstruction (noncommunicating). In early infancy before closure of the cranial sutures, head enlargement is the most common presentation, but in older children and adults with less elasticity in the skull, neurological symptoms usually relate to increasing pressure on structures of the brain. Symptoms in children may include headache relieved by vomiting, papilledema, strabismus, ataxia, irritability, lethargy, confusion, and difficulty communicating. Adults may have similar symptoms and may be misdiagnosed as having Alzheimer's. Treatment is a ventriculoperitoneal shunt, which is a catheter with a one-way valve to prevent backflow extending from the ventricles to the peritoneal cavity or the right atrium to drain excess fluid. Complications include infection characterized by a rapid rise in temperature, confusion, and neurological impairment and obstruction characterized by increasing signs of intracranial pressure. Prehospital: Provide supportive care. Elevate the patient's head for transport for surgical repair.

Types of dementia

Type of dementia	Characteristics
Alzheimer's disease	Progressive dementia beginning with short-term memory loss and difficulty remembering names. It progresses to impaired judgment; disorientation; confusion; behavioral changes; difficulty understanding, reading, and using language; dysphagia; incoordination and inability to walk; and incontinence.
Creutzfeldt-Jakob disease	Rapidly progressive prion disease with impaired memory, behavioral changes, and incoordination, leading to death.
Huntington's disease	Progressive genetic disorder characterized by involuntary movements, muscle rigidity, abnormal eye movement, ataxia, lack of impulse and behavioral control, increasing confusion, difficulty communicating, and depression.
Pick's disease (frontotemporal dementia)	Form of progressive dementia resulting in destruction of neurons with change of personality and lack of judgment and empathy. The loss of language may include the ability to understand and communicate.
Wernicke's encephalopathy	Inflammatory hemorrhagic encephalopathy due to thiamine deficiency, often associated with alcoholism. Symptoms include paralyzed eye muscles; double vision; ataxia; and a range of mental changes from forgetfulness to delirium tremens and Korsakoff's psychosis, which can lead to amnesia, disorientation, and hallucinations. Patients are able to produce language, although with some impairment, such as incorrect words or sounds, but they may have difficulty understanding.

Guillain-Barré syndrome (GBS)

Guillain-Barré syndrome (GBS) is an autoimmune disorder of the motor peripheral nervous system, resulting in demyelination of protective myelin sheaths, often triggered by a viral gastroenteritis or *Campylobacter jejuni* infection. As the myelin sheath becomes inflamed and demyelination occurs, the conduction of nerve impulses is blocked. In most cases, the axon remains intact and recovery occurs with remyelination; however, in severe cases, the axon is permanently damaged, and recovery is incomplete or death occurs. Symptoms include numbness and tingling with increasing lower extremity weakness that may ascend and become generalized, affecting the legs and then the arms, sometimes resulting in complete paralysis and an inability to breathe without ventilatory support. Deep tendon reflexes are typically absent, and some people experience facial weakness and ophthalmoplegia (paralysis of muscles controlling the movement of the eyes). Prehospital: Provide supportive care and oxygen as needed, and start an IV access line. If the patient is in respiratory failure, intubation and ventilation may be necessary.

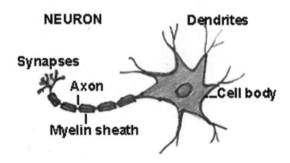

- 77 -

Meningitis and encephalitis

Meningitis is infection of the meninges (the lining around the brain and spinal cord), usually caused by bacteria. Pus covers the brain and invades and blocks the ventricles, obstructing the cerebrospinal fluid (CSF) and leading to increased intracranial pressure. Symptoms include abrupt onset, fever, chills, severe headache, nuchal (neck) rigidity, and alterations of consciousness with seizures, agitation, and irritability. Some may have rash, photophobia, hallucinations, and/or aggressive behavior, stupor, or coma. Infants may have incessant crying, floppiness, and bulging fontanels. Prehospital: Obtain a history of the symptoms and use contact/droplet isolation (masks). Provide supportive care and oxygen if the saturation level falls below 95%. Provide an IV access line. Keep the lights dim. **Encephalitis** is an infection of the brain tissue. A number of arboviruses, including West Nile virus, can cause flu-like symptoms that progress to viral encephalitis. Encephalitis can be a complication of Lyme disease, spread by infected ticks, and the herpes simplex virus. Onset usually involves flu-like symptoms with sore throat, headaches, muscle aches, fever and chills, myalgia, and rash. Progressive and advanced symptoms are similar to meningitis. Prehospital: Provide care similar to meningitis.

Multiple sclerosis (MS)

Multiple sclerosis (MS) is a central nervous system (CNS), immune-mediated, inflammatory, demyelinating disease believed to be triggered by an unidentified environmental source, such as a virus. The myelin sheath, primarily composed of lipids (fats), is white in appearance, creating the "white matter" of the brain. Impulses travel along the sheath, jumping from one node to another. With MS, an immune reaction causes killer T cells to attack the sheaths, which begin to demyelinate, leaving scarred areas along the axons, slowing nerve transmissions. Initially, symptoms come and go, and the sheaths undergo repair. Over time, however, cells cannot remyelinate and new cells don't develop adequately, so symptoms worsen. Symptoms vary widely, often beginning with muscle tingling and weakness, poor balance, and blurred/double vision. Patients may develop muscle spasticity, bladder and bowel problems, emotional changes, depression, and cognitive impairment. Advanced symptoms include difficulty speaking, breathing problems, tremor, seizures, and hearing loss. Prehospital: Provide IV hydration if the patient is dehydrated; assisted ventilation if he or she is in respiratory distress; and careful positioning to prevent injury, especially with spasticity.

Parkinson's disease (PD)

Parkinson's disease (PD) is an extrapyramidal movement motor system disorder caused by loss of brain cells that produce dopamine, resulting in decreased levels of dopamine. Symptoms appear when 60%–80% of neuronal cells are impaired and dopamine levels drop by 20%–50%. As dopamine levels fall, other areas of the brain function abnormally as well, further impairing motor function. Typical symptoms include tremor of the face and extremities, rigidity, bradykinesia (slow movement), akinesia (absence of movement), stooped posture, and lack of balance and coordination, causing increasing problems with mobility, talking, and swallowing. Some patients may suffer depression, mood changes, and dementia. Tremors usually present unilaterally in an upper extremity. Treatment includes symptomatic support, dopaminergic therapy (levodopa, amantadine, and carbidopa), and anticholinergics (trihexyphenidyl, benztropine). Patients may experience resistance to medications over time. Prehospital: Provide supportive care. Be aware of the risk of choking, especially with advanced Parkinson's disease, and look for signs. Place the patient in the recovery position to prevent aspiration.

Myasthenia gravis (MG)

Myasthenia gravis (MG) is an autoimmune disorder of the neuromuscular system in which acetylcholine receptors are damaged at neural synapses, preventing transmission of impulses to contract muscles. This results in the weakness of voluntary muscles, increasing with activity because the need for acetylcholine is not met. Muscles that are initially affected include those of the eye, neck, and face. Additionally, the thymus gland develops abnormalities, such as hypertrophy or thymoma, in about 90% of those with MG. Onset may be abrupt or gradual, and it occurs in women between ages 20 and 30 and men between ages 70 and 80. There are five classes of MG, depending on severity. Typical symptoms (which tend to worsen through the day) include drooping eyelids; double vision; difficulty speaking, chewing, and swallowing; weakened muscles of respiration; and weakened extremity muscles. Symptoms may exacerbate (worsen) with menstruation, infection, stress, or some medications. Treatment includes angiotensin converting enzyme (ACE) inhibitors, immunomodulating agents, IV immune globulin, plasmapheresis, and removal of the thymus. With myasthenic crisis, respiratory failure may occur. Prehospital: Provide the patient with supportive care, place in the recovery position, intubate and ventilate if he or she is in respiratory distress.

Cerebral palsy (CP)

Cerebral palsy (CP) is a nonprogressive motor dysfunction related to CNS damage associated with congenital, hypoxic, or traumatic injury before birth, during birth, or ≤2 years after birth. CP may include visual defects, speech impairment, seizures, and mental retardation.

Types of motor dysfunction

- Spastic: Constant hypertonia and rigidity lead to contractures and curvature of the spine.
- Dyskinetic: Tremors and twisting with exaggerated posturing and impairment of voluntary muscle control.
- Ataxic: Atonic muscles in infancy with lack of balance, instability of muscles, and poor gait.
- Mixed: Combinations of all three types with multiple areas of damage.

Characteristics of CP

Note: Characteristics may vary widely, depending upon the degree of CNS injury as follows:

- Hypotonia or hypertonia with rigidity and spasticity.
- Athetosis (constant writhing motions).
- Ataxia.
- Hemiplegia (one-sided involvement, more severe in the upper extremities).
- Diplegia (all extremities are involved, but it is more severe in the lower extremities).
- Quadriplegia (all extremities are involved with the arms flexed and legs extended).

Prehospital: Provide routine supportive care and position the patient to prevent injury.

Spina bifida and myelomeningocele

The terms **spina bifida** and **myelomeningocele** are often used interchangeably, but there is a distinction. Spina bifida is a neural tube defect with an incomplete spinal cord, and there often are missing vertebrae that allow the meninges and spinal cord to protrude through the opening.

There are five basic types, as follows:

1. <u>Spina bifida</u>: Defect in which the vertebral column is not closed with varying degrees of herniation through the opening.
2. <u>Spina bifida occulta</u>: Failure of the vertebral column to close, but there is no herniation through the opening, so the defect may not be obvious.
3. <u>Spina bifida cystica</u>: Defect in closure with an external sac-like protrusion with varying degrees of nerve involvement.
4. <u>Meningocele</u>: Spina bifida cystica with a meningeal sac filled with spinal fluid.
5. <u>Myelomeningocele</u>: Spina bifida cystica with a meningeal sac containing spinal fluid and part of the spinal cord and nerves.

Associated conditions can include hydrocephalus, brain damage, cerebral palsy, epilepsy, neurogenic bladder, and mental retardation. Prehospital: Provide routine supportive care according to the patient's needs and position him or her to prevent injury.

Gastrointestinal (GI) tract

Body part	Function
Mouth	Chews, moistens, begins carbohydrate hydrolysis (the breakdown of food by enzymes), creates a bolus of food. Connected to the esophagus by the pharynx.
Esophagus	Transports a bolus through the lower esophageal sphincter (which prevents backflow up the esophagus) to the stomach by peristalsis (wavelike contractions).
Stomach	Churns, secretes acids and enzymes, begins hydrolysis of proteins, and creates chyme (a more fluid substance).
Small intestine (about 20 feet long)	<u>Duodenum:</u> Accepts chyme and digests food to prepare for absorption. <u>Jejunum:</u> Absorbs most of the nutrients from the food, including vitamin B_{12}. Accepts bile from the liver and gallbladder to digest fats and pancreatic enzymes from the pancreas to digest proteins, fats, and carbohydrates. <u>Ileum:</u> Contains the ileocecal valve, which controls the flow of chyme into the large intestine.
Large intestine (about 5 feet long)	<u>Cecum:</u> Reabsorbs fluids and electrolytes. <u>Appendix:</u> Serves no function. <u>Ascending, transverse, descending colon:</u> Reabsorbs water, vitamin K, and electrolytes to form feces.
Rectum	Stores feces.
Anus	Contains sphincters that control the expelling of feces.

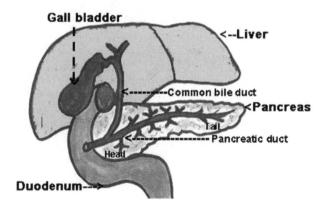

Gastrointestinal (GI) bleeding

Upper **gastrointestinal (GI) bleeding** (mouth to stomach) is characterized by nausea and hematemesis (vomiting of bright-red blood or partially digested, dark-brown, granulated ["coffee ground"] blood) and/or abdominal pain on palpation. With lower GI bleeding (small intestine to anus), the abdomen may be distended and tender and the patient may be passing blood through the anus. If bleeding has been slow and chronic, the patient may have only vague complaints of weakness and abdominal discomfort. In all cases, blood will mix with the stool. Melena (black-colored stool) usually indicates an upper GI bleed because the blood has been partially digested. Hematochezia (wine-colored stool or bright-red blood in the stool) indicates a lower GI bleed. Patients develop shock if blood loss is profound (≥40%). Prehospital: Examine the abdomen and note pain, monitor vital signs, and note signs of acute blood loss (fall in BP; increase in pulse; pallor; or cold, clammy skin). Provide suctioning if needed. Provide supplemental oxygen and ventilation as needed. Place the patient in the recovery position if he or she is vomiting. Place the patient flat with the feet elevated for shock. Provide shock treatment per protocol if necessary. Start an IV access line and administer fluids.

Trigeminal neuralgia (tic douloureux)

Trigeminal neuralgia (tic douloureux) is severe facial pain caused by pressure on or damage to the fifth cranial nerve. Trigeminal neuralgia may result from trauma (accidental, surgical), stroke, multiple sclerosis, or tumor. Patients may have intermittent severe stabbing, burning pain or, in some cases, continuous pain, generally on one side and one area of the face. Initial symptoms indicating damage to the fifth cranial nerve related to trauma may be numbness on one side of the forehead, cheek, and chin and the inability to smile. Treatment to control pain may include anticonvulsives such as carbamazepine and tricyclic antidepressants (TCAs) such as amitriptyline. Opioids are generally not effective for neuropathic pain. Prehospital: Evaluate facial trauma patients for potential injury to the fifth cranial nerve. If the patient is already diagnosed, avoid touching his or her face if possible and ask the patient what triggers an episode of pain. Blow-by oxygen may be needed if the patient cannot tolerate contact with a nonrebreather mask or nasal prongs.

Peritonitis

Peritonitis is a bacterial infection of the peritoneum (lining of the abdominal cavity) that can lead to septicemia and death. Patients with kidney failure (especially those patients on peritoneal dialysis), liver disease, or infection of the GI tract are especially at risk. Other causes include abdominal wounds, ruptured appendix, perforated colon, diverticulitis, abdominal surgery, and inflammatory bowel disease. Symptoms include signs of acute abdomen: abdominal pain and distension, rigid abdomen, nausea and vomiting, diarrhea, fever, and chills. Other symptoms may include decreased urine output, excessive thirst, and tachycardia (rapid pulse). Peritonitis may be associated with ulcerative diseases, such as Crohn's disease (open sores develop through all layers of the walls of any part of the GI tract, most commonly in the ileum and cecum) and ulcerative colitis (open sores develop in the inner lining of the colon). Prehospital: Obtain an accurate medical history, note the condition of the abdomen with gentle palpation, provide supplemental oxygen/ventilation as needed, and position the patient for comfort because he or she may be experiencing severe pain. Provide an IV access line.

Pediatric and geriatric patients with abdominal pain

Because **pediatric patients** (infants and small children) have large organs in relation to their size and very little protection with muscles or bone, organs such as the bladder, liver, and kidneys are more likely to suffer injury from abdominal trauma than they are in adults. Children have smaller rib cages and pelvic bones, so the abdomen is more vulnerable. Abdominal pain in the child may be associated with constipation (right lower quadrant pain) as well as appendicitis, which is characterized by right lower quadrant pain and a lack of appetite, but it may be hard to identify in children because they may not have appreciable or localized pain initially. Pain persisting for ≥48 hours usually indicates rupture of the appendix. Vomiting and diarrhea may rapidly deplete fluids because of the lower fluid volume, resulting in dehydration. **Geriatric patients** with acute abdomen may not exhibit typical abdominal rigidity or guarding. Additionally, abdominal pain may be an indication of a heart attack rather than a GI problem.

Acute abdomen

Acute abdomen is an acute intra-abdominal disorder that occurs with abrupt onset and usually requires emergency surgical intervention, although some patients may respond to other treatments, such as antibiotics. Acute abdomen may result from infection (peritonitis, pancreatitis, cholecystitis, appendicitis, diverticulitis), perforation, rupture of an internal organ (such as the spleen), aortic aneurysm, obstruction, or infarction (necrotic tissue resulting from a blood clot or obstructed blood supply). If the blood supply is interrupted, gangrene may occur within 6 hours. Acute abdomen is characterized by inflammation, distension (often including guarding and rigidity), and acute pain (moderate/severe of fewer than 7 days' duration). Abdominal pain is especially concerning in pediatric and geriatric patients and those with impaired immune systems (such as HIV/AIDS patients and those receiving chemotherapy). Acute abdomen in infants and children may indicate conditions not commonly found in adults such as pyloric stenosis, volvulus, and necrotizing enterocolitis. Prehospital: Obtain a medical history regarding the quality, location, and duration of pain as well as referred pain; place the patient in a comfortable position; administer oxygen; start an IV access line; and provide rapid transport.

Ulcerative diseases

Ulcerative colitis (UC) is superficial inflammation of the mucosa of the colon and rectum causing ulcerations ranging from pinpoint to extensive. Ulcerations may bleed and produce purulent material. The mucosa of the bowel becomes swollen, erythematous (red), and granular. Onset of UC is usually between ages 15 and 30. UC may affect only the rectum, the entire colon, or only the left colon. Indications of UC include abdominal pain (usually absent or mild unless the disease is severe), bloody diarrhea, rectal bleeding, fecal urgency, and tenesmus (a constant feeling of having to defecate). **Crohn's disease** is chronic inflammation of any area of the GI system but most commonly the small intestine and the beginning of the large intestine, resulting in ulcers that may involve the full thickness of the intestinal wall. An acute flare-up may mimic appendicitis. Indications include diarrhea (watery), rectal bleeding, abdominal cramping and pain (usually in the right lower quadrant), nausea, vomiting, fever, and night sweats. Prehospital: Provide supportive care, manage the patient's airway/ventilation/oxygen supplementation (to maintain an oxygen saturation of ≥94%), and provide shock treatment per protocol if necessary. Provide an IV access line and administer fluids.

Cholecystitis

Cholecystitis can result from obstruction of the bile duct with gallstones, sometimes causing pancreatitis from obstruction of the pancreatic duct. When the bile duct is obstructed, the gallbladder distends and becomes inflamed, preventing the flow of bile into the duodenum. Jaundice may occur if the common bile duct is obstructed and the bile is reabsorbed into the blood. The disease is most common in overweight women ages 20–40, but it can occur in pregnant women and people of all ages, especially diabetics or the elderly. Children may develop cholecystitis secondary to cystic fibrosis, obesity, or total parenteral nutrition. Symptoms range from asymptomatic to severe right upper quadrant or epigastric pain (especially after eating) persisting two to six hours per episode and flatulence. Disease of the biliary tract may cause radiation of pain to the back and nausea and vomiting. Prehospital: Take a careful medical history. Provide pain management, antiemetic, and supplemental oxygen if needed, and start an IV access line with acute abdomen.

Acute pancreatitis

Acute pancreatitis is related to chronic alcoholism or cholelithiasis in 90% of patients, but it may also be caused by viral infections, cysts, cystic fibrosis, drugs, trauma, and metabolic disorders. Pain is usually acute and is midepigastric, left upper abdominal, or more generalized and may radiate to the back. Nausea and vomiting and abdominal distension are common. Pancreatitis may result from direct injury to pancreatic cells or activation of pancreatic enzymes that essentially autodigest pancreatic tissue, resulting in edema, necrosis, and hemorrhage. Vasodilation and increased capillary permeability may result in hypovolemia as fluid shifts to the retroperitoneal space. Complications may include shock, acute respiratory distress syndrome, and multiorgan failure. Pancreatitis may range from mildly edematous to necrotizing. Chronic pancreatitis may develop over years, resulting in extensive tissue damage with symptoms occurring intermittently initially and then continuously. Oily, foul-smelling stools may occur. Prehospital: Take a complete medical history of the patient's complaints, provide pain management, antiemetics, and supplemental oxygen/ventilation as needed. Start an IV access line, and provide shock treatment per protocol if necessary.

Diverticulitis and appendicitis

Diverticulitis is inflammation of diverticula, which are bulging herniations in the intestinal wall, most commonly in the sigmoid colon, although they can occur anywhere within the GI tract from pharynx to anus. Diverticulitis may result in bowel obstruction, infection, perforation, or hemorrhage as undigested food and bacteria accumulate in diverticula, forming a fecalith (hard mass) that can impair circulation. Symptoms include acute pain (usually LLQ), abdominal distension, nausea, flatus, fever, constipation, and irregular bowel habits. **Appendicitis** is inflammation of the appendix resulting from bacterial infection and obstruction. Appendicitis is most common in adolescents and young adults. Typical symptoms include abdominal pain (often initially around the umbilicus [navel] and then localizing to the RLQ). Nausea and vomiting are common. With rupture, high fever and intense pain are common as the patient develops signs of peritonitis. Any movement may increase the pain. The patient may develop shock. Prehospital: Take a complete medical history, and position the patient for comfort with his or her knees flexed. Provide pain management, antiemetics, supplemental oxygen as needed, and an IV access line.

Bowel obstruction

Bowel obstruction occurs when there is a mechanical obstruction of the passage of intestinal contents because of constriction of the intestine, occlusion, or a lack of muscular contractions (paralytic ileus). Obstructions may be caused by congenital or acquired abnormalities/disorders. Small bowel obstruction may be caused by adhesions, surgical manipulation, cancer, or Crohn's disease, and large bowel obstruction may be caused by cancer, diverticulitis, or volvulus. Small bowel obstructions are usually corrected nonsurgically with a nasogastric (NG) tube and suction, whereas large bowel obstruction usually requires surgical intervention. Symptoms include abdominal pain, distension, and rigidity; nausea and vomiting; diminished or absent bowel sounds; severe constipation; respiratory distress (from the diaphragm pushing against the pleural cavity); shock; and sepsis. Untreated bowel obstruction may lead to infarction (ischemia and necrosis). Infarction has a high mortality rate even with surgery. Prehospital: Provide IV access and insert an NG tube (according to protocol). Provide pain management and a position of comfort. Monitor vital signs and provide supplemental oxygen/ventilation as necessary.

Hernias

Hernia repair (herniorrhaphy) is the most common surgery for infants and children and is also common in adults. Surgery is done to repair herniation of the peritoneum with a segment of bowel through the abdominal wall to prevent an incarcerated (twisted, ischemic, necrotic) hernia. There are three main types of hernias:

- Inguinal: Herniation in the inguinal canal. This is common in premature or low-birth-weight infants, usually males, and may occur bilaterally. It is also common in adult males.
- Femoral: Herniation posterior to the inguinal ligament. This is more common in females.
- Umbilical: Herniation in the umbilical ring.

Inguinal and femoral hernias are usually repaired early because of the danger of incarceration (tissue becomes stuck); however, umbilical hernias often heal over time in children without surgical repair. If incarceration has occurred prior to surgery, the affected segment of bowel is resected. Symptoms include obvious protrusion and mild discomfort. With incarceration, severe pain, inability to pass gas or stool, and nausea and vomiting are common, progressing to complete bowel obstruction, shock, and sepsis. Prehospital: Provide supportive care, IV access, and NS if perfusion is inadequate, and provide supplemental oxygen/ventilation as necessary.

Allergic reactions and anaphylaxis

Allergic reactions are a response of the body's immune system to an antigen (substance), such as peanuts or shellfish. The body produces antibodies (immunoglobulins, such as IgE or non-IgE) that can identify and try to neutralize or destroy antigens. Allergic responses may be mild (local rash, redness, itching, swelling, congestion), moderate (generalized itching, difficulty breathing), or severe (life-threatening anaphylaxis). With **anaphylaxis**, an antigen triggers the release of substances that affect the skin, cardiopulmonary system, and GI tract. Histamine causes initial redness and swelling by inducing vasodilation. In some cases, initial reactions may be mild, but subsequent contact can cause a severe, life-threatening response. Symptoms include a sudden onset of weakness, dizziness, and confusion; tachycardia; generalized swelling; itching; severe low BP leading to shock; airway obstruction; nausea and vomiting; hives; diarrhea; seizures; coma; and death. Prehospital: Inject epinephrine to the lateral thigh and repeat every 5–10 minutes as needed; provide an antihistamine (diphenhydramine) for itching, a vasopressor for hypotension, a

- 84 -

bronchodilator (salbutamol/magnesium sulfate) for respiratory distress, supplemental oxygen/ventilation, intubation if necessary, an IV access line, and immediate transport.

Collagen disease

Scleroderma is a diffuse connective tissue disorder in which insoluble collagen forms and accumulates in the tissues, leading to fibrotic changes, loss of elasticity, and impaired movement. The disorder starts in the hands and spreads systemically to the heart, lungs, and digestive system, eventually causing death. Scleroderma is characterized by the CREST syndrome: (**c**)alcium deposits in the skin, (**R**)aynaud's phenomenon (circulatory impairment in the hands and feet when exposed to the cold), (**e**)sophageal hardening, (**s**)clerodactyly, and (**t**)elangiectasia (capillary dilation that forms vascular lesions). Symptoms include generalized pain, stiffness, weakness, difficulty swallowing, nausea/vomiting, weight loss, shortness of breath, chest pain, and kidney failure, resulting in severe headache, vision problems, confusion, and hypertension. Prehospital: Care will vary depending on the presenting symptoms but may include pain management, supplemental oxygen/ventilation, and providing an IV access. If there is severe circulatory impairment in the hands or feet with Raynaud's syndrome, a calcium channel blocker (nifedipine) or topical nitroglycerin is indicated.

Systemic lupus erythematosus (SLE) is an autoimmune disorder. The immune system becomes unregulated, resulting in an abnormal overproduction of autoantibodies, leading to an immune complex and tissue damage (myopathy). The resultant inflammation stimulates increased the production of antigens, triggering the production of more antibodies in a repeating cycle. Manifestations include the following:

- Skin: Lesions, plaques, and a butterfly rash across the nose and cheeks.
- Mucosa: Oral ulcerations of the tongue or hard palate.
- Hematology: Anemia and iron deficiency.
- Cardiovascular system: Pericarditis and atherosclerosis are common.
- Kidneys: Progressive renal damage resulting in hypertension.
- Joints: Changes similar to those of rheumatoid arthritis.
- CNS: Changes in behavior and cognitive ability, depression, and psychosis may occur.
- GI: Nausea and vomiting.

Lupus may have inactive periods followed by flare-ups (mild to severe). In a lupus crisis, the patient may have kidney failure, fluid around the heart, swelling of the brain causing seizures, and respiratory distress. Prehospital: Assess for signs of infection; provide IV access and respiratory support with supplemental oxygen and intubation/ventilation if necessary.

Transplant-related problems

There is a wide range of solid organ **transplants,** including eye tissue, skin, heart, lungs, liver, pancreas, intestines, kidneys, bone, tendons, ligaments, and more recently uterus and face. The United Network for Organ Sharing (UNOS) has established allocation priorities for each type of transplant. The paramedic will likely have contact with patients who are potential donors and who are recipients. Because of immunosuppression required to prevent rejection of transplanted organs, patients are at risk of infection. Rejection may occur at any time after transplantation, although the risk is greatest in the first few weeks. Drugs for immunosuppression include azathioprine, corticosteroids, cyclosporine, tacrolimus, mycophenolate acid, and biologic agents such as polyclonal antibodies. Cyclosporine interacts with many drugs, and azathioprine may cause neutropenia, liver damage, and GI effects. Symptoms of rejection include weakness, fatigue, shortness of breath, pain, fever, hypotension, generalized edema, loss of appetite, decreased urinary output, and tachycardia. Prehospital: Record the patient's medications, observe for signs of infection and rejection, and provide supplemental oxygen/ventilation and IV access as indicated.

Infectious and contagious diseases

Infectious diseases, which may be communicable or noncommunicable, are those that are caused when microorganisms (such as bacteria, viruses, retroviruses, protozoa, helminths [worms], and fungi) invade the body and cause disease. Noncommunicable diseases may spread from an environmental source, such as contaminated water or food (such as with food poisoning), or from insects that carry the disease (such as with Lyme disease). However, they do not spread from person to person, so only standard precautions are needed when caring for these patients. **Contagious diseases** are infections that are communicable from person to person. They may be spread through direct physical contact and sneezing or coughing as well as through contact with blood or other body fluids (feces, semen, urine, or perspiration). With contagious diseases, the type of precautions needed depends on the mode of infection, and they may range from contact to droplet to airborne precautions; the type of PPE needed also varies.

Decontaminating an ambulance

Decontaminating an ambulance begins with removal of any debris with sharps being deposited in a sharps container and soiled linen being red-bagged. Then, the equipment and surfaces that have had contact with a patient or with contaminated materials must be cleaned, disinfected, or sterilized, depending on the type of equipment/surface and the type of contamination. Between patients, surfaces and equipment should be wiped down with a disinfectant, such as a 1:100 chlorine bleach solution or premixed wipes. Alcohol-based products are effective for many organisms, but not for *Clostridium difficile* (which is spread through fecal contamination). If equipment is left with a patient at a receiving facility, that facility must clean the equipment or place it in a red bag before returning it. At the end of the day, the entire ambulance should be cleaned. Various methods of sterilization, including the use of fogging agents and UV lights, are available. All cleaning procedures must be recorded for compliance purposes.

Human immunodeficiency virus/acquired immune deficiency syndrome (HIV/AIDS)

Human immunodeficiency virus (HIV) is the retrovirus that causes **acquired immune deficiency syndrome (AIDS)**. Diagnosis is determined by the CD4+ T-cell count with AIDS currently being diagnosed with a CD4+ count of <200 cells per mm^3. HIV is transmitted in bodily fluids (blood, semen, vaginal secretions, and breast milk) that contain free virions and infected CD4+ T-cells. The categories are as follows:

- Category A (CD4+ count <500): Asymptomatic or lymphadenopathy, sore throat, and fatigue.
- Category B (CD4+ count 200 to 499): Conditions include candidiasis, pelvic inflammatory disease, bacillary angiomatosis, fever, diarrhea, herpes zoster, low platelet count, weight loss, and peripheral neuropathy.
- Category C (AIDS) (CD4+ count <200): Invasive diseases are common. Conditions include cervical cancer, candidiasis, cytomegalovirus, encephalopathy, TB, *Pneumocystis jirovecii* pneumonia (formerly known as *P. carinii* pneumonia), Kaposi's sarcoma, toxoplasmosis, and wasting syndrome.

About 1.2 million people in the United States have HIV infection, but 13% are unaware of it. Risk factors include unprotected sex, especially males having sex with other males, and needle sharing. Prehospital: Provide supportive care, manage the airway, support ventilation, and provide IV access if necessary. Use droplet precautions for cough.

Hepatitis and fulminant hepatitis

Hepatitis, inflammation of the liver, is caused by bacteria, viruses, or exposure to toxic chemicals, including alcohol or drugs. However, viral infection is most common and may be foodborne or bloodborne, although only bloodborne diseases, hepatitis B and C, cause chronic liver disease. Symptoms include jaundice (yellowing of the skin, eyes) and clay-colored stool from impaired excretion of bile, dark urine, abdominal pain, flu-like symptoms, nausea and vomiting, loss of appetite, itching, and increased risk of bleeding. **Fulminant hepatitis** is an acute inflammation of the liver that may be caused by viruses, toxic substances, or overdose with acetaminophen and can result in encephalopathy, liver failure, and death within 1 to 72 days. Vaccinations are available for hepatitis A virus (HAV) and hepatitis B virus (HBV). Treatment for accidental exposure to HAV is prophylaxis with HAV immune globulin, and that for HBV is initiating vaccinations if the patient is unvaccinated or HBV immune globulin. Prehospital: Use standard precautions, provide supportive care as needed, manage the patient's airway/ventilation, and provide IV fluids if necessary.

Types of hepatitis infection

Type of hepatitis	Transmission	Characteristics
Hepatitis A (HAV)	Foodborne/oral-fecal, oral-anal sex	Usually mild infection (may be asymptomatic) lasting about 2 months.
Hepatitis B (HBV)	Bloodborne/ blood and body fluids/sex, needle sharing	It is the most common bloodborne hepatitis and very infectious. Most recover within 6 months, but up to 10% develop chronic disease, which can lead to liver failure or liver cancer, and they become carriers.
Hepatitis C (HCV)	Bloodborne/ blood and body fluids/sex/ needle sharing	Causes chronic infection and is the most common cause of liver transplantation. May be asymptomatic for 20 years.
Hepatitis D (HDV)	Bloodborne/ blood and body fluids/sex/ needle sharing	Co-infection with HBV and increases the risk of developing fulminant hepatitis and cirrhosis.
Hepatitis E (HEV)	Foodborne/oral-fecal, oral-anal sex	Usually found in travelers from South Asia or Africa from areas with poor sanitation. It is a mild form similar to HAV.
Hepatitis G (HGV-C)	Bloodborne/ blood and body fluids/sex/ needle sharing	Believed to be a variation of type C and can be a co-infection of HBV and HBC. Usually a mild infection, but it may be chronic.

Pneumonia

Pneumonia is inflammation of the lung, filling the alveoli with exudate and interfering with ventilation. It is common throughout childhood and adulthood. Pneumonia may be a primary disease, or it may occur secondary to another infection or disease, such as lung cancer. Pneumonia may be caused by bacteria, viruses, parasites, fungi, or toxins. Pneumonia is characterized by location (lobar, bronchial/lobular, interstitial). Symptoms include fever, chills, cough, purulent sputum, and difficulty breathing, chest pain on cough or deep inhalation, and headache. Bacterial pneumonia is treated with antibiotics, and viral pneumonia is treated with antivirals. Geriatric patients may exhibit confusion. Pediatric patients with undeveloped/poor immune systems or chronic illnesses (such as cystic fibrosis or asthma) have an increased risk. Prehospital: Use standard and droplet precautions, including wearing a protective face mask. Place the patient in a position of comfort (usually with his or her head elevated), manage the airway/ventilation, provide supplemental oxygen, and provide IV access line if indicated.

Tuberculosis (TB)

Tuberculosis (TB) is caused by *Mycobacterium tuberculosis* with airborne transmission. The bacteria multiply in the lungs. If the immune system walls off the organisms, latent TB develops and the patient has no symptoms and cannot spread the dormant disease. With active TB or reactivated dormant TB (associated with an impaired immune system), the bacteria multiply and form cavities, spreading throughout the lungs and sometimes to other parts of the body. Symptoms include cough (mucopurulent sputum or hemoptysis as the disease progresses), fever and chills, night sweats, general malaise and fatigue, anorexia and weight loss, and chest pain when breathing or coughing. Postexposure prophylaxis requires baseline testing immediately and in 8 to 12 weeks. Positive tests require 6 to 9 months of anti-tuberculosis medications for latent infection and 9 to 12 months for active infection. Prehospital: Use standard and airborne precautions, including an N95 or a high-efficiency particulate air (HEPA) filter mask. Provide supportive care and airway/ventilatory support with a high concentration of oxygen as needed. Mask the patient if possible and ensure that the ambulance is well ventilated, notify the receiving facility of the incoming TB patient.

Pediculosis (lice) and scabies

Pediculosis is infestation with lice, transmitted by direct contact as follows:

- Head lice (most common in children).
- Body lice (most common in transient populations, migrants, and homeless) feed on the body but live in clothing or bedding and are spread by sharing bedding, clothes, or towels.
- Pubic lice spread by sexual contact or (rare) sharing clothes or bedding and may infest the genital area, eyebrows, eyelids, lower abdomen, and beard.

Symptoms include itching and skin irritation. Treatment is with topical medication, such as permethrin 1% and manual removal of nits. **Scabies** is caused by microscopic mites that tunnel under the outer layer of the skin, raising small lines (burrows) a few millimeters long. Mites prefer warm areas, such as the webbing between the fingers and skin folds (waist, axillae, genital areas), but they can infest any area. Scabies causes intense itching, and subsequent scratching can result in excoriation and secondary infections. Scabies spreads easily through person-to-person contact. Treatment includes scabicide, such as permethrin 5% cream or oral ivermectin. Prehospital: Use standard and contact precautions.

Tetanus

Tetanus is a life-threatening, noncommunicable bacterial infection caused by a spore found in soil, dust, and animal feces. The bacteria produce an endotoxin affecting the central nervous system. Transmission is through puncture wounds/breaks in the skin or through the umbilical cord after birth. The incubation period is 2 days to months (usually 2 weeks). Symptoms include neck and jaw stiffness, facial spasms, difficulty chewing and swallowing, headache, sensitivity to noise, painful muscle contractions at the site of infection, opisthotonos (rigid hyperextension) positioning, and airway obstruction. Infants may be unable to suck. Complications include laryngospasm, respiratory distress, and death (30%). Preventive measures include tetanus immunizations and boosters every 10 years. After exposure, unimmunized patients

require tetanus immune globulin and tetanus toxoid. Prehospital: Use standard precautions, manage the airway/ventilation/intubation, and provide supplemental oxygen as needed, and an IV access line. Protect the patient from injury.

Infectious viral diseases

Disease	Vaccine	Characteristics/Considerations
Chickenpox (varicella)	Varicella or MMRV	Fever, flu-like symptoms, headache, and generalized vesicular rash. Complications: Viral encephalitis, meningitis, pneumonia, Reye syndrome. Use contact and airborne precautions until lesions are crusted over in 1–3 weeks.
Mumps	MMR or MMRV	Fever, earache, swelling of parotid gland(s), pain, stiff neck (15%). Complications: Spreads to testicles or other parts of the body (heart, kidneys, ovaries, pancreas, brain). There may be hearing impairment. Use standard and droplet precautions.
German measles (rubella)	MMR or MMRV	Low-grade fever, headache, sore throat, anorexia for 1–5 days and then a pink maculopapular rash on the face progressing to the neck, trunk, and legs. Complications: Encephalitis, arthritis (in adolescents). The disease is usually mild, but it poses a risk for the fetus if the mother is infected. Use standard and droplet precautions.
Measles (rubeola)	MMR or MMRV	High fever, conjunctivitis, cough, photophobia, Koplik spots in the mouth, and then a generalized dark-red maculopapular rash, subsiding in 4–7 days. Complications: Diarrhea, otitis media, bronchitis, pneumonia, encephalitis, death. Use airborne precautions while the patient is contagious.
Whooping cough (pertussis)	Dtap or tDap	Catarrhal stage (2 weeks): Nasal congestion, runny nose, low-grade fever, nonproductive cough. Paroxysmal stage (1–6 weeks): Severe "whooping" coughing spasms with thick sputum, especially at night. Infants may have apnea rather than whooping. Convalescent stage (up to 6 weeks): Gradual decrease in coughing. Treated with antibiotics. Use droplet precautions until 5 days after initiating antibiotics.

Influenza	Annual influenza	Abrupt fever, chills, aching, cough, runny nose, sore throat, and headache. Infants and young children: May have croup, conjunctivitis, nausea, vomiting, diarrhea, abdominal pain. Complications (most common in pediatric and geriatric patients): Otitis media, worsening of chronic lung conditions, pneumonia, myocarditis, encephalitis, Guillain-Barré syndrome, Reye syndrome. Use droplet and contact precautions.
Mononucleosis	N/A	Fever (2–3 days), sore throat, swollen tonsils, lymphadenopathy, enlarged spleen and liver, fatigue, malaise. Infants and young children may be asymptomatic. Symptoms usually last 2–3 weeks, although weakness may persist for months. Complications (rare): Encephalitis, meningitis, Guillain-Barré syndrome, ruptured spleen, low platelet count. Use standard precautions.
Herpes simplex 1		A blistering oral lesion or lesions on any other area of the skin. Cold sores typically occur at the border of the lip. Herpetic whitlow (infected finger) is from an infected child sucking a finger. Neonatal infection may be disseminated and may affect the liver, lungs, and brain. Herpetic gingivostomatitis syndrome includes fever, bilateral lymphadenopathy, and lesions in the mouth and tongue, progressing to open painful ulcers making swallowing difficult, so the patient drools. Symptoms usually last 1–2 weeks. Treatment is with acyclovir. Use standard precautions.
Hantavirus pulmonary syndrome		Hantavirus is transmitted through contact with the nesting material, feces, or urine of infected rodents or contaminated food. Initial symptoms are flu-like with fatigue, fever, and muscle aches. Half of those patients who are infected also experience headaches, chills, nausea and vomiting, diarrhea, and abdominal pain. Late symptoms occur within 4–10 days and include cough, shortness of breath, and a feeling of smothering progressing to pulmonary edema and respiratory failure. Prehospital: Use standard precautions, manage the airway/ventilation/intubation and supplemental oxygen as needed, provide an IV line access.
Lyme disease (*Borrelia burgdorferi*)		Tickborne bacterial disease with an incubation period of 1–55 days. <u>Phase I</u> (localized): Fatigue, malaise, headache, stiff neck, low-grade fever, muscle aches. Circular red rash (erythema migrans) at the bite site (50%), conjunctivitis, lymphadenopathy. <u>Phase II</u> (1–4 months after the bite, early disseminated): Multiple erythema migrans, pericarditis, arthralgia, myocarditis, cardiac conduction abnormalities, meningoencephalitis, cranial nerve palsies, peripheral neuropathy. <u>Phase III</u> (late disseminated): Chronic neurological impairment and Lyme arthritis. Prehospital: Use standard precautions. Provide supportive care, manage the airway/ventilation/supplemental oxygen as needed.

Rabies	Viral disease with a 30–90-day incubation period. It is transmitted through contact with the saliva of an infected animal (dog, cat, fox, skunks, raccoon, bat). The virus enters through open skin and travels along the nerves to the brain. Initial symptoms: Fever, chills, malaise, and pain at the bite site. Late: Anxiety, agitation, hallucinations, weakness, paralysis, hydrophobia, coma, respiratory failure, and death. Prehospital: Wash animal bites with soap and water and irrigate with povidone iodine. Notify the receiving facility of the possible need for rabies prophylaxis. Prehospital: Use standard and droplet precautions, provide supportive care, manage airway/ventilation/intubation/supplemental oxygen as needed, and provide an IV access line.

Sexually transmitted diseases

Disease	Characteristics/Considerations
Gonorrhea	Caused by the bacterial species *Neisseria gonorrhoeae*. Transmission is through anal, oral, or vaginal sex. The incubation period is 3 to 8 days. Male symptoms include painful urination, purulent discharge from the penis, and swollen testicles. Females are asymptomatic, or they may have mild difficulty urinating. Complications include prostatitis, orchitis, epididymitis, and sterility (males) and pelvic inflammatory disease and disseminated disease (females). It is treated with antibiotics. The infection may pass to a newborn during birth, causing gonorrheal eye infection and blindness unless eye prophylaxis is provided. Prehospital: Use standard precautions.
Chlamydia	Caused by the bacterial species *Chlamydia trachomatis.* Transmission is through anal, oral, or vaginal sex. It often occurs with gonorrhea. Symptoms: Many are asymptomatic, but the disease can spread and cause urethritis, proctitis, and epididymitis (males) and painful intercourse, pelvic inflammatory disease, fallopian tube damage, and vaginal bleeding (females). Complications include sterility and infertility. Treatment is with antibiotics. Prehospital: Use standard precautions.
Syphilis (*Treponema pallidum*)	Bacterial infection transmitted through oral, anal, or vaginal sex and needle sharing. The incubation period is 10 to 90 days. Primary symptoms (3–8 weeks): Chancres (very contagious). Secondary symptoms (1–2 years): Flu-like symptoms and rash, weight loss, and hair loss. Latent symptoms (>2 years): Asymptomatic. Noncontagious after 4 years. Treatment is antibiotics. Late/Tertiary symptoms: Gummas (lesions) in multiple organs, heart abnormalities, CNS impairment with psychosis, confusion, ataxia, and difficulty speaking. Prehospital: Standard precautions.
Genital herpes (herpes simplex virus 2)	Transmitted though oral, anal, or vaginal sex. The virus enters nerve endings, travels to the nerve ganglion, and stays dormant until reactivated by stress, immunosuppression, menstruation, sunburn, illness, or other triggers. Initial symptoms: Small vesicular lesions in the genital area that rupture and leave open crusting sores; painful urination; flu-like symptoms. Recurrent symptoms are less severe, lasting 8–12 days. Complications include dissemination to other areas of the body, aseptic meningitis, and damage to nerves resulting in atonic bladder, constipation, and impotence. Treatment is with antiviral agents. Prehospital: Use standard, contact, and airborne precautions until disseminated herpes is ruled out.

Gastroenteritis

Gastroenteritis is inflammation of the lining of the GI tract, including the stomach and intestines. It may be caused by bacteria (such as *Escherichia coli* and *Clostridium difficile*), viruses (such as rotaviruses), parasites (such as helminths [worms]), and protozoa (such as *Giardia lamblia*, also known as *Giardia intestinalis*). Symptoms include diarrhea, cramping, abdominal pain, nausea and vomiting, fever, general malaise, headache, abdominal distension, and dehydration if diarrhea or vomiting is severe. Blood tests include electrolytes (to evaluate fluid and electrolyte imbalance) and white blood cell count (it will be elevated with bacterial infection). Stool samples may show parasitic infection or bacteria (such as *C. difficile*). Prehospital: Monitor vital signs and assess for dehydration. Place an IV access line and administer IV fluids if the patient is dehydrated. Administer an antiemetic such as prochlorperazine (Compazine) for nausea and vomiting.

Note: Antidiarrheals are generally not recommended for emergent care because they may cause complications with some types of diarrhea. The use of antimicrobials depends on the causative organism.

Drug-resistant bacterial conditions

Drug-resistant bacterial conditions are an increasing problem because of the widespread use of antibiotics. Reasons for resistance to develop include the following:

- Failure to complete a course of antibiotics as prescribed, allowing for development of superinfections or resistant bacteria, or mismanaged or inappropriate antibiotic therapy, such as treating viral infections with antibiotics to placate patients.
- Prophylactic antibiotic use in livestock, poultry.
- Use of antibiotic soaps and lotions.

Patients who are hospitalized, have undergone surgery, have medical devices in place (such as urinary catheters or intravenous lines), are under the care of healthcare providers, and have been previously treated with antibiotics (particularly for long periods of time) or are immunocompromised are especially susceptible to developing drug resistance. Common drug-resistant infections include the following:

- Multidrug-resistant tuberculosis (MDR-TB).
- Extensive drug-resistant tuberculosis (XDR-TB).
- Methicillin-resistant *Staphylococcus aureus* (MRSA): Often seen in skin infections, wound infections, and pneumonia.
- Vancomycin-resistant *S. aureus* (VRSA): Infections are nonresponsive to methicillin or vancomycin, leaving few drugs to treat patients.
- Vancomycin-resistant enterococcus (VRE).

Endocrine system and hormones produced

Hypothalamus	Links the endocrine and nervous systems. Produces hormones that are stored in the posterior lobe of the pituitary gland, and stimulates the pituitary to release hormones.
Pineal gland	Secretes melatonin and dimethyltryptamine, which control sleep cycles and dreaming.

Pituitary gland	The posterior lobe secretes oxytocin (it stimulates uterine contractions/lactation) and vasopressin (aka antidiuretic hormone) (it raises BP and promotes water reabsorption). The anterior lobe secretes hormones that control cell growth (somatotropin), body growth (growth hormone), release of hormones by the thyroid (thyrotropin), release of steroids from the adrenal glands (corticotropin), and reproductive functions (follicle-stimulating hormone and luteinizing hormone).
Thyroid gland	Secretes hormones that control protein production, basal metabolic rate, and oxygen consumption (T3, T4, and calcitonin).
Parathyroid glands	Secretes parathyroid hormone, which controls the use of calcium.
Adrenal glands	Produce cortisol (roles in metabolism), aldosterone (water and sodium levels), and androgens (male hormones).
Ovaries	Secrete female hormones (estrogen and progesterone).
Testes	Secrete androgens (testosterone).

Diabetic conditions

Diabetes mellitus is a group of metabolic disorders that involve hyperglycemia (increased blood glucose [sugar]) because of defective production and/or action of insulin. Insulin metabolizes glucose to produce energy as fuel for body cells.

- Type 1: Autoimmune destruction of beta cells in the pancreas results in no or deficient insulin production. Treatment: Insulin. Symptoms: Rapid onset, increased thirst, frequent urination, increased hunger, delayed healing, weight loss, frequent infections, and blurred vision.
- Type 2: Insulin baseline may be normal or deficient, but there is no or an inadequate increase in response to a meal, so the glucose level rises but there is decreased uptake by the tissues. Insulin resistance occurs because there is decreased sensitivity to insulin by the tissues. Type 2 diabetes is often related to older age and obesity. Treatment is with oral diabetic agents. Symptoms include slow onset, increased thirst, increased urination, candidal (fungal) infections, delayed healing, and weight gain.
- Gestational: Beta cells in the pancreas are unable to produce adequate insulin during pregnancy, but normal production resumes after delivery. Treatment varies. Symptoms include being asymptomatic or having increased thirst and urinary frequency.

Hyperglycemia

Hyperglycemia is high blood glucose (sugar) with a level of greater than 130mg/dL after fasting for 8 hours or greater than 180 mg/dL 2 hours after eating. Hyperglycemia may occur in undiagnosed diabetic patients or in diabetic patients who have taken inadequate insulin; those who have eaten a diet too high in carbohydrates (sugars); or those who are ill, such as with an infection. Initial signs include polyuria (increased urine), polyphagia (hunger), polydipsia (increased thirst), headaches, lethargy, fatigue, and blurred vision, but if the blood sugar is very high (greater than 250 mg/dL), then patients may become increasingly somnolent, and he or she may develop diabetic ketoacidosis from the buildup of ketones as fat is broken down by the body for energy because sugar/glucose cannot be used. The patient may exhibit Kussmaul's breathing (fruity-smelling breath from ketones), could lapse into a coma, and could die if left untreated. Prehospital: Question the patient about diabetes and the use of diabetes medications. Check the patient's blood sugar level, and monitor the vital signs and oxygen saturation. Manage the airway and assisted ventilation as needed, and provide an IV access line and crystalloid fluids and regular insulin if indicated. Rapid transport is required with altered levels of consciousness.

Hypoglycemia

Hypoglycemia (low blood sugar/glucose) is most often caused by an insulin reaction (too much insulin for the amount of glucose/sugar intake) or an overdose of oral diabetes medications, which stimulate the overproduction of insulin. Hypoglycemia may occur if patients took insulin but skipped a meal, vomited, or exercised too strenuously, depleting the body of sugar/glucose while insulin levels remain high. Increased insulin levels cause glucose levels to fall to at or below 70 mg/dL, initially resulting in tremors, headache, blurred vision dizziness, and pallor leading to confusion, bizarre behavior, lack of coordination, combative behavior, personality changes, tachycardia, and irregular heartbeat. Severe hypoglycemia may lead to seizures, coma, and death. Hypoglycemia is life threatening if untreated. Infants may have dehydration and seizures; geriatric patients may have dehydration and stroke. Prehospital: Ask the patient about his or her diabetes status and use of diabetes medications. Check the patient's glucose level, and administer oral glucose tablets, one tablespoon of sugar, or a glass of orange juice if the patient is able to swallow; provide rapid transport for altered levels of consciousness.

Hyperglycemic hyperosmolar nonketotic syndrome (HHNS) or coma (HHNK)

Hyperglycemic hyperosmolar nonketotic syndrome (HHNS) or **coma (HHNK)** occurs in people without a history of diabetes or in people with mild type 2 diabetes but with insulin resistance resulting in persistent hyperglycemia, which causes osmotic diuresis. Fluid shifts from intracellular to extracellular spaces to maintain osmotic equilibrium, but the increased glycosuria and dehydration result in hypernatremia and increased osmolality (concentration). This condition is most common in persons 50–70 years old, and it often is precipitated by an acute illness such as a stroke, medications such as thiazides, or dialysis treatments. HHNS differs from ketoacidosis because although the insulin level is not adequate, it is high enough to prevent the breakdown of fat. Symptoms include polyuria, dehydration, hypotension, tachycardia, blood glucose >500 mg/dL, changes in mental status, hallucinations, seizures, and hemiparesis. Prehospital: Question the patient about his or her history of diabetes and use of diabetes medications. Check the patient's blood sugar level, monitor the vital signs and oxygen saturation, and provide supportive care and an IV access line as needed. Rapid transport is needed for altered levels of consciousness.

Insulin

Insulin is used to metabolize glucose when the pancreas does not produce insulin in cases of type 1 diabetes mellitus. Patients may need to take a combination of insulins (short and long acting) to maintain glucose control. The duration of action may vary according to the individual's metabolism, intake, and level of activity:

- Rapid acting (lispro [Humalog], aspart [Novolog], glulisine [Apidra]): Onset within 10–30 minutes, peaks between 30–90 minutes, and lasts 3–5 hours.
- Short acting (regular [R] [Humulin, Novolin, or Velosulin for insulin pump]): Onset within 30–60 minutes, peaks in 2–5 hours, and lasts 5–8 hours. Velosulin has an onset in 30 to 60 minutes, peaks in 1–2 hours, and lasts 2–3 hours.
- Intermediate acting (NPH [N]): Onset in 1–2 hours, peaks at 4–12 hours, and lasts 16–24 hours.

- Long acting (insulin glargine [Lantus/Basaglar] and insulin detemir [Levemir]): Lantus and Basaglar—Onset in 1–1.5 hours, no peak time, and lasts 20–24 hours. Levemir—Onset in 1–2 hours, peaks in 6–8 hours, and lasts up to 24 hours.
- Ultralong acting (insulin degludec [Tresiba]): Onset in 30–90 minutes, no peak, and lasts 42 hours.
- Combined/Premixed (NPH/Regular [70/30 or 50/50 or various other combinations]): Onset in 15–30 minutes, peaks at 2–12 hours (depending on the combination), and lasts 16–24 hours.

Oral antidiabetic drugs for type 2 diabetes mellitus

Sulfonylureas First generation: acetohexamide, chlorpropamide, tolazamide, and tolbutamide Second generation: glipizide, glyburide, glimepiride	These increase the production of insulin by the pancreas. They are more effective early in treatment, but they become less effective over time.
Meglitinides repaglinide, nateglinide	These increase the production of insulin by the pancreas. They are faster acting than sulfonylureas. They are taken 30 minutes prior to a meal up to the time of the meal so that they increase insulin production during and after the meal.
Biguanides metformin, metformin with glyburide	These reduce glucose production by the liver. They are often taken as part of combination therapy with another drug.
Biguanides metformin, metformin with glyburide	These reduce glucose production by the liver. They are often taken as part of combination therapy with another drug.
Alpha-glucosidase inhibitors acarbose	These slow the absorption of carbohydrates by the intestines. They are not effective for people with fasting hyperglycemia.
Thiazolidinediones pioglitazone, rosiglitazone	These improve insulin sensitivity, transport, and utilization. They are most effective for people with insulin resistance, but they do not increase the production of insulin, although they may be combined with another drug. Rosiglitazone has restricted use because of the risk of heart attack.

Hyperthyroidism and thyrotoxicosis/thyroid storm

Hyperthyroidism (thyrotoxicosis) usually results from excess production of thyroid hormones from immunoglobulins providing abnormal stimulation. Other causes include thyroiditis and excess thyroid medications. The most common cause of hyperthyroidism is Grave's disease, an autoimmune disorder that stimulates excess production of thyroid hormones. Symptoms of hyperthyroidism vary and include anxiety, tachycardia (90 to 160 bpm), atrial fibrillation, tremor, exophthalmos (bulging eyes), heat intolerance, dry itching skin (especially in geriatric patients), progressive weakness, and altered mental status progressing to coma. Treatment is with radioactive iodine or surgical removal of the thyroid.

Thyrotoxicosis/Thyroid storm is severe hyperthyroidism with sudden onset. It is precipitated by stress, such as injury, diabetic ketoacidosis, infection, heart failure, or surgery, in those untreated or inadequately treated for hyperthyroidism. If it is not promptly treated, it is fatal. Symptoms are similar to hyperthyroidism but more severe. Hyperthermia may be present (>38.5°C) with tachycardia (>130) and nausea, vomiting, and diarrhea. Prehospital: Initiate cooling procedures, provide an IV access line, manage the airway/ventilation/intubation/supplemental oxygen as necessary, provide cardiac monitoring, and provide rapid transport.

Hypothyroidism

Hypothyroidism occurs when the thyroid gland produces inadequate levels of thyroid hormones. Conditions may range from mild to severe myxedema (generalized swelling, including the face and lips). There are a number of causes, including the following:

- Chronic lymphocytic thyroiditis (Hashimoto's thyroiditis).
- Excessive treatment for hyperthyroidism.
- Atrophy of the thyroid gland.
- Medications such as lithium and iodine compounds.
- Radiation to the area of the thyroid gland.
- Diseases that affect the thyroid, such as scleroderma.
- Iodine imbalances.

Symptoms may include chronic fatigue, weight gain, constipation, menstrual disturbances, hoarseness, cold intolerance and subnormal temperature, bradycardia (slow pulse), hypotension, weight gain, thinning hair, thickening skin. Some dementia may occur with advanced conditions, resulting in misdiagnosis of Alzheimer's disease. Myxedema may be characterized by changes in respiration with hypoventilation and carbon dioxide retention resulting in coma. Treatment involves hormone replacement with synthetic levothyroxine. Prehospital: Manage the patient's airway/ventilation/supplemental oxygen and intubation if necessary. Monitor oxygen saturation and carbon dioxide levels, provide an IV access line, and administer a vasopressor or atropine for severe bradycardia if necessary.

Addison's disease and Addisonian crisis

Adrenocortical insufficiency (Addison's disease) is caused by damage to the adrenal cortex, related to a variety of causes, such as autoimmune disease, genetic disorders, infections, surgical removal of the gland, idiopathic atrophy, or tumor. Addison's disease may occur secondary to hypothalamus or pituitary malfunction if adrenocorticotropic hormone (ACTH) is not available to stimulate the adrenal cortex. Whatever the cause, the glucocorticoids, mineralocorticoids, and androgens normally produced by the adrenal cortex are deficient or absent. With Addison's disease, serum glucose and sodium levels decrease and serum potassium increases, and this can lead to severe dehydration and **Addisonian crisis**, characterized by circulatory shock, altered mental status, tachycardia, cardiac dysrhythmias, tachypnea, and hypotension. Addisonian crisis is life threatening. Prehospital: Manage the patient's airway/ventilation/supplemental oxygen as needed, provide IV access and IV fluids, and provide rapid transport because the administration of hydrocortisone is time critical. Calcium chloride and albuterol (per nebulizer) may help reduce potassium levels.

Cushing's syndrome/disease

Cushing's syndrome is characterized by excessive production of the steroid hormone cortisol (a "fight or flight" hormone). The most common cause is tumor of the pituitary gland, but it can also result from adrenal tumors; alcoholism; and steroid use, such as may occur with long-term steroid treatment for patients with COPD. **Cushing's disease** occurs when the following physical changes occur because of the increased cortisol level: Moon facies (round face), excessive weight gain and abdominal girth, excessive hair growth, abdominal stretch marks, bruising of the skin, generalized weakness, hypertension, severe insulin-dependent diabetes mellitus, decreased fertility, vision loss or impaired vision, and mood/behavioral or psychiatric problems. Treatment options may include surgery, radiation, or a change in medication, depending on the cause. Prehospital: Monitor patient's vital signs and general condition; if he or she is in diabetic ketoacidosis, provide an IV access line and insulin (per protocol). Manage the patient's airway/ventilation/supplemental oxygen as needed.

Assessing for risk of suicide

Suicidal ideation occurs frequently in those with mood disorders or depression (common in geriatric patients). Although females are more likely to attempt suicide, males actually successfully commit suicide three times more often, primarily because females tend to take overdoses from which they can be revived, whereas males choose more violent means (jumping from a high place, shooting, or hanging). This holds true for adolescents and adults. Risk factors include psychiatric disorders (schizophrenia, bipolar disorder, post-traumatic stress disorder [PTSD], and substance abuse), physical disorders (HIV/AIDS, diabetes, traumatic brain injury, spinal cord injury), and social problems (bullying). Passive suicidal ideation involves wishing to be dead or thinking about dying without making plans, whereas active suicidal ideation involves making plans. Patients at risk should be questioned about their feelings, problems, plans for suicide, and access to weapons. High-risk findings include the following:

- Violent suicide attempt (knives, gunshots) or access to a weapon.
- History of a suicide attempt and a suicide attempt with a low chance of rescue.
- Ongoing psychosis or disordered thinking.
- Ongoing severe depression and feelings of helplessness.
- Lack of a social support system.

Behavioral alterations

Behavioral alterations may include agitation, anger, throwing temper tantrums (children), acting aggressively (adolescents/adult), exhibiting poor judgment, and acting inappropriately. Behavioral alterations may result from psychiatric disorders (such as depression, schizophrenia, and bipolar disorder) and psychiatric medications as well as numerous other causes, including the following:

- Hypoglycemia/Low blood sugar (insulin reaction).
- Lack of adequate oxygen interferes with brain function.
- Shock (low BP; a rapid pulse results in inadequate blood supply to the brain).
- Mind-altering substances (cocaine, methamphetamine, lysergic acid diethylamide [LSD], Rohypnol [the date-rape drug]).
- Brain infection (meningitis, encephalitis, brain abscess).
- Seizure disorders (epilepsy, other causes of seizures).
- Poisoning/Overdose (lead poisoning, drug overdose).
- Malnutrition resulting in inadequate nourishment of brain tissue.
- Substance abuse (drug or alcohol abuse/withdrawal).
- Heat extremes (hypothermia/hyperthermia).

Indications of being a danger to self or others include severe agitation, hallucinations, delusional thinking, paranoia, self-destructive behavior (cutting, drug/alcohol abuse, promiscuity, risk-taking activities), depression, and suicide attempts. A patient may pose a risk to others if he or she is behaving in a threatening or violent manner and has a weapon (club, gun, knife, or baseball bat).

Calming patients with behavioral emergencies

Patients with **behavioral emergencies** are often agitated and may be confused, fearful, and/or aggressive, so the paramedic must remain calm and approach the patient slowly; remain at a safe distance; and avoid fast movements, threatening postures, or attempts at physical contact, acknowledging the patient's agitation and offering assistance ("I can see that you're upset, and I want to help") and maintaining eye contact (unless the person is violent and reacts aggressively). The paramedic should encourage the patient to talk about what is causing the behavior and should answer questions honestly while avoiding threatening, arguing, or challenging the patient. If the patient is suffering hallucinations or delusional thinking, the paramedic should avoid playing along ("I don't see what you do") but should also avoid contradicting the patient directly when responding. Family or friends may assist with intervention. The paramedic should not leave the patient unattended and should try to lower distressing stimuli (such as lights and noise) and consider contacting law enforcement. Restraints should be avoided if possible.

Agitated/excited delirium

Patients with **agitated/excited delirium** are often very combative, aggressive, violent, and uncooperative, and they may exhibit shouting, threaten violence, and behave bizarrely. The patient may experience hallucinations, disorientation, paranoia, and panic. Patients may be exceptionally strong and seem insensitive to pain. They are often hyperthermic (high temperature). Agitated/Excited delirium may be associated with hypoglycemia, brain damage, chemical imbalance, and substance abuse (methamphetamine, cocaine, phencyclidine [PCP—"angel dust"], and LSD). Patients often require restraints for their own or for others' safety, but they are at risk of death by asphyxiation or restraint (positional) because they fight desperately against the restraints. Prehospital: The paramedic should use active listening and try to establish rapport while assessing the patient's intellectual functioning, orientation, judgment and thought processes, language, mood, and appearance to determine if law enforcement or other assistance is needed. The patient may refuse care, but implied consent is legal for patients with abnormal behavior. The patient must be transported safely for treatment. The paramedic should look for medications or drugs on site and take them to the receiving facility.

Types of restraints

Patients needing restraints are often agitated, confused, and refuse care, but implied consent is legal for patients with abnormal behavior. **Restraints** include the following:

- Verbal: Try to calm the patient while being firm.
- Nonverbal: Use body language and a show of force (with a number of EMS personnel being present) to convince the patient.
- Physical: Use standard precautions; one person is assigned to each limb, while a fifth person reassures and tries to calm the patient. Apply multiple restraints as necessary, including across the trunk, being careful not to restrict the patient's breathing.
- Chemical: Use as a last resort (usually after physical restraints). Includes benzodiazepines (lorazepam) and neuroleptics (haloperidol).
- Tasers/Electrical stun guns: These may be used by law enforcement to subdue a severely agitated patient. They may cause burns, dart injuries, fall injuries, or cardiac arrest. Stun guns require direct contact, but Tasers may be shot from 20 feet away.

Document the reason for restraint, the types of restraints, the restraint technique, and the time the patient is restrained. Monitor the patient's condition continuously, including the heart rate, airway/ventilation/oxygen supplementation, and circulation.

Schizophrenia and psychosis

Schizophrenia, a thought disorder, causes psychotic episodes and distortion of reality and the inability to determine the line between fantasy and reality. The onset may be acute or more insidious. Symptoms are positive (delusions, hallucinations, disorganized or catatonic behavior, disorganized speech) or negative (flat affect/decreased emotional range, social isolation, poverty of speech, lack of interest and drive). Patients may have bizarre delusions (thought broadcasting) or hear voices (which they may try to drown out by turning the TV, radio, or music volume up loud). Patients may isolate themselves socially, exhibit poor hygiene, exhibit catatonia (a stiff, unmoving position), and have odd speech. Treatment is with typical and atypical antipsychotics and antidepressants (such as selective serotonin reuptake inhibitors [SSRIs]). **Psychosis** is not a disease but a description of a condition and may apply to various diagnoses (such as schizophrenia and bipolar disease). Psychosis is characterized by marked derangement of the personality and a distorted view of reality. Patients may experience hallucinations (seeing/hearing something not present), delusions (false or distorted beliefs), and illusions (false impressions). Prehospital: Provide supportive care.

Cognitive disorders

Cognitive disorders involve problems with memory and learning, including the following:

- Dementia: This is a condition (such as Alzheimer's) marked by memory loss, personality changes, and reasoning impairment. Patients may be unable to carry out activities of daily living or manage their own affairs. Dementia may range from mild (forgetful) to severe (fully dependent on others).
- Delirium: This severe state of agitation (agitated/excited delirium) may involve hallucinations, delusions, and bizarre violent behavior. Another form of delirium is common in older adults, especially those who are terminally ill, and it involves an acute sudden change in consciousness, language and memory disturbances, disorientation, confusion, audiovisual hallucinations, sleep disturbance, and psychomotor activity disorders. Symptoms are fluctuating.
- Amnesia: It may be a long- or short-term condition, and it is caused by trauma; severe stress; brain injury; and drugs, including illicit, sedative, and hypnotic drugs (barbiturates, benzodiazepines, cocaine, methamphetamine, Rohypnol). With retrograde amnesia, the patient cannot remember events before a particular time. With antegrade amnesia, the person cannot transfer short-term memories to the long term. Some may have a combined form.

Depression

Depression is a mood disorder characterized by profound feelings of sadness and withdrawal. It may be acute (such as after a death) or chronic with recurring episodes over a lifetime. The cause appears to be a combination of genetic (family history), biological (chemical imbalance), and environmental (abuse, substance abuse, medications, bullying, conflict, stress) factors. A major depressive episode is a depressed mood, profound and constant sense of hopelessness and despair, or loss of interest in all or almost all activities for a period of at least two weeks. Developmental hormone changes at puberty or hormone disruption from disease can also cause depression.

Depression can be mild, moderate, or severe, and it is characterized by a combination of the following symptoms that interfere with the ability to work, study, sleep, eat and enjoy once-pleasurable activities: persistent depressed mood, diminished interest in activities, weight gain or loss, insomnia or hypersomnia, constant fatigue, feeling of worthlessness, inability to focus, and suicidal ideation. Treatment is with antidepressants, such as SSRIs. Prehospital: Provide supportive care.

Bipolar disorder

Bipolar disorder is a mood disorder characterized by mania, depression, or both. The manic phase is a distinct period characterized by extremely elevated mood, energy, and unusual thought patterns, causing impairment in occupational functioning and social activities. Manic phases alternate with depressive phases that occur in varying patterns interspersed with periods of normal mood (euthymia). During the manic phase, patients may have grandiose beliefs, very rapid speech, racing thoughts, feeling "high," and acting recklessly. They may sleep little and have hallucinations and delusions. Depressive phases are the opposite of manic phases, although delusions and hallucinations may persist; additionally, suicidal ideation is common, so the person must be monitored carefully to prevent self-injury. Clients with bipolar depression often exhibit irritability, slow movement and speech, weight gain, and guilt. They may have impaired concentration and an inability to make decisions. Treatment is with mood stabilizers (such as lithium). Prehospital: Provide supportive care.

Mental status exam (MSE)

Mental status is usually assessed through normal interactions, and the **mental status exam** (MSE) can be used as a guide when assessing patients. Some components require only observation, whereas others require questioning. Components include the following:

- Appearance: Kempt, unkempt.
- Behavior/Attitude: Appropriate, inappropriate.
- Consciousness/Alertness: Conscious, arousable, able to focus.
- Orientation: Person, place, time, event.
- Speech/Language: Normal, abnormal, bizarre, tone, volume.
- Thought processes/content: Logical/Illogical thinking, delusions, hallucinations, paranoia, fixations, suicidal ideation.
- Affect: Flat (no expression), blunted (little expression), broad (a wide range of expressions), inappropriate (inconsistent), and restricted (one expression at all times).
- Mood: Happy, sad, depressed, elated, withdrawn.
- Attention span: Appropriate, short, scattered.
- Memory: Intact, short- or long-term memory loss.
- Judgment/Reasoning: Ability to make reasonable decisions and ability to understand and reason.
- Suicidal and/or homicidal ideation: Present/Absent.

Circulatory system

The **circulatory system** is responsible for the oxygenation of cells, perfusion (carrying blood with oxygen, glucose, and nutrients to the cells), and gas exchange (removing waste products, such as carbon dioxide). The circulatory system serves as a blood reservoir (5 L), maintains blood pH (7.35–7.45) through a buffer system, responds to infections, and facilitates coagulation (blood clotting). The heart is located between the lungs and under and to the left of the mediastinum (breastbone). The heart has four chambers: upper (right atrium, left atrium) and lower (right ventricle and left ventricle). The myocardium (heart muscle) receives blood from two major coronary arteries and their branches. The inner lining of the heart is the endocardium, and the lining that surrounds the heart is the pericardium, which has an inner double-layered serous membrane (visceral pericardium) and a fibrous outer layer (parietal pericardium). The cardiac cycle involves one complete heartbeat with systole (ventricular contraction) and diastole (relaxation) phases. Stroke volume is the volume of blood ejected from the left ventricle in one cardiac cycle (about 60–70 mL), and cardiac output is the heart rate times the stroke volume.

The venous system includes the veins, venules, and venous capillaries, and it brings blood back to the heart via the inferior and superior vena cava. The arterial system includes the coronary arteries, which branch from the aorta after it leaves the heart; arteries; arterioles; and arterial capillaries.

The **blood flows** as follows:

- Deoxygenated venous blood returns to the heart per the superior vena cava, inferior vena cava, and coronary sinus (bringing blood from the coronary arteries) into the right atrium, then it flows through the tricuspid valve into the right ventricle.
- From the right ventricle, blood flows through the pulmonic (semilunar) valve into the pulmonary artery and to the lungs to exchange carbon dioxide for oxygen.
- Oxygenated blood flows from the lungs through the pulmonary veins into the left atrium and through the mitral (bicuspid) valve into the left ventricle.
- From the left ventricle, blood flows through the aortic valve and into the ascending aorta, the coronary arteries, and the general circulation through the thoracic and abdominal aorta.

After the blood flows through the valves, they close to prevent backflow. Both atria and both ventricles contract simultaneously.

Components of the blood

Blood cells are produced in the bone marrow. Blood is a viscous, dark-red fluid comprised of cells, gases, and plasma (55%). Blood components include the following:

- Erythrocytes (red blood cells [RBCs]): RBCs carry hemoglobin, which transports oxygen. If the RBC count is low (such as from blood loss) or the oxygen-carrying capacity is impaired (such as with anemia), the patient may experience hypoxemia (low oxygen). The life cycle of RBCs is normally 120 days.
- Leukocytes (white blood cells [WBCs]): WBCs defend the body against invading organisms (viruses, bacteria, fungi, and parasites), and in the bloodstream and tissues, they respond to allergies. WBCs include lymphocytes (B, T, natural killer, and null cells), monocytes, eosinophils, basophils, and neutrophils.
- Thrombocytes (platelets): Platelets release clotting factors and have an active role in forming blood clots
- Plasma (55% of the blood): Plasma carries water, proteins, electrolytes, lipids (fats), blood cells, and glucose as well as clotting factors.

The primary blood types are A, B, AB, and O. Blood is either Rh– or RH+, and patients must receive transfusions of blood that are type and Rh compatible.

Normal findings of the complete blood count

Total erythrocytes (RBCs)	• Males >18 years: 4.5–5.5 million per mm³. • Females >18 years: 4–5 million per mm³.
Hemoglobin	Carries oxygen; it is decreased in anemia and increased in polycythemia. Normal values: • Males >18 years: 14–18 g/dL. • Females >18 years: 12–16 g/dL.
Hematocrit	Indicates the proportion of RBCs in a liter of blood (usually about 3× the hemoglobin number). Normal values: • Males >18 years: 45%–52% • Females >18 years: 36%–48%
Reticulocyte count (immature RBCs)	Measures marrow production and should rise with anemia. Normal values: • 0.5%–1.5% of total RBCs
Leukocytes (WBCs)	• Normal WBC for adults: 4800–10,000 • Acute infection: 10,000+ • Severe infection: 30,000+ • Viral infection: ≤4000 The differential provides the percentage of each different type of leukocyte. An increase in the WBC count is usually related to an increase in one type and often an increase in immature neutrophils, known as bands, referred to as a "shift to the left," an indication of an infectious process.

Heart sounds

First and second sounds	• The first heart sound (S1—"lub") is closure of the mitral and tricuspid valves (heard at the apex/left ventricular area of the heart). • The second heart sound (S2—"dub") is closure of the aortic and pulmonic valves (heard at the base of the heart). There may be a slight splitting of the S2.
Gallop rhythms	• S3 occurs after S2 in children and young adults, but it may indicate heart failure or left ventricular failure in older adults (heard with the patient lying on the left side). • S4 occurs before S1 and occurs with ventricular hypertrophy, such as from coronary artery disease, hypertension, or aortic valve stenosis.
Opening snap	Unusual, high-pitched sound occurring after S2 with stenosis of mitral valve from rheumatic heart disease.
Ejection click	Brief, high-pitched sound occurring immediately after S1 with stenosis of the aortic valve.
Friction rub	Harsh, grating sound heard in systole and diastole with pericarditis.
Murmur	Sound caused by turbulent blood flow from stenotic or malfunctioning valves, congenital defects, or increased blood flow.

Perfusion, oxygenation of tissues, and cardiac compromise

Perfusion depends on an adequate supply of RBCs, which carry oxygen. Perfusion may be impaired if the heart does not pump adequately, if the rate of heart contractions is too low or too rapid to be effective, and if the volume of blood and/or RBCs pumped is not adequate to provide oxygenation to the tissues. With adequate perfusion, **oxygenation of tissues** occurs when blood flows throughout the body, and gas exchange of carbon dioxide and waste products for oxygen occurs at the capillaries. **Cardiac compromise** results in inadequate circulation and/or perfusion of vital organs. Cardiac compromise may result from atherosclerosis (plaques/fatty deposits) in the arterial lumens, resulting in obstructed blood flow and inadequate dilation and constriction of arteries. Ischemia occurs with decreased blood flow and can damage tissues, but occlusion can result in the death of tissue. Cardiac compromise may result from heart damage causing an inadequate heart rate and/or pumping. Cardiac compromise may also result from an inadequate volume of circulating blood.

Acute coronary syndrome

Impairment of blood flow through the coronary arteries leads to ischemia of the cardiac muscle and **angina pectoris**—pain that may occur in the sternum, chest, neck, arms (especially the left arm), or back. The pain frequently occurs with crushing pain substernally, radiating down the left arm or both arms, although this type of pain is more common in males than females, whose symptoms may appear less acute and may include nausea, shortness of breath, and fatigue. Elderly or diabetic patients may also have pain in their arms, no pain at all (silent ischemia), or weakness and numbness in both arms. <u>Stable angina</u> episodes usually last for <5 minutes and are fairly predictable exercise-induced episodes caused by atherosclerotic lesions blocking >75% of the lumen of the affected coronary artery. Precipitating events include exercise; decrease in environmental temperature; heavy eating; strong emotions (such as fright or anger); or exertion, including coitus. Stable angina episodes usually resolve in less than 5 minutes by decreasing the activity level and administering sublingual nitroglycerin. Prehospital: Provide supportive care, oxygen, and nitroglycerin per protocol.

Unstable angina (also known as preinfarction or crescendo angina) is a progression of coronary artery disease, and it occurs when there is a change in the pattern of stable angina. The pain may increase, may not respond to a single nitroglycerin dose, and may persist for >5 minutes. Usually pain is more frequent, lasts longer, and may occur at rest when sitting or lying down. Unstable angina may indicate a rupture of an atherosclerotic plaque and the beginning of thrombus formation, so it should always be treated as a medical emergency with rapid transport because it may indicate a myocardial infarction. **Variant angina** (also known as **Prinzmetal's angina**) results from spasms of the coronary arteries; can be associated with or without atherosclerotic plaques; and is often related to smoking, alcohol, or illicit stimulants. Variant angina frequently occurs cyclically at the same time each day and often while the person is at rest. Nitroglycerin or calcium channel blockers are used for treatment. Provide supportive care, oxygen, and nitroglycerin per protocol.

Myocardial infarction (MI—heart attack) may occur after an episode of unstable angina caused by a rupture of an atherosclerotic plaque and thrombosis associated with coronary artery spasm, but it may also result from vasoconstriction, acute blood loss, decreased oxygen, and ingestion of cocaine. Symptoms may vary considerably, with males having the more "classic" symptom of a sudden onset of crushing chest pain. Elderly and diabetic patients may complain primarily of weakness.

Symptoms include the following:

- Angina with pain in the chest that may radiate to the neck or arms, crushing pain, tightness (often more than 30 minutes and unrelieved by rest or nitroglycerin).
- Hypertension or hypotension.
- Palpitations, tachycardia, bradycardia, and dysrhythmias.
- Dyspnea.
- ECG changes (ST segment and T-wave changes), tachycardia, bradycardia, and dysrhythmias.
- Pulmonary edema, peripheral edema, weak/absent peripheral pulses.
- Nausea and vomiting.
- Pallor, cold and clammy skin, diaphoresis.
- Neurological/psychological disturbances: Anxiety, light-headedness, headache, visual abnormalities, slurred speech, and fear.

Prehospital: Manage the patient's airway/ventilation/oxygen supplementation, provide supportive care, perform CPR/defibrillation if needed, provide rapid transport, start an IV access line, and give fluid resuscitation as needed.

ECG analysis and cardiac arrhythmias associated with myocardial infarction

Q wave

- Characterized by a series of abnormal Q waves (wider and deeper) on ECG, especially in the early morning (related to adrenergic activity).
- Infarction is usually prolonged and results in necrosis. This may indicate extensive transient ischemia.
- Usually transmural.

Non-Q wave

- Characterized by changes in the ST-T wave with ST depression (usually reversible within a few days).
- Usually reperfusion occurs spontaneously, so the infarct size is smaller. Contraction necrosis related to reperfusion is common.
- Usually nontransmural.

Myocardial ischemia results in ST-segment depression and T-wave inversion; myocardial injury, ST-segment elevation, T-wave inversion; myocardial infarction, in hyperacute T waves (initial stage), ST-segment elevation, T-wave inversion, and pathologic Q waves. Arrhythmias common to MI include sinus tachycardia (rapid heart rate), sinus bradycardia (slow heart rate), heart blocks, ventricular fibrillation, pulseless electrical activity (PEA), and asystole. Rapid transport is indicated for patients having no relief from medication, hypotension, hypoperfusion, and/or significant ECG changes/abnormalities. No transport is indicated only for patient refusal.

Management of a patient with chest pain

Management of a patient with chest pain begins with a thorough assessment, primary and secondary survey, and use of the OPQRST and SAMPLE methods of history taking. Patients are often very frightened, so the paramedic should provide clear feedback and reassurance. The patient should be placed in the semi-Fowler's position, especially if experiencing shortness of breath, and the oxygen saturation should be monitored. Respiratory compromise may require supplemental oxygen, BVM assistance, PEEP, CPAP/BiPAP, manually triggered ventilators (MTVs), or automatic transport ventilators (ATVs).

Pharmacological interventions (administer the medication according to protocol) may include the following:

- Aspirin (for suspected heart attack; Bayer, Heartline, ZORprin, Empirin): Provide 162 to 325 mg chewable (preferred). Contraindicated with GI bleeding, stroke.
- Nitroglycerin (for suspected angina; Nitrodur, Nitrolingual, NitroMist): Provide 0.4 mg sublingually repeated every 3–5 minutes up to three doses. Contraindicated if the patient has recently taken Viagra, had a stroke, or has excessive bleeding.
- Oral glucose (for suspected hypoglycemia/insulin reaction): Glucose tablets, solution.
- Nitrous oxide (50% nitrogen/50% oxygen): To relieve severe pain.
- Administer a 3- or 12-lead ECG that is recorded/transmitted during a pain episode.

All patients with chest pain should be transported because even mild chest discomfort may indicate that the patient is having a heart attack, especially in older patients and female patients, who often have atypical symptoms.

Conduction system of the heart

Normal **conduction of the heart** has the following four stages:

1. **Generation of an impulse at the sinoatrial (SA) node** (primary pacemaker) located at the junction of the right atrium and superior vena cava: The electrical impulse travels the cells of the atria along internodal pathways, causing electrical stimulation and contraction of the atria, including Bachmann's bundle, which stimulates the left atrium.
2. **Atrioventricular node conduction of impulse:** This occurs when the impulses from the SA node reach the AV node in the right atrial wall near the tricuspid valve. There is a slight delay (about one-tenth of a second), allowing the atria to empty.
3. **Atrioventricular bundle (bundle of His) conduction:** The AV node relays the impulse to the ventricles through the atrioventricular bundle—specialized conduction cells in the ventricular septum that branch to the right and left ventricles, carrying the electrical impulse.
4. **Purkinje fiber conduction:** Impulses are conducted down the AV bundles to the base of the heart where they divide into the Purkinje fibers, which stimulate the myocardial cells to contract the ventricles.

Heart failure

Heart failure (HF, aka congestive HF) includes disorders of contractions (systolic "left-sided" dysfunction) or filling (diastolic dysfunction) or both, which result in hypertrophy (thickening, enlarging, and stiffening) of the myocardium (heart muscle). The most common causes are coronary artery disease, myocardial infarction, systemic or pulmonary hypertension, cardiomyopathy, and valvular disorders. The incidence of HF correlates with age. Left-sided HF may cause pulmonary edema that impairs ventilation, leading to hypoxia, especially when the patient is lying in a supine position, and right-sided HF may cause abdominal and peripheral edema of the feet and legs. The circulatory time with HF decreases overall, so changes in oximetry to show hypoxia may be delayed. The autonomic nervous system's regulation of breathing to control oxygen levels may be impaired, resulting in periodic breathing patterns, Cheyne-Stokes breathing, or central sleep apnea. Medications used to treat HF include ACE inhibitors (captopril, lisinopril), angiotensin receptor blockers (ARBs) (losartan, valsartan), beta-blockers (metoprolol, carvedilol), aldosterone agonists (spironolactone), and diuretics (hydrochlorothiazide, furosemide).

Chronic heart failure develops insidiously over time as the heart muscles weaken and enlarge, so initially patients may only note fatigue, weight gain, and swelling in their feet and ankles. **Acute heart failure** is characterized by impairment of gas exchange and decreased cardiac output because of changes in preload, contractibility, and heart rhythm; symptoms are more acute and may include irregular heartbeat, chest pain, cough, and rapid breathing, wheezing, and cyanosis from lack of adequate oxygen. Patients may also suffer from anxiety, decreased activity tolerance, and disturbances in sleep patterns. Medical management is aimed at increasing cardiac function, providing support, and monitoring treatment. Patients often are acutely short of breath and sitting upright, with rales evident in their lungs. Assessment includes conducting primary and secondary surveys; taking a complete medical history including medication use/home oxygen use; and assessing the patient's level of consciousness, airway status (cough, sputum, labored breathing, tripod position), heart rate/rhythm, peripheral pulses, edema (pitting/nonpitting, ascites, sacral), and complications. Prehospital: Manage the patient's airway/ventilation/oxygen supplementation with a nonrebreather mask or BVM with high-flow oxygen, position for comfort, and suction if necessary.

Cardiogenic shock

Cardiogenic shock in adults is usually secondary to myocardial infarction damage of >40% of the left ventricle, reducing contractibility, interfering with the pumping mechanism of the heart, and decreasing oxygen perfusion. Characteristics include increased preload, increased afterload, and decreased contractibility. Together, these result in decreased cardiac output and an increase in the systemic vascular resistance (SVR) to compensate and protect vital organs. As the cardiac output decreases, the tissue perfusion decreases, coronary artery perfusion decreases, fluid backs up, and the left ventricle fails to adequately pump the blood, resulting in pulmonary edema and right ventricular failure.

Symptoms	Usual Treatment
• Hypotension with systolic BP <90 mm Hg • Tachycardia >100 bpm with weak, thready pulse and dysrhythmias • Decreased heart sounds • Chest pain • Tachypnea and basilar rales • Cool, moist skin; pallor	• IV fluids • Inotropic agents (norepinephrine, dopamine) • Anti-dysrhythmics (lidocaine, procainamide) • Intra-aortic balloon (IAB) pump or left ventricular assist device

Prehospital: Manage the patient's airway/ventilation/oxygen supplementation/intubation as needed; provide an IV access line with fluid resuscitation; monitor ECG vital signs, and cardiac status; and provide inotropic/vasopressor (norepinephrine, dopamine) support as indicated.

Dissecting aortic aneurysm

A **dissecting aortic aneurysm** occurs when the wall of the aorta is torn and blood flows between the layers of the wall, dilating and weakening it until it risks rupture (which has a 90% mortality rate). Aortic aneurysms are more than twice as common in males as females, but females have a higher mortality rate, possibly because they are often older at presentation. **Thoracic aortic aneurysms** are usually related to atherosclerosis, but they may also result from Marfan syndrome, Ehlers-Danlos syndrome, and connective tissue disorders. Aneurysms are often asymptomatic but may cause substernal pain, back pain, dyspnea and/or stridor (from pressure on the trachea), cough, distension of the neck veins, and edema of the neck and arms. Rupture usually does not

- 106 -

allow time for emergent repair. **Abdominal aortic aneurysms** (these are not usually palpable until they are 5 cm/diameter) may cause mild constant or intermittent pain, but rupture results in severe abdominal pain, hypotension, and a palpable mass, and a 50% death rate. Prehospital: Manage the airway/ventilation/intubation/oxygen as needed. Provide antihypertensives (esmolol/labetalol), an IV access line, and fluids.

Cardiac dysrhythmias

Sinus bradycardia is characterized by a regular pulse <50 to 60 bpm with P waves in front of QRS, which are usually normal in shape and duration. The PR interval is 0.12–0.20 seconds, the QRS interval is 0.04–0.11 seconds, and there is a P:QRS ratio of 1:1. Prehospital: Monitor, provide an IV access line, perform a 12-lead ECG, administer atropine (per protocol), and/or perform transcutaneous pacing if the patient is hypotensive or hypoperfusing. Administer epinephrine or dopamine if necessary.

Sinus tachycardia (ST): The sinus node impulse increases in frequency. ST is characterized by a regular pulse >100 bpm with P waves before QRS, but sometimes they are a part of the preceding T wave. The QRS is usually of normal shape and duration (0.04–0.11 seconds), but it may have consistent irregularity. The PR interval is 0.12–0.20 seconds, and there is a P:QRS ratio of 1:1. The rapid pulse decreases the diastolic filling time and causes reduced cardiac output with resultant hypotension. Prehospital: Stable—Monitor, provide supportive care, vagal maneuvers, an IV access line, and 12-lead ECG. Narrow—administer adenosine (per protocol). Wide—consult a cardiac expert. Unstable—perform cardioversion.

Sinus arrhythmia: Irregular impulses from the sinus node, often paradoxical (increasing with inspiration and decreasing with expiration) because of stimulation of the vagal nerve during inspiration; it rarely causes a negative hemodynamic effect (common in both children and young adults and often lessens with age, but it may persist in some adults). Prehospital: No treatment unless associated with severe bradycardia.

Supraventricular tachycardia (SVT): The heart rate is >100 bpm. SVT may have a sudden onset and result in congestive heart failure. The heart rate may increase to 200–300 bpm. SVT originates in the atria rather than the ventricles, but it is controlled by the tissue in the area of the AV node rather than the SA node. The rhythm is usually rapid but regular. Prehospital: Monitor, oxygen supplementation, adenosine (per protocol) if unstable.

Atrial flutter: The atrial rate is faster, usually 250–400 bpm, than the AV node conduction rate, so not all of the beats are conducted into the ventricles, effectively blocked at the AV node, preventing ventricular fibrillation, although some extraventricular impulses may go through. Prehospital: Monitor, provide defibrillation, and administer an antiarrhythmic (amiodarone) if necessary.

Atrial fibrillation (AF): Conditions that cause atrial fibrillation are coronary artery disease, valvular disease, pulmonary disease, heavy alcohol ingestion, and cardiac surgery. AF is characterized by atrial rates of 250–400 with ventricular rates of 75–150, with the ventricular rate usually being regular. P waves are saw-toothed (referred to as F waves), the QRS shape and duration (0.4–0.11 seconds) are usually normal, PR interval may be hard to calculate because of F waves, and the P:QRS ratio is 2–4:1. Prehospital: Monitor, provide defibrillation, or administer antiarrhythmics (amiodarone) if necessary to convert the unstable AF to a sinus rhythm (per protocol).

Ventricular tachycardia: is ≥3 premature ventricular contractions (PVCs) in a row with a ventricular rate of 100–200 beats per minute. A detectable rate is usually regular, and the QRS complex is ≥0.12 seconds and is usually abnormally shaped. The P wave may be undetectable with an irregular PR interval if a P wave is present. The P:QRS ratio is often difficult to ascertain because of the absence of P waves.

Prehospital: Monitor, provide defibrillation, start an IV access line, and administer epinephrine. If there is failure to convert, administer amiodarone (per protocol).

Ventricular fibrillation: Rapid, very irregular ventricular rate >300 bpm with no atrial activity observable on the ECG, caused by disorganized electrical activity in the ventricles. The QRS complex is not recognizable because the ECG shows irregular undulation.

Prehospital: Monitor, provide defibrillation, start an IV access line, and administer epinephrine. If there is failure to convert, administer amiodarone (per protocol).

Second-degree AV block, type II (Mobitz): Only some of the atrial impulses are conducted unpredictably through the AV node to the ventricles. The PR intervals are the same if impulses are conducted, and the QRS complex is usually widened. The P:QRS ratio varies 2:1, 3:1, and 4:1. Prehospital: Monitor: May progress to complete heart block, requiring transcutaneous pacing.

Third-degree AV block: There are more P waves than QRS with no clear relationship between them and an atrial rate 2–3 times the pulse rate, so the PR interval is irregular. With SA node malfunction, the AV node fires at a lower rate. With AV node malfunction, the pacemaker site in the ventricles takes over at a bradycardic rate; thus, with complete AV block, the heart still contracts, but often ineffectually. Prehospital: Monitor. May progress to complete heart block, requiring transcutaneous pacing.

First-degree AV block: Atrial impulses are conducted through the AV node to the ventricles at a slower rate than normal. The P and QRS are usually normal, but the PR interval is >0.20 seconds, and the P:QRS ratio is 1:1. Prehospital: Monitor. It usually requires no specific treatment.

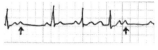 **Second-degree AV block, type I (Wenckebach):** Each atrial impulse in a group of beats is conducted at a lengthened interval until one fails to conduct (the PR interval progressively increases), so there are more P waves than QRS, but the QRS complex is usually of normal shape and duration. Prehospital: Monitor. Usually does not cause significant problems unless it is associated with a myocardial infarction.

Pulseless electrical activity and asystole

Pulseless electrical activity is any rhythm without a palpable pulse (this is common after defibrillation). Identifying and correcting the underlying cause is critical for treatment. Common causes include the following:

Five H's

1. Hypokalemia/Hyperkalemia
2. Hypoxia
3. Hypothermia
4. Hypovolemia
5. Hydrogen ion (acidosis)

Five T's

1. Toxins
2. Tamponade (cardiac)
3. Tension pneumothorax
4. Thrombosis (lungs)
5. Thrombosis (heart)

Prehospital: Begin CPR, start an IV access line, administer epinephrine (per protocol) every 3 to 5 minutes, provide intubation and ventilation, and give oxygen as indicated. Provide rapid transport.

Asystole ("flatlined") is the absence of an audible heartbeat, palpable pulse, and respirations. The ECG may show some P waves initially. The QRS complex is absent, although there may be an occasional QRS "escape beat." Prehospital: Check leads, begin CPR, start an IV access line, administer epinephrine (per protocol) every 3 to 5 minutes, provide intubation and ventilation, and give oxygen as indicated. Provide rapid transport.

Transcutaneous pacing

Transcutaneous pacing is used temporarily to treat bradydysrhythmia that doesn't respond to medications (atropine) and results in hemodynamic instability. Generally, an arterial line is placed and the patient is provided oxygen before the pacing. The placement of pacing pads (large self-adhesive pads) and ECG leads varies somewhat according to the type of equipment, but usually one pacing pad (negative) is placed on the left chest, inferior to the clavicle, and the other (positive) is placed on the left back, inferior to the scapula. The heart is sandwiched between the two pads such that the myocardium is depolarized through the chest wall. Lead wires attach the pads to the monitor. The rate of pacing is usually set between 60 and 70 bpm. Current is increased slowly until capture occurs—a spiking followed by a QRS sequence—then the current is readjusted downward if possible just to maintain capture. Demand and fixed modes are available, but the demand mode is preferred. Patients may require analgesia, especially if a higher current setting is needed.

Endocarditis, pericarditis, and myocarditis

Endocarditis (infection of the heart's endothelial surface and valves) is caused by organisms entering the bloodstream (such as from a surgery, catheterization, or IV drug abuse) and migrating to the heart, forming vegetations (verrucae), collagen deposits, and platelet thrombi. The heart valves frequently become deformed, but the organisms may also invade other tissues. Symptoms are usually nonspecific and include fatigue, intermittent fever, arthralgia, and petechiae on the upper trunk. Untreated, it may develop into left-sided heart failure, heart abscess, and cardiac dysrhythmias. **Pericarditis** (infection of the pericardium [the sac enclosing the heart] by a pathogen) may be acute or chronic. The pericardium becomes inflamed and fills with exudate. As the infection subsides, fibrosis and scarring may occur. Complications include pericardial effusion (accumulation of fluid), which can lead to cardiac tamponade. Acute symptoms include an abrupt onset of sharp, sternal, radiating, angina-like pain, increasing with inspiration and relieved by sitting up and leaning forward, and dyspnea. **Myocarditis** is inflammation of the heart muscle caused by a viral infection or autoimmune reaction. Symptoms typically include fatigue, palpitation, and shortness of breath.

Congenital heart disease

Congenital heart disease is one of the leading causes of death in children within the first year of life. There are two main types of congenital heart disease: acyanotic and cyanotic. They may also be classified according to hemodynamics related to the blood flow pattern.

Acyanotic congenital defects
Increased pulmonary blood flow:

- Atrial septal defect
- Atrioventricular canal defect
- Patent ductus arteriosus
- Ventricular septal defect

Obstructed ventricular blood flow:

- Aortic stenosis
- Coarctation of the aorta
- Pulmonic stenosis

Cyanotic congenital defects
Decreased pulmonary blood flow:

- Tetralogy of Fallot
- Tricuspid atresia

Mixed blood flow:

- Hypoplastic left heart syndrome
- Total anomalous pulmonary venous return
- Transposition of the great arteries
- Truncus arteriosus
- Ebstein's anomaly

Hypertensive crisis

Hypertensive crisis (aka malignant hypertension) is a marked elevation in BP than can cause severe organ damage if left untreated. Causes include encephalopathy, intracranial hemorrhage, aortic dissection, eclampsia, and heart failure. Classifications are as follows:

- **Hypertensive emergency**: Acute hypertension, usually >120 mm Hg diastolic; it must be treated immediately to lower the BP in order to prevent damage to vital organs, such as the heart, brain, or kidneys.
- **Hypertensive urgency**: Acute hypertension must be treated within a few hours, but the vital organs are not in immediate danger. The BP is lowered more slowly to avoid hypotension, ischemia of vital organs, or failure of autoregulation with a one-third reduction in 6 hours.

Symptoms include headache, dizziness, dyspnea, weakness, visual disturbances, anxiety, chest pain (atypical), heart failure, acute coronary syndrome, and stroke. Prehospital: Asymptomatic hypertension requires referral to a physician, whereas severe symptoms require rapid transport. Interventions include airway support/ventilation with oxygen supplementation, IV line access, and advanced life support as needed. Patients with severe dyspnea and pulmonary edema may need CPAP.

Cardiac tamponade

Cardiac tamponade occurs when fluid, usually blood, accumulates in the pericardial sac. If the fluid accumulates rapidly, the walls of the pericardial sac do not have time to stretch to accommodate the fluid, so the patient may quickly develop pulseless electrical activity (PEA) with fluid accumulation of 50 to 250 mL. If fluid accumulates slowly, such as with pericardial effusions associated with cancer, patients may tolerate up to 2 L of fluid before symptoms become acute. Cardiac tamponade compresses the heart and limits the venous return to the heart and blood flow into the ventricles, thereby reducing cardiac output. Symptoms: Beck's triad includes decreased arterial BP, increased jugular venous distension, and muffled heart sounds. Patients may be anxious, dyspneic, dizzy, and have angina-like pain. Prehospital: Manage airway/high concentration oxygen, monitor the ECG, provide an IV access line and fluids as indicated, and provide rapid transport for pericardiocentesis.

Thromboembolism and pulmonary embolism

Thromboembolism includes the formation of a thrombus (such as in the heart with atrial fibrillation and in the deep veins with immobilization) and an embolism in which a clot breaks off and travels through the circulatory system. Although thromboembolism may cause a heart attack or stroke, the most common presentation is a **pulmonary embolism (PE)** resulting from deep vein thrombosis. The patient may or may not complain of pain at the thrombus site, which may be swollen and erythematous (red), typically in a lower extremity. When the patient develops PE, the usual presentation is acute onset of dyspnea and tachycardia and sitting in the tripod position. Some patients may have ECG abnormalities, frothy sputum, cough, fever, hemoptysis, and jugular vein distension. Prehospital: Provide supportive care, manage the patient's airway/ventilation/intubation as needed with oxygen to maintain oxygen saturation >94%, establish an IV access line, administer up to 1 L of NS, and give norepinephrine if indicated. If protocol permits, administer heparin for PE.

Jugular venous pressure

Jugular venous pressure (neck vein) is used to assess the cardiac output and pressure in the right heart because the pulsations relate to changes in pressure in the right atrium. This procedure is usually not accurate if the pulse rate is >100. This is a noninvasive estimation of the central venous pressure and waveform. Measurement should be done with the internal jugular if possible; otherwise, the external jugular may be used.

- Elevate the patient's head to 45° (and to 90° if necessary) with the patient's head turned to the opposite side of the examination.
- Position the light at an angle to illuminate the veins and shadows.
- Measure the height of the jugular vein pulsation above the sternal joint, using a ruler.
  - The normal height of the jugular vein pulsation is ≤4 cm above the sternal angle.
  - Increased height (>4cm) indicates increased pressure in the right atrium and right heart failure. It may also indicate pericarditis or tricuspid stenosis. Laughing or coughing may trigger the Valsalva response and also cause a pressure increase.

Carbon monoxide poisoning

Carbon monoxide poisoning occurs when people breathe in carbon monoxide, usually related to industrial or household accidents or suicide attempts. Carbon monoxide binds to hemoglobin 200 times more readily than oxygen, and once the carbon monoxide binds to hemoglobin (creating

- 111 -

carboxyhemoglobin), the hemoglobin can no longer bind to or transport oxygen, resulting in hypoxemia. Symptoms vary depending on the percentage of saturation. At 10%, patients may complain of headache and nausea. At >20%, a patient becomes increasingly weak and confused with alterations in mental status. At >30%, a patient may have dyspnea, chest pain, and increased confusion. When the level continues to increase, a patient may experience seizures, coma, and death. Skin color may be cyanotic, pink, or bright cherry red (but this is not a reliable sign). Prehospital: Manage the patient's airway/ventilation/oxygen supplementation with 100% oxygen with a nonrebreather mask. Note: Pulse oximetry cannot distinguish carbon monoxide from oxygen.

Poison control resources

The **National Capital Poison Center** provides a website with an online tool— webPOISONCONTROL—(https://triage.webpoisoncontrol.org/#/exclusions) and a telephone number (1-800-222-1222) for people who swallow (ingest) or come into contact (absorbed, inhaled, injected) with poisonous (toxic) substances.

- webPOISONCONTROL: Can be used for patients (ages 6 months to 79 years and nonpregnant women) who are asymptomatic and unintentionally swallowed a single drug or medication, household product, or berries over a short period of time (minutes to a few hours) and are otherwise healthy.
- Telephone contact: Is used for all other situations, including a patient with symptoms, pregnant women, nonswallowing contact, those ages <6 months or >79, or those who swallowed materials or substances other than those listed for online assistance. Telephone contact can be made for any poisoning if it is preferred to online assistance.

This service is free and usually requires about 3 minutes for a response. When calling, be prepared to describe the substance (include the product name and dosage for medications), amount swallowed, age of patient, weight of patient, time since exposure, and the patient's ZIP Code and email address. If unsure of the amount of poison or the weight of the victim, estimates are acceptable.

Methods of poisoning

Ingestion	Drugs, overdose, toxic/caustic liquids (bleach, cleaning solution, antifreeze, gasoline), mouse/rat poison, pesticides, some plants, and alcohol	Wide range of symptoms, depending on the substance; anaphylaxis, lethargy, constricted pupils, mouth burns, nausea and vomiting, pain, diarrhea, difficulty breathing, confusion, seizures, and coma. (Toddlers are particularly at risk.)
Inhalation	Toxic gases, smoke, hair spray, carbon monoxide, chlorine, halogens	Difficulty breathing, lethargy, confusion, nausea, vomiting, headache, cyanosis, seizures, slurred speech, and coma.
Injection	Heroin, morphine, drug overdose	Local irritation, lethargy, confusion, slurred speech, nausea, vomiting, difficulty breathing, seizures, and coma. (Adolescents are prone to experimentation with drugs.)
Absorption	Cleaning products, various chemicals	Local irritation, anaphylaxis, burns, tissue damage, rash, nausea, vomiting, shortness of breath, and confusion.

Prehospital: Treatment varies according to the severity. Contact a poison control center if necessary, provide supportive care, remove the substance residue from the patient's mouth, place the patient in the recovery position, manage the patient's airway/ventilation/oxygen supplementation, provide CPR as necessary, induce vomiting or administer activated charcoal only if advised by the poison control center or another expert, and provide rapid transport. If the contamination is by inhalation, remove the patient from the source as soon as possible. If the contamination is by absorption, remove the contaminated clothes and wash the patient's skin with large amounts of soap and water and flush the affected eyes with water or NS .

Poisoning by nerve agents/cholinergics

Nerve agents/Cholinergics are toxic chemicals (organophosphates) that damage the nervous system and bodily functions, leading to death in a short time. Nerve agents include tabun (GA), sarin (GB), soman (GD), and VX, and they are used in terrorist attacks. GA, BG, and GD persist in the environment for 10 minutes to 24 hours during the summer and 2 hours to 3 days during the winter (cold weather), and they have very fast action. VX persists longer in the environment and is more lethal. Symptoms of exposure (gas/aerosol) include salivation, lacrimation, urination, defecation, GI upset, and emesis (SLUDGE); runny nose; pupil contraction; vision impairment; slurred speech; chest pain; hallucinations; respiratory distress; and coma. High doses may cause immediate seizures and death. Prehospital: Move away from the area quickly or shelter in place, remove the patient's clothing, and wash the patient's body with large amounts of soap and water. Use an autoinjector for atropine and pralidoxime (separate injections [Mark I] or combined dose [DuoDote]), unless there is only mild tearing or runny nose, and use diazepam for seizures. Provide airway/ventilation/oxygen supplementation and circulation support.

Safe use and disposal of autoinjectors

Autoinjectors are spring-loaded syringe/needle devices that contain preloaded doses of medication and can be easily administered by following the directions on the devices. Autoinjectors are available for nerve agent treatment for emergency medical personnel—Mark I and DuoDote.

- Atropine autoinjector: For symptoms of nerve damage (increases heart rate, dries secretions, dilates pupils, and reduces GI upset).
- Pralidoxime (2-PAM chloride) autoinjector: For symptoms of nerve damage, twitching, and difficulty breathing.
- Diazepam autoinjector: For convulsions associated with nerve agents.

Wear appropriate PPE, remove the safety cap, cleanse the skin with alcohol, and (holding the device perpendicular to the skin) apply firm pressure with the tip of the injector against the skin in the outer thigh until the device fires the needle into the muscle tissue (avoid jabbing). Then, hold the autoinjector in place for at least 10 seconds to ensure that the medication is completely injected. Carefully remove the needle from the skin. Avoid touching the needle, and do not attempt to recap it. Dispose of the intact device in a sharps container.

Indicators of substance abuse

Many people with **substance abuse** (alcohol or drugs) are reluctant to disclose this information. Common agents include cannabis (marijuana), hallucinogens (LSD), stimulants (cocaine, methamphetamine), barbiturates (secobarbital [Seconal], amobarbital [Amytal]), sedatives (zolpidem [Ambien], eszopiclone [Lunesta], hypnotics/benzodiazepines (alprazolam [Xanax], diazepam [Valium], lorazepam [Ativan]), and opiates (heroin, morphine, fentanyl, oxycodone, hydrocodone)

A number of indicators are suggestive of substance abuse, including the following:

Physical signs

- Needle tracks on arms or legs
- Burns on fingers or lips
- Pupils abnormally dilated or constricted, eyes watery
- Slurring of speech, slow speech
- Lack of coordination, instability of gait
- Tremors
- Sniffing repeatedly, nasal irritation
- Persistent cough
- Weight loss
- Dysrhythmias (abnormal pulse)
- Pallor, puffiness of face

Other signs

- Odor of alcohol/marijuana on clothing or breath
- Labile emotions, including mood swings, agitation, and anger
- Inappropriate, impulsive, and/or risky behavior
- Lying
- Missing appointments
- Difficulty concentrating/short term memory loss, disoriented/confused
- Blackouts
- Insomnia or excessive sleeping
- Lack of personal hygiene

Ethanol (alcohol) abuse and withdrawal

Ethanol (the alcohol that is found in alcoholic beverages, flavorings, and some medications) is a multisystem toxin and CNS depressant. It is often the drug of choice of teenagers, young adults, and those >60 years old. Ethanol overdose affects the CNS and other organs. If patients are easily aroused, they can usually safely sleep off the effects, but if a patient is semiconscious or unconscious, emergency medical treatment is needed. Young children frequently ingest alcohol in products such as perfumes and cleaning solutions, which are often more toxic than alcoholic beverages.

Infants/Young children

- Seizures, coma, death
- Respiratory depression and hypoxia
- Hypoglycemia (especially infants and toddlers)
- Hypothermia

Teenagers/Adults

- Altered mental status, coma, circulatory collapse, death
- Hypotension, bradycardia with arrhythmias
- Respiratory depression and hypoxia
- Cold, clammy skin or flushed skin
- Acute pancreatitis/abdominal pain

Chronic abuse of ethanol (alcoholism) is associated with alcohol withdrawal syndrome (delirium tremens) with abrupt cessation of alcohol intake, resulting in hallucinations, tachycardia, diaphoresis, sometimes psychotic behavior, and a high mortality rate. Prehospital: Manage the patient's airway /ventilation/oxygen supplementation and provide CPR if necessary, start an IV access line if indicated, maintain body temperature, and reduce noise/light.

Abuse and overdose of narcotics

Narcotics include opiates (drugs derived from opium) and opioids (synthetic narcotics). Drugs frequently abused include heroin and many prescription drugs, such as morphine, meperidine, fentanyl (pills and patches), oxycodone, hydrocodone, buprenorphine, and methadone. Patients

- 114 -

often crush pills and snort or inject them to increase their effects. Because tolerance to the drugs occurs, patients tend to take higher and higher doses, resulting in addiction and an increasing risk of overdose. Narcotics reduce pain and provide a feeling of euphoria or well-being as well as drowsiness. Symptoms of overdose may include slurred speech, pupil (pinpoint) constriction, nausea, hypotension, vomiting, lack of coordination, alterations of consciousness, coma, respiratory depression, cyanosis, and cardiac arrest (death). Patients may have a runny, irritated nose from snorting drugs or needle marks from injecting. Prehospital: Manage the patient's airway/ventilation/oxygen supplementation, and provide CPR if necessary. Provide an IV access line and fluids. Administer naloxone (an opioid reversal agent) per autoinjector or nasal spray (according to protocol).

Antidotes and treatments for toxic ingestions

Treament for **toxic ingestions** includes the following:

- **Administration of a reversal agent** (antidote) if the toxic substance is known and an antidote exists. Antidotes for common toxins include the following:
- Opiates: Naloxone (Narcan).
- Acetaminophen: N-acetylcysteine.
- Calcium channel blockers, beta-blockers: Calcium chloride, glucagon.
- Tricyclic antidepressants: Sodium bicarbonate, physostigmine.
- Ethylene glycol and toxic alcohols: Fomepizole and ethanol infusion (and, later, dialysis).
- Iron: Deferoxamine.
- Digitalis/Digoxin: Digibind.
- Cyanide: Methylene blue, glyceryl trinitrate.
- Benzodiazepines: Flumazenil.
- Beta-blockers/Calcium channel blockers: Glucagon.
- Warfarin (Coumadin): Phytomenadione (vitamin K).
- **GI decontamination** at one time was standard procedure (syrup of ipecac and gastric lavage followed by activated charcoal). It is no longer advised for routine use, although selective gastric lavage may be appropriate if done within 1 hour of ingestion.

Activated charcoal (1 g/kg/wt) orally or per NG tube binds to many toxins if given within 1 hour of ingestion. It may also be used in multiple doses (every 4–6 hours) to enhance elimination.

Nonnarcotic medication overdose

Drug	Overdose symptoms
Acetaminophen (Tylenol)	Toxicity occurs with dosage >140 mg/kg in one dose or >7.5g in 24 hours:

6. (Initial) Minor gastrointestinal upset.
7. (Days 2–3) Hepatotoxicity (liver damage) with right upper quadrant pain.
8. (Days 3–4) Hepatic failure with metabolic acidosis, coagulopathy, kidney failure, encephalopathy, nausea, vomiting, and possible death.
9. (Days 5–12) Recovery period (survivors). Prehospital: Manage airway/ventilation/oxygen, Recovery position if nauseated, supportive care.

Prehospital: Manage the patient's airway/ventilation/oxygen supplementation. Use the recovery position if the patient is nauseated. Provide supportive care.

NSAIDs/Salicylates	Toxicity (4–48 hours after ingestion) includes headache, nausea, abdominal pain, tinnitus (ringing in the ears), diaphoresis, hypertension, fluid in the lungs, alterations in mental status, cardiac dysrhythmias, seizures, and respiratory arrest. Prehospital: As above.
Dextromethorphan (cough syrup/cold medications)	Mild: Restlessness and euphoria and signs of intoxication. Moderate: Slurred speech, lack of coordination, memory loss, hallucinations and "stoned" appearance. Severe: Altered state of consciousness, impaired vision, hearing, emotional detachment, and an inability to comprehend spoken words, leading to hallucinations, delusions, tachycardia, temporary blindness, and respiratory arrest. Some patients exhibit violent or psychotic behavior. Prehospital: As above; restrain if necessary.
Cardiac	Digitalis (digoxin) toxicity may cause (initially) increasing fatigue, lethargy, depression, nausea, "halo" vision, and vomiting, progressing to a sudden change in heart rhythm, such as an irregular rhythm, palpitations, heart block, tachycardia, and, later, bradycardia. Prehospital: Manage the patient's airway/ventilation/oxygen supplementation and circulation as needed.
Psychiatric	Benzodiazepine toxicity may result from accidental or intentional overdose with such drugs as Xanax and Valium. Indications are often nonspecific neurological changes such as lethargy, dizziness, alterations in consciousness, and ataxia. Respiratory depression and hypotension are rare complications. Prehospital: Provide supportive care.
	Mild lithium toxicity (Eskalith, Lithobid) can include severe vomiting and diarrhea, increased muscle tremors and twitching, lethargy, body aches, ataxia, ringing in the ears, blurry vision, vertigo, or hyperactive deep-tendon reflexes. More severe symptoms can include elevated temperature, low urine output, hypotension, heart abnormalities, decreased level of consciousness, seizures, coma or death. Prehospital: Manage the patient's airway/ventilation/oxygen supplementation and circulation as needed.

Respiratory conditions

Respiratory condition	Assessment/Findings	Prehospital
Asthma	An immune response causes constriction of bronchi and inflammation and increased secretions in the lower airways. Symptoms include cough, wheezing, diminished breath sounds, dyspnea, and difficulty speaking. Children's symptoms are often intermittent, whereas adults' tend to be persistent. Death from asthma is most common in those older than 65. Geriatric patients are most at risk from influenza, pneumonia, and pneumococcal pneumonia.	Administer albuterol (nebulized/metered dose) per protocol and oxygen (6–8 LPM), and provide airway management/ventilation. Provide CPAP for moderate/severe cases. Severe: Provide rapid transport.
Pneumonia	Infection of the lungs (bacterial, viral, fungal, or parasitic) resulting in fever, chills, cough, purulent sputum, difficulty breathing, chest pain on cough or deep inhalation, and headache. Infants may exhibit sternal retraction, decreased feeding, and irritability. Adolescents may have vomiting, diarrhea, sore throat, and earache along with typical symptoms.	Use standard and droplet precautions, including wearing a protective face mask. Place the patient in a position of comfort (usually with the head elevated), and manage the patient's airway/ventilation/oxygen supplementation. Severe: Provide rapid transport.
Pertussis (whooping cough)	Severe persistent "whooping" cough, thick sputum, postcough emesis, petechiae on the upper body, and sclera from exertion. Infants may develop CNS damage, apnea, or pneumonia; children may develop hernia or muscle damage; and adults may develop hernia or a fractured rib.	Use standard and droplet precautions, provide the patient a position of comfort, and manage the patient's airway/ventilation/oxygen supplementation as needed.
Cystic fibrosis	Progressive congenital disease that particularly affects the pancreas and lungs, causing the production of thick mucus that clogs the lungs and causes recurrent bacterial infections of the lower respiratory tract. Symptoms include severe cough, sputum, fever, and dyspnea.	Use standard and droplet precautions, and provide the patient a position of comfort. Manage the patient's airway/ventilation/oxygen supplementation. Start an IV access line. Severe: Provide rapid transport.

Chronic obstructive pulmonary disease (COPD)	Disease with limitations of airflow, narrowing airways, exertional dyspnea, chronic cough, right-sided heart failure (cor pulmonale), damaged and distended alveoli, barrel chest, and clubbed fingers. Symptoms include severe dyspnea, cough, sputum, cyanosis, and the tripod position.	Manage the patient's airway/ventilation and provide oxygen per nasal cannula or Venturi mask to maintain oxygen saturation >90%, provide the patient with a position of comfort or capnography near 35–45 mm Hg, peak flow, and consider CPAP. Administer a beta-agonist bronchodilator (albuterol) according to protocol. Severe: Provide rapid transport.
Chronic bronchitis (one form of COPD)	Chronic inflammation of bronchial passages with cough and sputum production, resulting in narrowed airway passages and dyspnea. Symptoms usually persist for more than 3 months per year.	
Emphysema (one form of COPD)	Chronic inflammation of the alveoli of the lungs results in ruptures and large, distended air sacs that trap air. Symptoms include dyspnea, cyanosis, difficulty exhaling, barrel chest, altered mental status, and pursed-lip breathing.	

Spontaneous pneumothorax

Spontaneous pneumothorax is air in the pleural space that causes the lung to collapse but without an obvious cause. Symptoms include an abrupt onset of sharp chest pain on the affected side, dyspnea, difficulty breathing, and decreased/absent respirations on the affected side.

- Primary (no underlying lung disease): It is most common in tall, thin adolescents and young adults and is associated with cigarette smoking. It often resolves without treatment and rarely progresses to tension pneumothorax.
- Secondary (underlying lung disease): It is most common in those with chronic obstructive pulmonary disease (COPD), cystic fibrosis, and severe asthma, and it poses a risk of death because of respiratory compromise. Patients may develop hypoxemia, altered mental status, coma, and tension pneumothorax.

Prehospital: Manage the patient's airway/ventilation/oxygen supplementation, place the patient in a position of comfort, and transport. A large spontaneous pneumothorax will require catheter aspiration of air or insertion of a chest tube.

Pulmonary edema

Pulmonary edema occurs when the alveoli in the lungs fill with fluid.

- Cardiogenic: The left ventricle weakens, so the heart cannot pump adequate amounts of blood, resulting in back pressure in the left atrium and the vessels in the lungs, forcing fluid into the alveoli. Left ventricular damage can result from coronary artery disease, cardiomyopathy, myocardial infarction, defective heart valves, and uncontrolled hypertension.

- Noncardiogenic: Damage to the capillaries in the lungs causes them to leak fluid into the alveoli. Conditions causing noncardiogenic pulmonary edema include acute respiratory distress syndrome (ARDS), adverse drug reactions, pulmonary embolism, lung injury, viral infections, nervous system conditions, toxin exposure, smoke inhalation, near drowning, and high-altitude pulmonary edema (HAPE).

Symptoms include severe dyspnea, orthopnea, tachycardia, cough, and chest pain. Prehospital: Manage airway/ventilation and supplemental oxygen/CPAP or intubation with PEEP, and start an IV access line. Medications may include dopamine, dobutamine, nitroglycerin, and furosemide (per protocol). Severe cases require rapid transport. HAPE: Immediately descend to a lower altitude (500–1000 m), provide supplemental oxygen and a portable hyperbaric chamber, and administer acetazolamide or dexamethasone (per protocol).

Epiglottitis

Acute epiglottitis (supraglottitis) occurs in children primarily from 1 to 8 years old and in young adults. Acute epiglottitis requires immediate medical attention because it can rapidly become obstructive. The onset is usually very sudden and often occurs during the night. The patient may awaken suddenly with a fever, but he or she usually does not have a cough.

Symptoms include the following:

- Tripod position: Sits upright, leaning forward with the chin out, mouth open, and tongue protruding.
- Agitation: Appears restless, tense, and agitated.
- Drooling: Excess secretions combined with pain or dysphagia and a mouth-open position cause drooling.
- Voice: No hoarseness, but the voice sounds thick and "froglike."
- Cyanosis: Color is usually pale and sallow initially but may progress to frank cyanosis.
- Throat: On examination, the epiglottis appears bright red and swollen. Note: The patient's throat should not be examined with a tongue blade unless intubation and tracheostomy equipment is immediately available because the examination can trigger an obstruction.

Prehospital: Provide rapid transport, administer high-flow oxygen with a blow-by mask, or provide slow ventilation with a BVM.

Metered-dose inhaler (MIDI/MDI) and the small-volume nebulizer

The paramedic may administer or assist the patient with use of a metered-dose inhaler (MIDI/MDI) or a small-volume nebulizer for medications such as albuterol, according to protocol, as follows:

- The **MIDI/MDI** is a pressurized cartridge that is used for the administration of a specific dose of an aerosolized medication. Shake the medication vigorously before use, prime if it is the initial use, position 4 cm (two finger widths) away from the patient's mouth or between the lips, have the patient exhale and breathe in slowly and completely while the MIDI is activated, and then have the patient hold the breath for 10 seconds, waiting 1 minute between puffs. Stop the treatment if the patient becomes shaky, dizzy, coughs uncontrollably, has palpitations, or has a pulse increase of ≥ 20 bpm. Resume slowly after 5 to 10 minutes.

- A **small-volume nebulizer** includes a nebulizer cup that holds 2–4 mL of medication, air tubing, a compressor to aerosolize the medication, and a T-piece and mouthpiece or face mask for delivery. Dilute the medication with sterile water or NS, not tap water, if necessary. Have the patient sit upright for treatment, breathing normally through the mouth, using the mouthpiece or face mask.

Capnography and end-tidal CO_2 (ETCO$_2$) readings and peak flow meter

Capnography provides a visual display of end-tidal carbon dioxide (ETCO$_2$/PETCO$_2$) levels in inhalation and exhalation. Capnography is recommended to establish the correct placement of an endotracheal tube, to assess the effectiveness of CPR, to evaluate respiratory distress (asthma, COPD, overdose), and to assess the patient's response to treatment. Normal ETCO$_2$ is 35–45 mm Hg. Hypercarbia (a measurement of >45 mm Hg) occurs with hypoventilation (overdose, sedation, postseizure, head trauma, stroke), and hypocarbia (a measurement of <35 mm Hg) with hyperventilation (anxiety, bronchospasm, pulmonary edema, decreased cardiac output). ETCO$_2$ levels are less accurate with sidestream measurement used for the nasal cannula and face mask than with the mainstream sensor used with an endotracheal tube, so it's important to keep the sensor close to the mouth and secured.

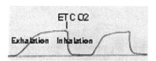

The **peak flow meter** is a handheld device that is used to determine the maximum flow rate of air on a forceful exhalation. Peak flows are used to monitor asthma and COPD. Peak flow measures are taken three times, with the highest flow rate being recorded. Optimal levels are individualized for all patients.

Sickle cell disease and crises

Sickle cell disease is a recessive genetic disorder of chromosome 11, causing defective hemoglobin so that the red blood cells (RBCs) are sickle-shaped and inflexible, resulting in their accumulating in small vessels and causing painful blockages. Although normal RBCs survive for 120 days, sickled blood cells may survive only 10–20 days, stressing the bone marrow that cannot produce RBCs fast enough and resulting in anemia. Different types of **crises** occur (aplastic, hemolytic, vaso-occlusive, and sequestering), which can cause infarctions in organs, severe pain, damage to organs, and rapid enlargement of the liver and spleen. Vaso-occlusive crisis is common in adolescents and adults, and it can be triggered by sickness, stress, dehydration, temperature changes, and high altitude. Young children are prone to splenic sequestration (RBCs trapped in the spleen, causing it to enlarge and sometimes rupture) resulting in pain in the left abdomen. Acute chest syndrome is most common in children 2–4 but is more severe in adults (cough, pain, fever, and dyspnea). Prehospital: Manage the patient's airway/ventilation/oxygen supplementation and circulation, start an IV access line and give fluids as indicated, provide analgesia and emotional support, and provide rapid transport for severe symptoms.

Clotting disorders

Clotting disorders include the following:

- Hemophilia is an inherited disorder in which the person lacks adequate clotting factors, which results in bleeding with trauma, bruising, spontaneous hemorrhage (often in the joints), and epistaxis. There are three primary types: A (80%–90%), B, and C.
- Disseminated intravascular coagulation (DIC) (consumption coagulopathy) is a secondary disorder that is triggered by another event, such as trauma, congenital heart disease, necrotizing enterocolitis, sepsis, and severe viral infections. DIC triggers coagulation (clotting) and hemorrhage through a complex series of events, with clotting and hemorrhage occurring simultaneously, putting the patient at risk of death.
- Von Willebrand's disease is a group of congenital bleeding disorders (inherited from either parent) affecting 1%–2% of the population, associated with deficiency or lack of von Willebrand factor (vWF), a glycoprotein.

Prehospital: Monitor for signs of bleeding, and manage the patient's airway/ventilation/oxygen supplementation. For all: Provide an IV access line and rapid transport for hemorrhage or acute blood loss resulting in hypotension.

Transfusion-related complications

Transfusion-related complications can include the following:

- Infection: Bacterial contamination of blood can result in severe sepsis with chills, fever, diarrhea, hypotension, and shock.
- Transfusion-related acute lung injury (TRALI): Occurs ≤6 hours. Characterized by noncardiogenic pulmonary edema. There may be severe dyspnea and arterial hypoxemia. TRALI may be fatal, but it usually resolves in 12–48 hours with supportive care.
- Circulatory overload: Excess fluid volume, especially with heart failure. Characterized by cough, dyspnea, orthopnea, headache, hypertension, tachycardia, jugular venous distension, and signs of pulmonary edema.
- Allergic reaction: Reactions to foreign proteins may be mild (itching, flushing, urticaria) to severe (anaphylaxis).
- Febrile (nonhemolytic): Reaction to white blood cells in packed red blood cells or platelets. Characterized by a sudden onset of chills, fever, headache, anxiety, and muscle aches.
- Acute hemolytic: In incompatible blood transfusions, antibodies destroy donor red blood cells (most common with ABO incompatibility), usually resulting from errors in labeling blood. Characterized by chills, fever, tachycardia, chest pain, lumbar pain, hypotension, uncontrolled bleeding, and blood in the urine.

Hematological conditions

Anemia   Anemia occurs when there are deficient numbers of RBCs or the hemoglobin doesn't bind to sufficient oxygen to meet body demands. Anemia results in a decrease in oxygen transportation and decreased perfusion throughout the body, causing the heart to compensate by increasing cardiac output. The types include iron-deficiency (inadequate iron), blood-loss, hemolytic (red cells destroyed), aplastic (bone marrow damaged), and pernicious (vitamin B_{12} deficiency) anemia.

Leukopenia	A low WBC count (<4000) makes the patient vulnerable to infection. Causes include chemotherapy, autoimmune disorders, cancer, viral infections, medications (such as antibiotics), radiation, HIV/AIDS, and TB.
Lymphomas	Cancer of the lymphocytes (the WBCs involved in the immune response). Two main types are Hodgkin's and non-Hodgkin's lymphoma.
Polycythemia	Excessive RBC count, resulting in viscous (thick) blood and an increased risk of clots.
Multiple myeloma	Cancer of the plasma cells, resulting in tumor in the bone marrow, bone pain, anemia, kidney failure, and infection.
Thrombocytopenia	Low platelet count, increasing the risk of bruising and bleeding.

Hemodialysis

Hemodialysis is used primarily for those who have progressed from renal insufficiency to uremia with end-stage renal (kidney) disease (ESRD). With hemodialysis, blood is circulated outside of the body through a dialyzer (a synthetic semipermeable membrane), which filters the blood and removes waste products and excess fluids. A vascular access device, such as a catheter, fistula, or graft, must be established for hemodialysis, with fistulas and grafts usually being placed in an arm and a catheter being placed in the upper chest (into the superior vena cava). Tubing from the dialysis machine attaches to the access device for treatments, which are usually done for 4 hours three times weekly. Emergent conditions include low BP, nausea/vomiting, irregular pulse, cardiac arrest, bleeding from the access site, and difficulty breathing. Missed treatments may result in electrolyte excess, weakness, and pulmonary edema. Prehospital: Manage the patient's airway/ventilation/oxygen supplementation, apply pressure to stop any bleeding, position the patient flat if he or she is in shock, and position upright if there is difficulty breathing. Provide an IV access, but avoid placing the IV and measuring the BP on the arm with the access site.

Peritoneal dialysis

Peritoneal dialysis is used to remove waste products and excess fluids from those with ESRD. A catheter is placed into the peritoneal cavity of the abdomen. The peritoneum comprises the visceral peritoneum (the lining of the gut and other viscera), which makes up about 80% of the total peritoneal surface area, and the parietal perineum (lining the abdominal cavity), which is the most important for peritoneal dialysis. A dialysate solution is instilled (usually about 2 L for adults but less for children, taking about 10 minutes) through the catheter, the catheter is clamped, and the solution (dwell) is left in place for 3–6 hours. The solution is then drained (usually for about 20 minutes), and the process is repeated with new dialysate. Peritoneal dialysis increases the risk of obesity, peritonitis, hernia, malnutrition, hypertriglyceridemia, and back pain. Obesity, older adulthood, and lack of social support are contraindications for peritoneal dialysis. Prehospital: Manage the patient's airway/ventilation/oxygen supplementation, use contact precautions if there is purulent drainage from the catheter site, and position the patient for comfort.

Urinary catheter management

A **urinary catheter** is inserted through the urethra and into the bladder to drain urine. Straight catheterizations are done with sterile catheters periodically to empty the bladder or to relieve urinary retention, whereas retention catheters (Foley) have a balloon that inflates to keep the catheter in place for continuous drainage. Foley catheters may be indicated for patients with neuromuscular disorders, incontinence, urinary retention, dementia, or urinary disorders. Catheters may also be inserted suprapubically (above the pubis bone) directly into the bladder, especially for males with long-term catheterization. Urinary collection bags should be kept below the level of the bladder, and the tubing is secured so that the catheter is not inadvertently pulled out, causing trauma to the urethra, especially in males. Thick, cloudy urine may indicate infection. Scant urine and lower abdominal pain/distension may indicate blockage of the catheter. Milking the catheter may help relieve a blockage. When removing a Foley catheter, the balloon must first be deflated. Prehospital: Provide supportive care, start an IV access line, and give fluids to keep the vein open if there is severe abdominal pain.

Renal (kidney) and urinary calculi

Renal (kidney) and urinary calculi (stones) occur frequently, more commonly in males, and they can be related to diseases (hyperparathyroidism, renal tubular acidosis, and gout) and lifestyle factors, such as sedentary work. Their incidence is highest between ages 35 and 45. Additionally, some medications can precipitate calculi. Calculi can form at any age, most are composed of calcium, and they can range in size from very tiny to >6mm. Stones of <4mm can usually pass in the urine easily.

Symptoms
Symptoms occur with obstruction and are usually of sudden onset and acute.

- Severe flank pain radiating to the abdomen and labia or testicle on the same side as the stone (adolescents and adults), abdominal or pelvic pain (young children)
- Nausea and vomiting
- Diaphoresis
- Hematuria (blood in urine)

Prehospital
- Analgesia: Opiates and NSAIDs as needed (per protocol).
- Provide supplemental oxygen if needed.
- Start an IV access line and give fluids if indicated.
- Transport.

Renal (kidney) failure

Acute renal (kidney) failure is abrupt and is an almost complete failure of kidney function, occurring over a period of hours/days. It most commonly occurs in hospitalized patients, but it may occur in others as well. Causes include MI, heart failure, sepsis, anaphylaxis, burns, trauma, infections, transfusion reactions, medications (NSAIDs and ACE inhibitors), and obstruction. Symptoms include reduced or absent urinary output, increased nocturia (nighttime urination), altered mental status, tinnitus, a metallic taste in the mouth, tremors, seizures, flank pain, abdominal pain, hypertension, increased bruising. **Chronic renal failure** occurs after years of disease that damages the kidneys, often being essentially asymptomatic until the damage is severe. Early symptoms may include anorexia, general malaise, headaches, itching, and weight loss. Later symptoms include fluid retention (pulmonary edema, peripheral edema, ascites), headache, bruising, dry skin, muscle cramping, bone pain, weakness, breath odor, excessive thirst, frequent hiccups, dyspnea, vomiting (especially in the morning), and hypertension. Prehospital: Manage the patient's airway/ventilation/oxygen, provide an IV access line (if the patient is hypotensive or if there is evidence of pulmonary edema), and transport.

End-stage renal disease (ESRD)

Acute and chronic liver failure may progress to **end-stage renal disease (ESRD)** when the kidneys are no longer able to function and the patient needs dialysis or a kidney transplant. The patient may develop uremic syndrome, which results in decreased production of red blood cells and platelets, electrolyte imbalances, bone disease, multiple endocrine disorders, cardiac problems (especially congestive heart failure), anorexia, and malnutrition. Symptoms include altered mental status, hallucinations, and confusion from the accumulation of waste products in the blood; increasing edema and shortness of breath from accumulated fluids; chest and bone pain; severe pruritus; nausea, vomiting, and diarrhea; tremors, muscle twitching, and seizures; and increased bruising and discoloration of the skin. Prehospital: Manage the patient's airway/ventilation/oxygen, start an IV access line (if the patient is hypotensive or if there is evidence of pulmonary edema), and transport.

Urinary tract infections

Cystitis is an infection (usually bacterial) of the bladder resulting in urinary frequency, urgency, and burning. Urine may be cloudy, bloody, and/or foul smelling. Other symptoms include lower abdominal discomfort and low-grade fever. Young children may have daytime wetting, and older adults may exhibit confusion. If the infection spreads to the kidney, **pyelonephritis** may develop. Pyelonephritis is a potentially organ-damaging bacterial infection of the kidney. Pyelonephritis can result in abscess formation, sepsis, and kidney failure. Treatment requires a prolonged period of antibiotics.

Symptoms of pyelonephritis
Symptoms vary widely, but they can include the following:

- Dysuria with frequency, hematuria (blood in urine), and flank and/or low back pain
- Fever and chills
- Costovertebral angle (between the 12th rib and vertebrae) tenderness
- Changes in feeding habits (infants)
- Changes in mental status (geriatric)

Younger women often exhibit symptoms associated more often with lower urinary infection, so the condition may be overlooked.

Prehospital
Provide supportive care, an IV access line, and fluids if there is high fever and/or abdominal pain.

Male genital tract conditions

Condition	Characteristics	Prehospital
Epididymitis/ Orchitis	Inflammation of the epididymis/testicle. Swelling of the testicle, scrotum, and/or groin area, pain worsening with bowel movement, fever, urethral discharge.	Provide supportive care and analgesia as needed.
Fournier's gangrene	Severe infection of the male genitalia resulting from injury, genital piercing, penile implants, instrumentation, or rectal foreign body. Beginning with erythema and pain and progressing to swelling with crepitus, cyanosis of tissues, purulent discharge, fever, severe pain, and enlarging necrosis.	Manage the airway, ventilation and oxygen, start an IV access line, administer crystalloids for patients in shock, and provide rapid transport.

Phimosis/ Paraphimosis	Phimosis: Constricted prepuce over the tip of the penis. Uncircumcised young boys and older adults are especially at risk. It may cause difficulty urinating. Paraphimosis: Foreskin retraction/constriction causing swelling of the glans, can result in necrosis and gangrene with severe pain.	Provide supportive care, cold compresses to reduce any swelling, and rapid transport (for paraphimosis).
Testicular mass	This may indicate a cancerous tumor or swelling from another condition (such as testicular torsion, epididymitis, orchitis). It may or may not be painful, depending on its cause.	Provide supportive care.
Priapism	Erection lasting >4 hours, most common in males in their 30s with leukemia and sickle cell disease. May occur with medications (Viagra), alcohol, and illicit drugs. Ischemic: Increasing penile pain with rigid shaft but soft glans. Nonischemic: Not painful; the penis is erect but not rigid.	Provide supportive care and transport for possible surgical intervention.
Benign prostatic hypertrophy (BPH)	Enlarged prostate, most common in males over 50 and caused by hormone changes. It results in compression of the urethra with difficulty urinating and urinary retention; nocturia.	BPH is rarely an emergent condition. Provide supportive care.
Testicular torsion	The testicle cord twists, resulting in a twisted spermatic cord and reduced blood flow; it is most common in adolescents and may result from trauma. Abrupt severe scrotal pain and swelling scrotal mass, nausea, vomiting, fever, bloody semen, abdominal pain.	Provide supportive care, analgesia, and rapid transport.
Blunt trauma	Severe pain, penile, testicular swelling, bloody discharge from penis. May be associated with pelvic fracture and shock.	Manage the airway, ventilation, and oxygen; start an IV access line; administer crystalloids for patient in shock; provide cold compresses and rapid transport.

Vaginal bleeding

Vaginal bleeding may indicate heavy menstrual bleeding (menorrhagia) or abnormal bleeding between cycles (metrorrhagia). Vaginal bleeding may also be an indication of an ectopic pregnancy or spontaneous abortion; in postmenopausal women, it may be a sign of endometrial cancer. Menorrhagia may result from hormonal imbalance, clotting disorders, uterine fibroids, and endometrial polyps. Metrorrhagia may result from infection, cancer, and cervical/endometrial polyps. Symptoms may include cramping and abdominal pain, depending on the cause. It's important to determine when the bleeding started and about how much blood had been lost (the number of sanitary pads that are saturated per hour, for example) as well as the presence or absence of pain. If the blood loss is excessive, the patient may exhibit signs of shock. Prehospital: Use standard precautions, manage the patient's airway, ventilation, and oxygen as needed. Monitor vital signs. Position the patient flat for shock, and provide IV access and fluids

Female reproductive system

The **female reproductive system** includes the ovaries, fallopian tubes, uterus, cervix, vagina, vulva, labia minora, labia majora, clitoris, and breasts. Functions include ovulation, fertilization, menstruation, pregnancy, and lactation. <u>Menarche</u> (onset of menses) is usually between 9 and 15, but it may occur in younger girls and should be considered as a possibility with younger girls. <u>Menopause</u> occurs at approximately age 50, usually following a period of about 10 years of irregular periods during which time the person may become pregnant. The normal menstrual cycle is 28 days, but it may be up to 45 days in adolescents. Assessment should include abdominal or vaginal pain, vaginal bleeding or discharge, fever, nausea and vomiting, and dizziness. Patients should have their privacy protected during an examination, and the paramedic should communicate openly, asking for permission to touch the patient. The paramedic should consider the possibility of pregnancy or sexually transmitted disease with any abnormal condition.

Gynecological conditions

Condition	Characteristics	Prehospital
Ovarian cyst/ Ovarian torsion	An ovarian cyst is a fluid-filled cyst that develops in the ovary and can rupture. Ovarian torsion is twisting of the ovary, impairing circulation, sometimes as the result of a mass or hemorrhage. Symptoms may include severe pain, nausea, vomiting, and abdominal distension.	Provide supportive care and an IV access line if the condition severe; manage the airway, ventilation, and oxygen; and provide transport.
Endometriosis	Tissue that usually lines the uterus migrates to other parts of the reproductive system and abdomen, causing chronic abdominal pain or severe pain during menses.	Provide supportive care.
Prolapsed uterus	The uterus protrudes through the vagina. It may occur after childbirth (with a risk of hemorrhage) or in older females (usually with little risk of hemorrhage). Patients may complain of vaginal pressure, low back pain, and difficulty urinating.	After childbirth: Using sterile gloves, try to push the uterus back into place; provide supportive care and rapid transport. Older adult: Provide supportive care.
Pelvic inflammatory disease (PID)	Inflammation of reproductive organs from sexually transmitted disease, leading to abscess, ectopic pregnancy, severe chronic pelvic pain, and infertility. Symptoms: Vaginal discharge, fever, painful intercourse, and abdominal pain.	Provide supportive care, a position of comfort, and an IV access line if there is a high fever.
Bartholin's cyst	If the Bartholin glands at the vaginal entrance become blocked, painless cysts and swelling occur. If they become infected, an abscess may develop with swelling and severe pain.	Provide supportive care and a position of comfort.

Vaginitis, vulvovaginitis	Inflammation, itching, burning, discharge, and pain of vagina or vagina and vulva. It is often associated with infection (fungus, bacteria, or protozoa), and it is common with diabetes. May indicate sexual abuse in children.	Provide supportive care.
Vaginal foreign body	Various items may be inserted into the vagina, including vaginal suppositories in their wrapper, forgotten tampons, and sex toys; these may cause vaginal discharge, pain, and inflammation.	Position supine with the knees bent; do not attempt to remove item. Transport.

Sexual assault and legal issues

The crime scenes associated with a **sexual assault** include the patient (body, injuries, clothing, and emotional response) and the place the assault occurred. A victim of sexual assault has the right to consent to or refuse each element of a sexual assault evaluation, although some states may mandate reporting of sexual assault to the authorities. The paramedic should wear disposable gloves when handling clothing, and clothing should be handled gently so that evidence, such as strands of hair or other materials, is not lost in transfer. Documenting the assault should be done in detail with direct quotations. If the patient refuses transport, the best approach is to point out services that could benefit the patient, such as prophylaxis to prevent STDs and pregnancy. Patients are often frightened and confused, so pressuring them to protect others or trying to frighten them more by suggesting that they might be pregnant or develop an STD is a negative approach that may backfire.

Musculoskeletal system

The **musculoskeletal system** includes 203 bones including long bones (e.g., the femur in the thigh), short bones (e.g., the carpal bones in the fingers), and flat bones (e.g., the sternum). The outer hard shell of the bone is the cortex, and the inner porous area is the trabecular bone. The vertebrae lack the cortex layer. Long bones have three parts: The middle section is the diaphysis, followed by the metaphyses, and then the epiphyses (the bone ends). In growing children, an epiphyseal plate of cartilage separates the metaphyses and epiphyses, allowing bone growth. This plate closes in adults, but damage to this area in a child may impair bone growth. The middle part of the short bones contains yellow bone marrow (fatty tissue). Red bone marrow, which produces blood cells, is found in the middle of the flat bones (pelvis, sternum, ribs, and scapula) and at the ends (epiphyses) of the long bones. The skeletal system is connected by cartilage and tendons, and it is protected, supported, and allowed movement by about 700 soft-tissue muscles.

Musculoskeletal conditions

Condition	Characteristics	Prehospital
Osteomyelitis	Infection of the bone (usually with *Staphylococcus aureus*). It is most common in children and adolescents. Symptoms: Pain, erythema, swelling, general malaise, purulent discharge, fever, and chills.	Use standard and contact precautions; splint the bone if necessary.
Osteoarthritis	Damage to the cartilage between bones (usually from an old injury) and bone spurs, causing pain on movement, joint crepitus, joint enlargement, and limited mobility, especially in the morning.	Provide supportive care.

Rheumatoid arthritis	Autoimmune disorder that causes the synovial lining of the joints to swell, with onset between ages 20 and 40, eventually causing joint erosion/deformity. May affect the eyes, heart, lungs, and vessels as well. Symptoms: Enlarged joints, inflammation, limited range of motion, skeletal deformities, pain, and limited mobility.	Provide supportive care.
Gout	Metabolic disorder in which uric acid crystals accumulate in the joints (big toe, thumb) and can lead to kidney stones. Symptoms include swollen, red joints and pain.	Provide supportive care; give NSAIDS for inflammation and pain (avoid aspirin).
Degenerative disc disease	Most common in the lumbar region, resulting in chronic low back pain and stiffness with pain sometimes radiating down one or both hips and legs as well as numbness and tingling. Pain tends to lessen in older adults because the inflammatory proteins associated with pain decrease.	Provide supportive care and analgesia if necessary and a position of comfort.
Cauda equina syndrome	Compression and inflammation of the nerve roots at the distal (tail) end of the spine where the peripheral nervous system connects to the CNS, resulting in severe low back pain, leg numbness or weakness (one- or two-sided), numbness in the saddle area, bowel and bladder dysfunction, and sexual dysfunction. (It requires surgical decompression within 48 hours.)	Provide supportive care, analgesia if necessary, and a position of comfort.
Sprain/Strain	Sprain: Stretching/Tearing of ligaments (most commonly in the ankle) resulting in pain, swelling, bruising, limited mobility. Strain: Stretching/Tearing of muscles and/or tendons, resulting in pain, swelling, muscle spasms, and limited mobility.	Provide supportive care and RICE (rest, ice, compression, and elevation).

Nontraumatic fractures

Nontraumatic fractures occur when the bone weakens and can no longer support the body, such as may occur with a cancerous tumor of the bone or osteoporosis. Common fractures associated with osteoporosis include fractures of the vertebrae and hip. Osteoporotic fractures are most common in older adults, but they may also occur in adolescents with eating disorders. Infants and young children with multiple nontraumatic, nonabusive fractures may have a genetic disorder, such as osteogenesis imperfecta. Assessment of suspected fractures includes evaluating pain/tenderness, swelling around the fracture site, loss of sensation or movement, circulatory impairment (note the color of the skin, pallor or cyanosis), and deformity (especially noticeable in limb fractures). Prehospital: Splint extremity fractures; manage the patient's airway, ventilation, and circulation as needed; and transport for treatment.

Nosebleed (epistaxis)

Recurrent **nosebleed (epistaxis)** is common in young children (ages 2–10), especially boys, and it is often related to nose picking, dry climate, trauma, or central heating. Its incidence also increases between 50 and 80 years of age and may be associated with NSAIDs, hypertension, and anticoagulants. Patients abusing cocaine may suffer nosebleeds because of damage to the mucosa.

The anterior nares have plentiful blood vessels and may bleed easily, usually from one nostril. Bleeding in the posterior nares is more dangerous and can result in considerable blood loss. Blood may flow through both nostrils or backward into the throat, and the person may be observed swallowing and may vomit blood. The blood may block the airway in unconscious patients Prehospital: Sit the patient in an upright position, leaning forward so blood doesn't flow down the throat if the patient is conscious; pinch the nostrils together firmly for at least 10 minutes; and advise the patient to avoid sniffing or blowing the nose.

Eyes and eye conditions

The **eyes** fit into sockets (orbits) in the skull. The eyelid and sclera are lined with **conjunctiva** (clear tissue). The outer layer of the eye is the cornea, which focuses light. The pupil (at the center) dilates or constricts to control light coming into the eye. The iris (colored part) adjusts the size of the pupil. The lens is behind the pupil and allows the eyes to focus. The vitreous humor is the gel-like substance in the middle of the globe. The retina at the back of the eye transmits visual images to the brain. The sclera (white part) contains blood vessels and protects the eye.

Condition	Characteristics	Prehospital
Burns	Chemical/Fire: Pain, tearing, difficulty opening the affected eye.	Irrigate with NS or sterile water for 20–30 minutes.
Corneal abrasion (scratch)/ Foreign body	Often associated with a failure to use safety glasses or wearing contact lenses. A foreign body may remain in the eye(s). Symptoms: Blurred vision, pain, tearing, photophobia, and squinting (muscle spasms).	As above. Do not attempt to remove a foreign body; patch both eyes to prevent movement.
Conjunctivitis	Allergic response or bacterial or viral (most common) infection of the conjunctiva. Symptoms: Pain, itching, and redness.	Use standard and contact precautions for viral/bacterial infection. Use a warm compress for 10–15 minutes to relieve discomfort and promote healing.
Retinal detachment	The retina detaches from the back of the eye, interfering with blood supply. Most common in patients over 50 and may result from injury, aging, and diabetes. Symptoms: Floaters, impaired vision, and flashes.	Provide supportive care and immediate transport for surgical intervention to save the vision.
Hyphema	Blood collects between the cornea and iris, covering all or part of the visible eye, often after a traumatic injury. Symptoms: Pain, visible blood, and impaired vision.	Provide supportive care. Tell the patient to avoid aspirin (which may increase any bleeding).
Eyelid inflammation	Chalazion is swelling and inflammation from a blocked oil gland in the eyelid. Hordeolum (stye) is an acute infection of the eyelid glands. Symptoms: Redness, swelling, and pain.	Provide supportive care and a warm compress for 10–15 minutes.

Ear anatomy and ear conditions

The outer part of **the ear** (pinna/auricle) opens into the ear canal, where vibrations travels to the tympanic membrane and into the middle ear (malleus, incus, stapes) and through the oval window, which connects to the inner ear and labyrinth where semicircular ducts connected to nerves and the cochlea relay information about the position of the head and balance. The cochlea sends signals to the brain. The auditory canal extends from the middle ear to the nasopharynx to drain excess fluid.

Ear conditions

Condition	Characteristics	Prehospital
Foreign body in the ear canal	Frequently found with small children (nuts, screws, sticks, rocks).	Provide supportive care. Do not attempt to remove. Needs a physician's attention.
Impacted cerumen	Earwax impacts into the ear canal, often covering the eardrum and impairing hearing. Common in older adults.	Same as above.
Ménière's disease, labyrinthitis	Damage to the inner ear or inflammation causes vertigo, dizziness, lack of balance, hearing impairment, nausea, and vomiting.	Provide supportive care, place in the supine position (unless vomiting), keep lights dim.

Shock and Resuscitation

Shock

Shock is a life-threatening condition that occurs when the tissues do not receive adequate oxygen, such as with severe bleeding or fluid loss, severe infection, heart failure, or abnormal dilation of the blood vessels. Indications of shock include extreme thirst; anxiety and restlessness; weak, rapid pulse; altered mental status progressing to loss of consciousness; rapid, shallow respirations; hypotension (low BP—often a late sign); and cool, clammy, pale skin with mottling sometimes on the extremities from inadequate perfusion. If left untreated, shock may lead to cardiac arrest. Note that geriatric patients may have a higher baseline respiration and heart rate and an irregular pulse. Prehospital: Apply pressure to control the bleeding, perform spinal stabilization if needed, place the patient in the shock position (flat with feet elevated above the level of the heart, 8 to 12 inches), manage the patient's airway/ventilation and administer high-concentration oxygen, provide warming blankets to maintain the body temperature, provide reassurance, apply a pneumatic anti-shock garment (PASG), insert an IV access line, and administer fluids for hemorrhage/severe hypotension. Provide rapid transport if needed.

Shock generally occurs in stages as the body tries to compensate. Compensated shock occurs in the early stage while the body speeds up the heart rate and respirations and diverts blood to the vital organs (resulting in pale, cool skin) to maintain adequate perfusion and BP. Decompensated shock occurs when the body can no longer compensate and the BP falls and symptoms worsen. With irreversible shock, recovery is no longer possible because of cell damage caused by inadequate oxygenation and perfusion. Types of shock include the following:

Type	Cause
Cardiogenic	Heart failure, myocardial infarction, drug overdose, dysrhythmia, congenital heart disease.
Distributive	Anaphylaxis, drug overdose.
Hypovolemic	Hemorrhage, severe vomiting and/or diarrhea, severe burns, dehydration.
Obstructive	Pneumothorax, pericardial tamponade.
Neurogenic	Spinal cord injury (a form of distributive shock because of decreased vascular tone.).
Septic	Sepsis, severe infections. (This is also a form of distributive shock.)

Signs and symptoms are similar for all types of shock even though the mechanisms are different.

Hypovolemic shock

Hypovolemic shock occurs when the total circulating volume of fluid decreases, leading to a fall in venous return that in turn causes a decrease in ventricular filling and preload. This results in a decrease in stroke volume and cardiac output. This in turn causes generalized arterial vasoconstriction, increasing afterload (increased systemic vascular resistance), and causing decreased tissue perfusion.

Hypovolemic shock is classified according to the degree of fluid loss as follows:

- Class I: <750 mL or ≤15% of total circulating volume (TCV). (This is usually well tolerated.)
- Class II: 750–1500 mL or 15%–30% of TCV. (Tachycardia, anxiety, narrow pulse pressure, and increased respirations.)

- 131 -

- Class III: 1500–2000 mL or 30%–40% of TCV. (Hypotension, pallor, cold, clammy skin, delayed capillary refill, severe tachycardia, and altered mental status.)
- Class IV: >2000 mL or >40% of TCV. (There is severe shock, a weak thready pulse, cyanosis, and death without aggressive resuscitation.)

Prehospital: Control the patient's bleeding; insert two large-bore, short IV catheters; give 250–500 cc of warm isotonic boluses (20–30 mL/kg); keep the patient warm; maintain the patient's airway/ventilation/oxygen supplementation to maintain oxygen saturation at 90%–92%; maintain the systolic BP at 70–90 mm Hg; place him or her in the shock position; and provide rapid transport.

Complications of shock

Acute respiratory distress syndrome (ARDS)	Damage to the vascular endothelium and the increase in permeability of the alveolar-capillary membrane cause pulmonary edema as the alveoli fill with blood and protein-rich fluid and collapse. Atelectasis with hyperinflation and areas of normal tissue occur as the lungs "stiffen." Hypoxemia and tachypnea increase as the body tries to compensate to maintain a normal $paCO_2$. Symptoms occur within 72 (usually 24–48) hours of serious injury. Untreated, this condition results in respiratory failure, multiorgan failure, and a mortality rate of 5%–30%. (PEEP is used for ventilation.)
Acute renal failure	The renal tubules are damaged, and the kidneys are unable to filter out the waste products of metabolism.
Multiple-organ failure/dysfunction syndrome (MOFS/MODS)	MOFS/MODS is a progressive deterioration and failure of two or more organ systems with mortality rates of 45%–50% with two organ systems involved and up to 80%–100% if there are three or more systems failing. Trauma patients and those with severe conditions, such as shock, are particularly vulnerable, especially in those >65 years old.

Respiratory failure/arrest

Respiratory failure occurs when ventilation is insufficient for adequate gas exchange so that levels of carbon dioxide in the blood increase and levels of oxygen decrease. Respiratory failure may result from respiratory infection (pneumonia, tuberculosis), heart failure, chronic respiratory illness (asthma, chronic bronchitis, COPD), trauma, and depression of the CNS (usually from medications or trauma). Respiratory failure may be acute with sudden onset or chronic, developing over time. If untreated, respiratory failure can lead to **respiratory arrest**, which in turn leads to cardiac arrest. Indications of respiratory failure include altered mental status, cyanosis, labored breathing (dyspnea and orthopnea), coughing, fatigue, diminished breath sounds, and the presence of rales (crackles) and rhonchi (snoring/whistling sound). Patients may have hemoptysis (bloody sputum). The patient's oxygen saturation level is lower than 90% per pulse oximeter. Prehospital: Manage the patient's airway/ventilation/oxygen supplementation; positive-pressure ventilation may be needed. Place the patient in a position of comfort (usually high Fowler's).

Heimlich maneuver for choking

The universal sign of choking is when a person clutches his or her throat and appears to be choking or gasping for breath. If the person can speak ("Can you speak?") or cough, the **Heimlich maneuver** is not usually necessary. The Heimlich maneuver can be done with the victim sitting, standing, or supine. The Heimlich maneuver for children (≥1 year) and adults is as follows:

- Wrap your arms around the victim's waist from the back if sitting or standing. Make a fist and place the thumb side against the victim's abdomen slightly above the umbilicus. Grasp this hand with the other and thrust sharply upward to force air out of the lungs.
- Repeat as needed.
- If the victim loses consciousness, ease him or her into a supine position on the floor, place your hands similarly to CPR but over the abdomen while sitting astride the victim's legs. Repeat upward compressions five times. If no ventilation occurs, attempt to sweep the mouth and ventilate the lungs mouth to mouth. Repeat compressions and ventilations until recovery or emergency personnel arrive.

Indications of choking in infants of younger than 1 year old include lack of breathing, gasping, cyanosis, and the inability to cry. The procedure for **Heimlich chest thrusts** includes the following:

- Position the infant in the prone position along your forearm with the infant's head being lower than the trunk, being sure to support the head so the airway is not blocked.
- Using the heel of the hand, deliver five forceful upward blows between the shoulder blades.
- Sandwich the child between your two arms, and turn the infant into the supine position and drape over your thigh with his or her head lower than the trunk and the head supported.
- Using two fingers (as for CPR compressions), give up to five thrusts (about 1.5 inches deep) to the lower third of the sternum.
- Only do a finger sweep and remove a foreign object if the object is visible. Repeat five back blows, five chest thrusts until the foreign body is ejected.
- If the infant loses consciousness, begin CPR. If a pulse is noted but spontaneous respirations are absent, continue with ventilation only.

Emergency defibrillation with a manual defibrillator

Emergency manual defibrillation is for acute ventricular fibrillation or ventricular tachycardia with no audible or palpable pulse (it is ineffective for asystole or PEA).

- Immediately start CPR while other EMS personnel set up the defibrillator and start an IV. Minimize CPR interruptions.
- Put the power on, set the energy level (200 joules for biphasic; 360 joules for monophasic), and charge.
- Apply conductive gel and place the pads with adhesive (interferes less with CPR) or by hand. Anterior/Posterior placement (is the most effective and is used for children): Posterior—below the scapula, lateral to the spine, center at T7. Anterior—below the clavicle on the right midclavicular line, lateral to the sternum. Anterior/Lateral placement: First—right side of the sternum below the clavicle (2nd–3rd intercostal space). Second— left midaxillary line (4th–5th intercostal space).
- Verify shockable rhythm. Announce "CLEAR"; deliver the shock.
- Continue CPR beginning with compressions for 2 minutes/five cycles between defibrillations.
- If pulseless ventricular tachycardia or ventricular fibrillation continues, administer epinephrine 1 mg every 3–5 minutes while continuing CPR.

If the patient is wet, dry off the chest, remove any transdermal patches on the chest, and shave any excessive hair before applying the pads. Place the pads at least 1 inch (2.5 cm) away from an implanted device.

Cardiopulmonary resuscitation (CPR) for cardiac arrest

Cardiac arrest of unknown cause in adults or children is usually treated as though it were ventricular fibrillation or pulseless ventricular tachycardia, but the protocol varies. **Cardiopulmonary resuscitation (CPR)** involves the following components:

- Immediate defibrillation is performed according to protocol with an AED/manual defibrillator (preferred) followed by CPR, beginning with compressions (30:2 compression to ventilation at the rate of 100–120 per minute at least 2 inches deep; two-finger compressions, to one-third of the chest depth for infants and children) for 2 minutes/five cycles and repeat defibrillation.
- Repeat cycles of 2 minutes of CPR and defibrillation. (Laypeople may use compression-only CPR.)
- If a defibrillator is not readily available, CPR may begin first. Note that if a BVM is used, the break in compressions should not exceed 10 seconds. If an advanced airway/intubation is in place, ventilation should be at the rate of 8 to 10 per minute, maintaining oxygen saturation ≥94% but <100% with ventilation between compressions.
- The $ETCO_2$ value should be 10–20 mm Hg if chest compressions are adequate, increasing to 35–45 mm Hg with the return of spontaneous circulation (ROSC).

Termination of resuscitation efforts

Criteria for **termination of resuscitation efforts** include the following considerations:

- ≥18 years.
- Arrest is cardiac-related and not a condition that may respond to hospital treatment.
- Endotracheal intubation was successful and maintained throughout resuscitation efforts.
- Standard advanced cardiac life support efforts were used.
- Resuscitation efforts were maintained for 25 minutes or asystole through four rounds of drugs.
- At the time of the decision to terminate, the patient exhibits asystole or an agonal rhythm (the bizarre, ineffective, wide ventricular rhythm associated with dying).
- Official DNR order.
- Newborn: No heartbeat detected after 10 minutes of CPR.

Note: Older age, quality of life, and time of collapse prior to EMS arrival are not criteria for termination. Generally, resuscitation efforts are continued until arrival at the receiving facility on those patients younger than 18 unless the child has a terminal disease and an advance directive that limits resuscitation efforts. Prior to termination, the paramedic should have direct communication with medical oversight and the family members that are present should be consulted/advised. Family resistance must be noted and reported. Criteria for withholding resuscitation include DNR status, obvious signs of death (such as rigor mortis/lividity), or conditions that are unsafe for the rescuer.

Post-resuscitation return of spontaneous circulation (ROSC)

If a patient undergoing resuscitation has **return of spontaneous circulation (ROSC)**, his or her ventilation and oxygenation must be supported to maintain the oxygen saturation ≥94% but less than 100% to avoid hyperoxia. Ventilation should be maintained at 10–12 breaths per minute with an ETCO$_2$ value at 35–40 mm Hg. Hyperventilation must be avoided. Hypotension (systolic BP <90 mm Hg) should be treated with an IV bolus (1–2 L saline) and vasopressor infusion. Treatable causes (the five H's and five T's) should be addressed, and a 12-lead ECG should be used to monitor the patient's condition. If the patient is nonresponsive, therapeutic hypothermia (to 32–24° C) for 12–24 hours may be considered as a neuroprotective measure. If the patient is responsive and able to follow commands, he or she should be immediately transported to the appropriate receiving facility: the ICU or cardiac cath lab for acute myocardial infarction (AMI) or ST-elevated myocardial infarction (STEMI) for percutaneous coronary intervention (PCI). Note: Brain damage begins within 4–6 minutes of cardiac arrest, and it is irreversible after 8–10 minutes.

Impedance threshold device (ITD)

The **impedance threshold device** (such as the ResQPOD ITD) is a small, single-use device that fits into the airway circuit (face mask or advanced airway) with CPR. During CPR, compressions generate positive pressure that promotes cardiac output and, when released completely, negative pressure (a vacuum) within the thorax that refills the heart, so adequate negative pressure ensures better filling. During compressions with an ITD, a valve in the device allows air to escape, but, when the compressions are released, the valve closes to prevent the intake of air, increasing negative pressure and improving circulation on subsequent compressions; however, the device allows the paramedic to ventilate the patient, and it has flashing timing lights every 6 seconds (so 1 ventilation with every flash equals 10 per minute). The ITD may double the blood flow to the heart and double the systolic BP as well as increase cerebral perfusion.

Mechanical piston-driven chest compression device and a load-distributing band or vest CPR

With **automated chest compression devices** for CPR, manual CPR should be started while the equipment is obtained and readied. These devices are only intended for adults and nontraumatic arrests, and they must be removed for defibrillation.

- Piston-driven device (Thumper): Uses pneumatic (air) power on a piston device set at a prescribed compression depth. The backboard must first be secured with straps, the device is slid into a slot in the backboard, the massager pad is placed over the sternum, the device is turned on, and the compression depth is then set. The device can also control ventilations and tidal volume.
- LUCAS device: It is also piston driven and is similar to the Thumper, but it applies decompression suction on recoil to increase negative pressure and it does not provide for ventilations.
- Load-distributing band/Vest CPR (AutoPulse): A device that contains a backboard and fits like a vest around the patient's chest and applies compression to the chest and around the thorax, increasing perfusion pressure. It can be set for continuous compressions or 30:2, and it automatically adjusts to the patient's size.

Special arrests and peri-arrest situations

Drowning	For water rescue, start with ventilation because compressions are ineffective. On land, open the patient's airway and check for breathing (respiratory arrest may occur before cardiac arrest). If there are no respirations, ventilate twice and check his or her pulse. If there is no pulse, begin CPR at a 30:2 ratio and defibrillate as soon as possible for VT/VF or follow asystole protocol, depending on the situation. If the patient vomits (common), turn him or her to one side, clear the mouth/suction, and resume CPR.
Electrical shock/Lightning	Begin CPR following standard protocol. Early intubation may be necessary if face, mouth, or neck burns are present. Maintain spinal stabilization because of the risk of back/neck injury. Provide an IV access line and fluids for extensive tissue injury after resuscitation.
Pregnancy	Begin CPR following standard protocol. If the fundus height is at or above the umbilicus, use lateral uterine displacement (LUD) during CPR to relieve aortocaval compression. Alert resources for immediate peri-mortem C-section (in the second half of a pregnancy) if ROSC is not achievable or resuscitation is futile.
Hypothermia	If no pulse or respiration is detectable, begin immediate CPR (30:20) and defibrillate as soon as possible. Remove any wet clothing (during resuscitation if possible) and begin with warming protocols. Manage the patient's airway/ventilation/oxygen supplementation with warm, humidified oxygen. After ROSC, warm the patient to 32°C–34°C. Treat the underlying cause, such as drug overdose. Do not consider terminating efforts until the patient is rewarmed.
Electrolyte imbalance	Sodium, magnesium (except for extreme hypermagnesemia), and calcium abnormalities rarely lead to cardiac arrest. However, hyperkalemia (high potassium) (>6.5 mEq/L/mmol/L) may be lethal. Stabilize the heart cells with 5–10 mL of 10% calcium chloride or 10–20 mL of 10% calcium gluconate; shift potassium to the cells with 1 mEq/kg sodium bicarbonate and 25 g 50% glucose (unless he or she is hyperglycemic) with 10 U regular insulin (if available) and 2.5 mg albuterol (per nebulizer); and provide diuresis with 20–40 mg furosemide (per protocol).
Trauma	Follow standard protocol, but the patient may require cervical spine stabilization and advanced airway/ventilation or cricothyrotomy, depending on the injuries. Use barriers to protect yourself from blood. Note: A chest blow may cause VF, requiring rapid defibrillation.

Trauma

Blunt trauma

Motor vehicle crashes	Result in 30%–40% of accidental deaths and half of closed-head and spinal cord injuries with injuries usually more serious with ejection, lateral (T-bone) impacts, and unrestrained patients, although lap belts increase the risk of abdominal injury (bowel injury in children). Shoulder belts may cause vascular injuries. Injuries include crush (compression), shear (tearing), and burst (rupture from sudden increase in pressure). The risk of death increases if another vehicle occupant dies. Most frontal collisions result in injuries from impact with steering wheel, dashboard, windshield, or floorboards. More severe injuries occur at speeds of >25 mph.
Motorcycle crashes	Approximately 75% of deaths are from head injuries, but injuries to the spine, pelvis, and extremities, including limb loss, are common.
Pedestrian/ motor vehicle impacts	Often results in Waddell's triad (tibiofibular or femur fracture, trunk injury, and head/face injury). Small children are often run over, and adults are thrown over the car by the impact. Intra-abdominal injury and pelvic fractures may occur from fender contact with the hips.
Falls	The most common cause of accidental death in geriatric patients is by falling. Anticoagulants increase the risk of injury with falls. The degree of injury depends on the patient's weight and the fall distance. Injuries are most severe with a fall distance of >20 feet for adults and >10 feet for children. A three-story fall results in 50% mortality; the mortality is almost 100% for five-story falls. Horizontal landings cause fewer injuries (hand, wrist, head/face, and abdominal) than feet-first landings, which often result in fractures of the heel, leg, pelvis, and/or vertebrae.
Sports injuries/ Play	Injuries vary depending on the type of injury but can include head injuries, musculoskeletal injuries, and abdominal injuries. Helmet or knee contact to the flank area may cause kidney injury. The most common injuries are strains, sprains, and knee injuries.
Assaults	Assaults are most common in young males and include facial and head injuries. Severe torso injuries may occur with kicking/stomping. If the patient is intoxicated and has altered consciousness, then he or she is treated as having a head injury. Assaults include domestic violence and child abuse, with distinctive patterns of injury.

Fractured ribs and flail chest

Fractured ribs usually result from severe blunt trauma (motor vehicle accident, physical abuse). Underlying injuries should be expected according to the area of fractures as follows:

- Upper two ribs: Injuries to the trachea, bronchi, or great vessels.
- Right-sided ≥ rib 8: Liver trauma.
- Left-sided ≥ rib 8: Spleen trauma.

Pain may be the primary symptom of rib fractures, resulting in shallow breathing. **Flail chest** (more common in adults and adolescents than children) occurs when at least three adjacent ribs are fractured, anteriorly and posteriorly, so that they float free of the rib cage. Variations include the sternum floating with ribs fractured on both sides. With flail chest, the chest wall cannot support changes in intrathoracic pressure, so paradoxical respirations occur with the flail area contracting on inspiration and expanding on expiration. Ventilation decreases. Prehospital: Manage the patient's airway/ventilation/oxygen supplementation (PPV with BVM or intubation). Provide cardiac monitoring, an IV access line, and supportive care. Observe for signs of tension pneumothorax or hemothorax.

Blunt cardiac trauma

Blunt cardiac trauma most often occurs as the result of motor vehicle accidents, falls, or other blows to the chest, which can result in respiratory distress as well as hypovolemia from rupture of the great vessels of the heart and/or cardiac failure from cardiac tamponade or increasing intrathoracic pressure. The heart is particularly vulnerable to chest trauma, with the right atrium and right ventricle being the most commonly injured because they are anterior to the rest of the heart. *Commotio cordis*, an often-lethal dysrhythmia from a blow to the pericardial area, may occur (most common in young males with sports injuries). Cardiac trauma may be difficult to identify because of other injuries, but if it is suspected, an ECG should be done and any abnormalities (dysrhythmias, ST changes, sinus tachycardia, or heart block) should be noted. Decreased cardiac output and cerebral oxygenation may result in severe agitation with combative behavior. Prehospital: Provide CPR and defibrillation if indicated; manage the patient's airway/ventilation/oxygen supplementation; provide an IV access line with severe injury; and monitor changes in the patient's level of consciousness.

Penetrating trauma

Gunshot wounds	Solid organs (brain, liver, spleen) often suffer more damage than more elastic tissues (fat, lungs). If a bullet is not deformed after entering the tissue, it tends to tumble (180°), creating a tunnel of injury (permanent cavity) and damage to the surrounding tissue (temporary cavity). If the bullet is deformed, it causes more severe localized tissue damage. Bullets usually have a straight trajectory, but they may be deflected if they strike bone. Shotgun blasts within 15 feet cause more damage than other gunshot wounds, but they are usually less severe at a distance.
Stab wounds	Stab: Includes hand-driven objects (knives, glass shards, ice picks, or pieces of metal/wood). Surface puncture wounds are often small, but their depth varies according to the instrument used, which should be removed surgically. Slash: These are usually long but not deep lacerations. Impalement: This usually results from objects larger than a knife, often from a fall onto an object, but it can include arrows and nails from pneumatic tools.

Revised trauma score (RTS) and primary assessment of trauma patients

The r**evised trauma score (RTS)** uses the Glasgow Coma Scale (GCS) score, systolic BP, and respiration rate to establish a score for triage (START). Scores may range from 0 to 12. For triage purposes, an RTS of 12 indicates delayed treatment; 11 indicates urgent, and a score of 3 to 10 indicates that immediate treatment is required. Scores of less than 3 indicate death. However, the scores are weighted differently, with the GCS score having the greatest weight (RTS = 0.9368 GCS + 0.7326 BP + 0.2908 R), so a reference chart must be used to determine the actual score based on the initial assessment of the patient.

Primary assessment of trauma patients should include evaluation of circulation, the airway, breathing, and circulation (including observing for deviated septum, changes in chest wall motion, fractures, sucking chest wounds, and crepitation [of the neck and chest] from air), as well as an assessment of disability with a brief neurological exam (pupils, limb movement) and GSC/RTS. Removing the patient's clothing for examination and logrolling him or her are part of the assessment.

GCS (score)	Systolic BP (score)	Respirations (score)
13-15 (4)	>89 (4)	10-29 (4)
9-12 (3)	76-89 (3)	>29 (3)
6-8 (2)	50-75 (2)	6-9 (2)
4-5 (1)	1-49 (1)	1-5 (1)
3 (0)	0 (0)	0 (0)

Types of bleeding

Types of bleeding	Characteristics	Prehospital
Arterial	Bright-red spurting blood that is difficult to control; it lessens as the BP falls.	Using standard precautions and PPE as indicated, apply sterile gauze dressing and pressure with the fingertips if it is a small bleed or apply direct hand pressure if it is more copious. As dressings saturate, add new dressings but don't remove the old ones. A tourniquet may be needed if bleeding is uncontrolled. Maintain the patient in the shock position, especially with an arterial bleed or severe blood loss, and keep him or her warm. Avoid giving food or fluids, and transport immediately for severe bleeding. Severity relates to the rate of blood loss volume and the age and health of patient. The blood volume is less with pediatric patients. Moving the injured area, a change in body temperature, medications, and the removal of bandages may impair clotting.
Venous	Dark-red blood flowing in a steady stream; it may be copious, but it is easier to control than an arterial bleed.	
Capillary	Oozing; it usually clots spontaneously.	
Internal	Usually evidenced by increasing signs of shock and/or discolored swollen, painful tissue, guarding, coughing up blood, or rectal bleeding. Long-bone fractures (femur) and pelvic fractures may result in severe blood loss.	

Chest wounds

Type	Characteristics	Prehospital
Sucking	This is an open pneumothorax in which air sucks into the thoracic cavity, deflating the lung, usually through a penny-size or larger wound. Patients will exhibit respiratory distress, absent breath sounds on the affected side, wound gurgling on inspiration, and bubbling of blood around the wound.	Apply an occlusive dressing with an Asherman Chest Seal dressing or with Vaseline gauze covered with secured (taped on three sides) plastic wrap or aluminum foil and place the patient in a position of comfort.
Impalement	This is a penetrating wound with an object impaled into the chest. Symptoms may be similar to those listed above, depending on the site of impalement and the depth. Impalement may cause hemothorax, tension pneumothorax, or pericardial tamponade.	Expose the wound area, and secure the object manually with a bulky dressing. Do not remove the object unless it is necessary for performing chest compressions (CPR). Control any bleeding.

- 139 -

Special considerations of fluid resuscitation

Special considerations of **fluid resuscitation** include the following:

- Geriatric patients: Underlying hypertension may result in shock with systolic BP >100 mm Hg. Even small amounts of bleeding may lead to shock, especially if the patient has anemia and is less able to tolerate excessive fluids because of underlying anemia or electrolyte imbalances.
- Pediatric patients: Infuse up to 20 mL/kg of warmed isotonic solution, and start a second or third infusion if he or she is nonresponsive to the first infusion. Use continuous infusion for uncontrolled hemorrhage to maintain perfusion en route. It's important to manage temperature control to maintain perfusion. Use an age-specific vital sign chart to monitor vital signs.
- Pregnant patients: Shock results in shunting of maternal blood away from the fetus to the mother's vital organs, so it's critical to maintain the patient's BP as close as possible to normal.

Hemothorax

Hemothorax occurs with bleeding into the pleural space, usually from major vascular injury such as tears in the intercostal vessels, lacerations of the great vessels, or trauma to the lung tissue. Hemothorax is most common with penetrating wounds. A small bleed may be self-limiting and seal, but a tear in a large vessel can result in massive bleeding, followed quickly by hypovolemic shock from decreased circulating blood. The pressure from the blood may result in the inability of the lung to ventilate and a mediastinal shift. Clots in the chest area may trigger fibrinolysis, which breaks down clots and increases bleeding. Often a hemothorax occurs with a pneumothorax, especially in severe chest trauma. Further symptoms include severe respiratory distress, decreased breath sounds, unequal breath sounds, dullness on auscultation, jugular venous distension, and shock. Prehospital: Manage the patient's airway/ventilation/oxygen supplementation, provide an IV access line and fluid bolus for shock but avoid aggressive fluids because of the risk of hemodilution, provide the patient a position of comfort (the shock position if necessary), and provide rapid transport.

Tension pneumothorax

If not treated promptly, a sucking chest wound (open pneumothorax) may progress to a **tension pneumothorax,** especially if mechanical ventilation is used. A tension pneumothorax occurs when pressure in the pleural space exceeds that of the atmosphere, causing a mediastinal shift (which is usually difficult to assess visually) with displacement of the trachea away from the affected site, putting pressure against the great vessels (decreasing cardiac output), and putting pressure against the heart (resulting in tachycardia). Patients are usually in severe respiratory distress with jugular vein distension, absent breath sounds on the affected side, narrow pulse pressure, pulsus paradoxus, and unequal chest rise. Prehospital: Place an airtight seal or Asherman Chest Seal over the open wound, manage the patient's airway/ventilation/oxygen supplementation to an oxygen saturation level of ≥94%, provide cardiac monitoring, start an IV access line, and provide rapid transport. Tension pneumothorax will require needle decompression or insertion of a chest tube (according to protocol).

Diaphragmatic rupture

A **ruptured diaphragm** is usually caused by blunt trauma, often associated with rib fractures and/or a ruptured spleen. Injuries to the left diaphragm are more common because the liver provides some underlying protection on the right. Symptoms may be overlooked initially, so a careful abdominal examination should be done. Symptoms include respiratory and circulatory impairment and herniation of abdominal organs into the chest cavity that is often associated with nausea and vomiting and abdominal pain, sometimes radiating to the left shoulder from pressure on the phrenic nerve. Prehospital: Manage the patient's airway/ventilation/oxygen supplementation and provide supportive care.

Traumatic asphyxia occurs when severe crushing pressure on the chest pushes against the heart, forcing blood from the right side of the heart back into the venous system (superior vena cava), including the neck and head veins, resulting in inadequate oxygenation to the upper extremities, face, and brain. Symptoms include altered mental status, seizures, swollen tongue, subconjunctival hemorrhages in the eyes, and cyanosis of the arms. Prehospital: Manage the patient's airway/ventilation/oxygen supplementation, provide supportive care, provide cardiac monitoring, and start an IV access line with fluid bolus for shock.

Peritoneal spaces and the anatomy of the abdominal and genitourinary systems

The **peritoneum** lines the abdominal cavity. The anterior (front) area is the intraperitoneal space, which contains the stomach, the first part of the duodenum, the small intestines, and part of the large intestines and rectum as well as the liver, bile ducts, spleen, ovaries, part of the pancreas and ureters, and bladder. The posterior (back) retroperitoneal space contains part of the duodenum, the ascending and descending colon, and part of the rectum as well as part of the pancreas and ureters, the kidneys, the adrenal glands, the uterus, and the fallopian tubes. The ovaries, uterus, and fallopian tubes comprise the female reproductive system. Solid organs include the liver, spleen, ovaries, uterus, pancreas, kidneys, and adrenals. Hollow organs include the bile ducts, stomach, large and small intestines, fallopian tubes, ureters, and bladder.

Eviscerations and impaled objects

Eviscerations occur with open abdominal wounds, such as opening incisions or traumatic injuries, which allow the internal organs (often the intestines) to protrude externally. Surgical repair is required to reinsert the organs into the abdomen. The patient may go into shock, especially if the evisceration is part of other major injuries (common in trauma cases). Prehospital: Provide supportive care; cover the eviscerated organs with thick, sterile gauze dressings moistened with NS, but do not attempt to reinsert them; manage the patient's airway/ventilation/oxygen supplementation as needed; and provide rapid transport. **Impalements** occur when an object penetrates the abdomen and remains in place and may be associated with multiple internal injuries and bleeding. Prehospital: Do not remove the object, but do expose the abdomen and manually secure the object with bulky dressings and control any bleeding. Provide supportive care, manage the patient's airway/ventilation/oxygen supplementation as needed, and provide rapid transport.

Blunt wounds

Abdominal trauma may result in **blunt wounds**, which may occur as the result of motor vehicle accidents, motor cycle accidents, pedestrian injuries, sports injuries, falls, blast injuries, and assaults. Blunt injuries comprise crush (compression), shear (tearing), and burst (sudden increased pressure) injuries. Motor vehicle accidents often result in liver injury in the passenger with impact on that side of the vehicle and spleen injury in the driver with impact on the driver's side. Other injuries from blunt trauma include damage to the diaphragm; retroperitoneal hematomas; and intestinal injuries, including perforation. Symptoms of internal injuries include pain, guarding, abdominal distension, discoloration, tenderness on movement, and evidence of lower rib fractures. Some patients may exhibit rectal bleeding and/or vomiting of blood. Prehospital: Provide airway/ventilation/oxygen supplementation as needed, place in a position of comfort, treat for shock if indicated (especially with suspected internal bleeding), and provide rapid transport for patients in an unstable condition.

Penetrating wounds

Abdominal trauma may result in **penetrating wounds**, which are almost always related to gunshot wounds (high energy), shotgun wounds (medium energy), or knife wounds (low energy). Gunshot and shotgun wounds tend to cause more extensive damage than stab wounds, especially to the colon, liver, spleen, and diaphragm, and they may have an exit wound. Interior injuries may be extensive because the bullet damages tissues and may ricochet off of bone. Hemorrhage and peritonitis (especially with perforation of the intestines) are common complications. Pain is often more acute with injury to hollow organs than to solid organs, although blood loss may be severe with injury to the liver, spleen, or kidneys, and blood collecting in the retroperitoneal space may not be evident on inspection, palpation, or auscultation. Prehospital: Control external bleeding, manage the patient's airway/ventilation/oxygen supplementation, mobilize the spine if indicated, and apply a pneumatic antishock garment (PASG) if indicated for shock or pelvic fracture (contraindicated with difficulty breathing, pregnancy [second and third trimesters], evisceration, an impaled object, and open fractures).

Vascular injuries

Vascular injuries usually result from penetrating injuries, which may partially or complete transect a vessel, or blunt injuries, which may damage the wall or dissect the vessels. Acceleration/deceleration may result in shearing injuries. Indications of vascular injuries include pulsatile bleeding, enlarging hematoma, and ischemia distal to the vascular injury, as noted by the six P's (pain, pallor, pulseless, paresthesia, poikilothermia [unstable core body temperature], and paralysis) as well as audible bruit or palpable thrill and signs of increasing shock or compartment syndrome. Abdominal vessel injuries are most common in the aorta and inferior vena cava (45% mortality), but additional injuries, such as to the hepatic veins and portal vein, increase mortality rates (90%). Internal venous hemorrhage may be more severe than arterial. Prehospital: Control external bleeding, manage the patient's airway/ventilation/oxygen supplementation, start an IV access line with fluid bolus if needed for shock (but beware of hemodilution with bleeding), and provide rapid transport (surgical repair within 1 hour is critical).

Hepatic (liver) injury

Hepatic (liver) injury is the most common cause of death (mortality rates of 8%–25%) from abdominal trauma and is often associated with multiple organ damage, so symptoms may be nonspecific. Liver injuries are classified according to the degree of injury, as follows:

I.   Tears in the capsule with hematoma.
II. Laceration(s) of the parenchyma (<3 cm).
III. Laceration(s) of the parenchyma (<3 cm).
IV. Destruction of 25%–75% of a lobe from burst injury.
V.   Destruction of >75% of a lobe from burst injury.
VI. Avulsion (tearing away).

Hemorrhage is a common complication of hepatic injury. Treatment often includes intravenous fluids for fluid volume deficit as well as blood products (plasma, platelets) for coagulopathies. Prehospital: Manage the patient's airway/ventilation/oxygen supplementation, control external bleeding, treat signs of shock, start an IV access line with fluid bolus if indicated (but beware of hemodilution), provide rapid transport for an unstable patient.

Splenic injury

The spleen is the most frequently injured solid organ in blunt trauma because it's not well protected by the rib cage and it is very vascular. Symptoms may be very nonspecific. Kehr's sign (radiating pain in the left shoulder) indicates intra-abdominal bleeding, and Cullen's sign (ecchymosis around the umbilicus) indicates hemorrhage from a ruptured spleen. Some may have right upper abdominal pain, although diffuse abdominal pain often occurs with blood loss, associated with hypotension. **Splenic injuries** are classified according to the degree of injury, as follows:

- Tear in splenic capsules or hematoma.
- Laceration of parenchyma (<3 cm).
- Laceration of parenchyma (>3cm).
- Multiple lacerations of parenchyma or burst-type injury.

Treatment may be supportive if the injury is not severe; otherwise, suturing or removal of the spleen may be needed. Prehospital: Control external bleeding, manage the patient's airway/ventilation/oxygen supplementation, treat signs of shock, start an IV access line with fluid bolus if indicated (but beware of hemodilution), and provide rapid transport for an unstable patient.

Pneumatic antishock garment (PASG)

The **pneumatic antishock garment (PASG)** is indicated for hypovolemic shock and hypotension associated with and stabilization of pelvic and bilateral femur fractures. PASG is contraindicated with respiratory distress, pulmonary edema, pregnancy (second and third trimesters), heart failure, myocardial infarction, stroke, evisceration, abdominal or leg impalement, head injuries, and uncontrolled bleeding above the garment.

The procedure for PASG use is as follows:

- Place the garment flat on the patient-transport device/stretcher and transfer the patient onto the garment.
- If the patient is already on the stretcher, place the garment under his or her legs first and then lift the patient's buttocks and slide the garment upward until the upper garment edge is 1 inch below the bottom ribs.
- Secure the legs first and then the abdominal section with the Velcro straps. Attach the pump hoses to each leg and the abdominal section at the valves and close the stopcocks.
- Open the stopcock for each leg and abdominal section one at a time, and inflate them one at a time.

After inflating each section, close the stopcock and check the vital signs. Stop inflating if the systolic BP≥ 90 mm Hg. If the systolic BP is still <90 mm Hg, then proceed to filling the next section or sections until all three are filled.

Traumatic injuries to genitalia

Site	Characteristics	Prehospital
Penis	Blunt, penetrating, crushing, or amputating injuries as well as urethral penetration. Pain and bleeding may be severe.	Control external bleeding, do not removed the impaled object. Provide pain management, an ice pack to reduce swelling, and emotional support.
Scrotum	Blunt, penetrating, or crushing injury may result in severe pain and swelling.	As above but do not attempt to relieve scrotal pressure except with ice packs.
Vagina	May have external bruising and tearing (especially with sexual assault) at the vaginal opening. There may be pain, swelling, and bleeding.	Control external bleeding, and provide emotional support, but do not remove impaled objects.
Vulva	May include blunt, penetrating, or crushing injury as well as bite marks (with sexual assault) with pain, swelling, and bleeding.	As above. Report sexual assaults according to protocol.

Orthopedic trauma

Fractures usually result from trauma (falls, auto accidents), but <u>pathologic fractures</u> can result from minor force to diseased bones (osteoporosis or cancerous lesions). <u>Stress fractures</u> are caused by repetitive trauma (forced marching). <u>Salter-Harris fractures</u> involve the cartilaginous epiphyseal plate near the ends of long bones in children who are growing, and this can impair bone growth. Fracture types are listed as follows:

- Open fractures with soft-tissue injury and a break in the skin overlying the fracture, including puncture wounds from external forces or bone fragments; these can result in osteomyelitis (bone infection).
- Closed fractures involve a broken bone but no break in the skin.

Symptoms include pain, deformity or angulation, swelling, bruising, inability to move the joint or bear weight, grating on movement, and impaired function or circulation. Isolated fractures are usually not life threatening, but pelvic and femur fractures may involve severe blood loss. Prehospital: Cover open wounds with sterile dressings, manually stabilize and immobilize the fracture area, but do not replace protruding bones, apply a cold pack, and place the patient in a position of comfort.

Subluxation (partial dislocation of a joint) and **luxation** (complete dislocation of a joint) can cause neurovascular compromise, which can be permanent if reduction is delayed. This is especially a problem with <u>hip dislocations</u>, which most commonly occur in automobile accidents when the person's knees impact the dashboard. <u>Elbow dislocations</u> often result from athletic injuries and may cause nerve damage. <u>Shoulder dislocations</u> are the most common type and also often result from athletic injuries. They may become chronic. <u>Knee dislocations</u> may result in severe injury to the popliteal artery, and this can lead to amputation, so rapid transport and emergent surgical repair are indicated. Differentiating between fractures and dislocations can be difficult because the symptoms and appearance are often similar. A deformity may not be evident, or it may be obscured by edema, or edema may give the appearance of a deformity. Extensive bruising may occur with all types of injuries, and pain may occur even with minor soft-tissue injuries. Prehospital: Splint and immobilize the area, and place the patient in a position of comfort.

- 144 -

Amputations may be partial or complete and result from crush, guillotine (cutting), or avulsion (twisting) injuries. A <u>simple amputation</u> requires no extrication and other injuries or shock are absent, but a <u>complex amputation</u> may involve multiple injuries, shock, and delayed treatment because of extrication. The amputated limb should be treated initially as though it could be reattached, although single digits (except the thumb) and lower limbs are not usually reattached. The part should be irrigated with normal saline (NS) to remove debris; wrapped in NS-moistened gauze; and placed in a sealed plastic bag, which should be immersed in ice water. The body part should not freeze and should not be placed directly on ice. Prehospital: Manage the patient's airway/ventilation/oxygen supplementation; control bleeding by direct pressure or, if there is severe hemorrhage, by applying a BP cuff proximal to (above) the injury 70 mm Hg greater than the systolic BP for <30 minutes; irrigate the stump with NS if it is dirty; cover the open area with NS-moistened gauze; and elevate the stump.

Strains and sprains

A **strain** is an overstretching of a part of the musculature ("pulled muscle") that causes microscopic tears in the muscle, usually resulting from excess stress or overuse of the muscle. The onset of pain is usually sudden with local tenderness on use of the muscle. A **sprain** is damage to a joint, with a partial rupture of the supporting ligaments and/or tendons, usually caused by wrenching or twisting that may occur with a fall. The rupture can damage blood vessels, resulting in edema, tenderness at the joint, and pain on movement with pain increasing over 2–3 hours after the injury. An avulsion fracture (the bone fragment is pulled away by a ligament) may occur with strain. Prehospital: Immobilize the area for transport, use rest, ice, compression, and elevation (the RICE protocol), and monitor the patient's neurovascular status (especially for sprains) by checking the pulse, capillary refill, color, and sensation distal to (below) the injury.

Types of fractures

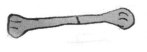
Transverse: Usually occurs in long bones and is at risk of displacement unless it is splinted to prevent movement. Most often occurs from direct impact, such as sports injuries. May suggest abuse if occurring in small children.

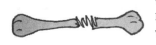
Comminuted: Usually result from high-impact trauma, such as with motor vehicle accidents, and it is more common in older adults or those with weakened bones. This fracture is very painful and is often accompanied by swelling and muscle spasms.

Spiral: Common in toddlers who fall on an extended leg, breaking the tibia, but it may also occur with abuse in small children as a result of jerking on or twisting an extremity (usually the arm).

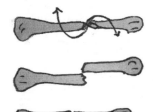
Displaced: Poses a risk of damage to surrounding tissues, including nerves and blood vessels and may lead to an open fracture if not properly splinted. Usually the deformity is evident.

Greenstick: Most common in children whose bones are less hard. It is usually quite painful but without deformity.

The femur is the long bone in the thigh. Although any part of the femur may fracture, fractures in the upper femur are common and are generally referred to as hip fractures. **Femur fractures** in young patients usually result from high-impact trauma, such as motor vehicle or pedestrian/motor vehicle accidents, whereas femur fractures in geriatric patients are most often from falls and are associated with osteoporosis. Patients may have many comorbidities and may present with dehydration and blood loss. Mortality rates for **hip fractures** are high, with 10% during the initial treatment and 25% over the next year. Symptoms of femur fractures include pain and deformity at the fracture site and an inability to walk or bear weight. A hematoma may be present. Prehospital: Splint the leg in the position it was found in with a traction splint (Hare Traction Splint/Sager Emergency Traction Splint), flush open fractures with NS to remove debris, and apply an NS-moistened sterile gauze dressing, monitor vital signs and neurovascular status, and assess soft tissue for damage. Provide an IV access and fluids if indicated.

Pelvic fractures represent about 3% of total fractures, but they pose a greater risk than most other types of fractures. Pelvic fractures most often result from a motor vehicle accident (50%–60%) in adults and a pedestrian/motor vehicle impact (60%–80%) in children. Pelvic fractures may be accompanied by major injuries to soft tissue and internal organs, especially the bladder, urethra (especially in children and women), and colon. A fracture on one side often results in a fracture on the other side as well. The primary cause of death after a pelvic fracture is hemorrhage with between 50% and 70% of patients with unstable fractures requiring multiple transfusions. Geriatric patients have higher mortality rates than do younger patients. Symptoms include pain and tenderness, bloody urine, rectal bleeding, vaginal bleeding, retroperitoneal bleeding, hematoma over the fracture site, pain on hip motion, and signs of shock (with blood loss). Prehospital: Monitor vital signs for indications of shock, position supine, apply PASG or a pelvic wrap device (per protocol) to stabilize and prevent excessive movement, and monitor the patient's airway/ventilation/oxygen supplementation. Provide an IV access (large bore) and fluid as indicated.

Prehospital management of fractures

Fracture	Prehospital
Tibia/Fibula (lower leg)	Manually immobilize during splinting. Splint the joint above and below the fracture(s) (upper thigh to ankle) with a padded rigid long-leg splint or a pneumatic splint, and then secure it to the other leg for additional support.
Shoulder	Apply a sling to the affected side and secure the patient's arm against the body with a swathe to limit movement.
Knee	If the pulse below the fracture is adequate and there is no deformity, splint with the knee straight. If there is deformity, splint the leg in the position it was found. If there is no pulse below the fracture, consult with medical assistance immediately. Never use a traction splint.
Clavicle (upper chest)	Apply a sling to the affected side. (Common in young children who fall with an arm outstretched.)
Humerus (upper arm)	Apply a sling to the affected side and swathe the arm to the body to limit movement.
Radius/Ulna (forearm)	Splint from the elbow to the wrist and secure above and below the fracture. Elevate the arm.
Elbow	Apply a sling to the affected side 30 to 60 seconds (often results from a fall).

Fat embolism

Fat embolism, a life-threatening complication of fractures, can occur when fat enters the venous circulatory system, typically lodging in the pulmonary microvasculature, causing increased pulmonary vascular resistance. Patients most at risk are the young with multiple injuries, the elderly, and those with preexisting disease (pulmonary hypertension, right ventricular disorder, or metastatic cancer). Preventive methods include stabilizing fractures of long bones or pelvis within

24 hours of injury. Signs of fat embolism include abrupt bradycardia, hypertension, jugular venous distension, hypoxemia, decreased $ETCO_2$ concentration, chest and upper extremity petechiae, fat globules in the retina, and various cardiac irregularities such as dysrhythmias. As the pulmonary artery pressure increases, cardiac output decreases. Prehospital: Immediate treatment includes 100% oxygen with mechanical ventilation per endotracheal tube with adequate IV fluids. Epinephrine or related drugs may be used for hemodynamic support per protocol.

Musculoskeletal injuries and the types of splints

Assessment of musculoskeletal injuries should include the following:

- Palpation/Inspection for tissue damage, swelling, deformity, and tenderness.
- Comparison with the opposite side if a limb is involved.
- Assessment of neurovascular status (pulse, color, sensation, and function) distal to (below) the fracture.
- Assessment of the six P's: Pain (site of pain, degree, character), pallor (below the fracture or generalized), paresthesia (impaired sensation below fracture), distal pulses (intact, weak, absent), paralysis (with or without impaired sensation), and pressure (often associated with swelling and pain).
- Assessment of age and general condition (geriatric patients are more likely to have fractures from relatively minor injuries because of osteoporosis).

If a fracture or dislocation is suspected, then the area should be splinted or immobilized for transport. **Types of splints** include rigid (should be padded), nonrigid (moldable), traction, air (pneumatic devices), pillow/blanket, short spine board, and long spine board. Splinting procedures are similar for adults, pediatric patients, and geriatric patients.

Compartment syndrome

Compartment syndrome occurs when muscle perfusion is inadequate because of constriction caused by a cast or tight dressing or because of an increase in the contents of the enclosed compartment of a muscle sheath resulting from edema or hemorrhage, which increases pressure and compression, often related to fractures, crush injuries, burns, rhabdomyolysis, and snakebites. Compartment syndrome most often affects the forearm and leg muscles. Symptoms include severe throbbing pain unrelieved by opiates, numbness and tingling as pressure on the nerves increases, cyanosis and decreased or absent pulse distal to injury, limb paralysis, and edema (with tissue often being rigid). Necrosis and permanent damage may occur within 4 hours if treatment is inadequate or delayed. Prehospital: Remove the constriction (cast, splint, or dressing), elevate the limb, apply an ice compress, provide pain management, and provide rapid transport because the patient may need surgical fasciotomy to relieve the pressure.

Achilles tendon

Tendons are fibrous tissues that connect muscles to bones. The **Achilles tendon** (the largest in the body) attaches the muscles of the lower leg to the heel and is strong but inflexible, so it can easily become inflamed from chronic irritation, such as from sports (hill running, jumping), resulting in tendinitis. If tendinitis is untreated, it can result in a tear in the tendon and eventual rupture. Rupture can also result from sudden blunt trauma.

Pain and stiffness in the back of the heel is common with tendinitis; but with tear or rupture, the area may become bruised and swollen, and walking may be difficult (although it is not usually impossible) and very painful. The patient is able to place the foot into plantar flexion (foot pointing downward) if the tendon is completely or partially intact but cannot do so if it is ruptured (a positive sign for rupture). Severe tendinitis, tear, or rupture may require surgical repair. Prehospital: Provide RICE therapy.

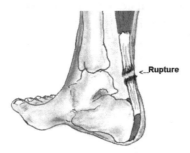

Knee/Patella injury

The **patella** is anterior to the knee joint and embedded within the quadriceps tendon. The patella protects the underlying bones of the joint and facilitates knee extension. Ligaments (patellar, medial tibial, and lateral fibular) form a fibrous capsule to surround and support the joint. The anterior and posterior cruciate ligaments lie within the joint in a crisscross fashion from femur to tibia to maintain the position of the tibia in the joint. The lateral collateral ligament connects the femur to the fibula and stabilizes the knee. The medial collateral ligament connects the femur to the tibia and prevents excessive extension, stabilizes the knee, and allows rotation. Injury may occur with twisting (common in sports), torsion, and hyperextension.

Knee/Patella injury	Characteristics
Compression syndrome	Results from weak quadriceps muscles or knee injury (as from a direct blow to knee). Knee pain without swelling, worsens after long sitting, when standing, and walking up or down hills/stairs. The knee may catch or give way. Prehospital: Provide RICE therapy.
Anterior cruciate ligament (ACL) injury	Usually rupture results from violent impact/trauma and may cause severe pain and hemarthrosis, swelling, and a slightly flexed position. May require knee aspiration. Prehospital: Provide RICE therapy.
Posterior cruciate ligament (PCL) injury	Injury usually occurs from a direct blow to the knee when the knee is flexed. Symptoms are similar to ACL injury. Prehospital: Provide RICE therapy.
Lateral collateral ligament injury	Injury usually results from forceful bending of the knee toward the midline, most often tearing the attachment to the fibula. Tenderness is present, and there is sometimes joint crepitus. Injury may occur to the peroneal nerve, impairing the ability to move the anterior and lateral leg muscles. Prehospital: Provide RICE therapy.
Medial collateral ligament injury	Injury usually results from forceful bending of the knee away from the midline, most often tearing the attachment to the femur. With a tear, pain is often severe but function remains. With a rupture, lateral movement is lacking and pain and swelling are evident. Prehospital: Provide RICE therapy.

Shoulder injuries

Sternoclavicular sprain results from tearing of the ligaments that connect the sternum to the clavicle, usually resulting from a direct blow or twisting of an arm extended backward. Symptoms

- 148 -

include pain near the top of the chest (below the neck). The pain increases on activity (such as lifting) and when lying on the affected side. Prehospital: Provide a protective sling.

The **rotator cuff** comprises the muscle and ligaments of the shoulder joint. The bones in the joint include the scapula and humerus. Muscles (subscapularis, supraspinatus, infraspinatus, spines minor) and tendons anchor to the head of the humerus so that the arm can move in all directions, and ligaments connect the bones. Part of the rotator cuff is under the scapula. The most common injury to the rotator cuff is a tear in the supraspinatus tendon, so that the tendon is separated from its attachment, resulting from violent pull on arm, abnormal rotation, or fall on outstretched hand. Prehospital: Provide a protective sling.

Open soft-tissue injuries

Injury	Characteristics	Prehospital
Abrasion	Painful superficial scraping of the outermost layer of skin. There is little or no bleeding.	Irrigate with water or NS to remove debris and cover with nonadherent dressing.
Laceration	A cut or break in the skin from impact with a sharp object. Bleeding may vary from mild to severe.	Apply pressure to control the bleeding, irrigate to remove debris if necessary, and cover with a dry sterile gauze dressing.
Puncture	Wound from impact with a sharp pointed object (knife, bullet); it may exhibit little external bleeding but major internal bleeding and soft-tissue damage. An exit wound may be present.	Apply pressure to control any bleeding, manage the patient's airway/ventilation/oxygen supplementation, and provide rapid transport if the patient's condition is unstable.
Impaled object	Penetrating object remains in wound.	Leave the object in place and pad with bulky dressings.
Foreign body in eye(s)	Patient has pain; tearing; redness; and blurred or impaired vision from dirt, dust, chemicals or other materials in the eye(s).	Cover both eyes loosely (avoiding pressure) to prevent movement. If it is chemical contamination, flush the eye(s) with copious amounts of NS or water.
Avulsions	The skin and underlying soft tissue are torn away, such as with a degloving injury, from any part of the body, although lower extremity injury is the most common. Bleeding may be severe, especially if vessels are torn or exposed.	Flush with sterile water or NS to remove debris if necessary, apply pressure and dressings to control bleeding and protect tissue, apply an ice pack, seal the avulsed skin and tissue in a plastic bag, and place in ice water for possible reimplantation or skin grafts. Return loose flaps to their anatomic positions.
Blast injury	Involves varying degrees of soft-tissue injury and sometimes amputations, fractures, impalements, traumatic brain injuries, ruptured eardrum, pulmonary injury, perforated bowel, and burns.	Manage the patient's airway/ventilation/oxygen supplementation; control bleeding and shock; and provide CPR if necessary, supportive care, and rapid transport.

- 149 -

Closed soft tissue injuries

Injury	Characteristics	Prehospital
Contusion	Results from blunt or compressive pressure to a muscle and is a common sports injury. These may include other injuries, such as sprains, strains, fractures, and damage to internal organs. Symptoms include tenderness, pain on movement, and bruising. If bruising is in the shape of an instrument, it usually indicates abuse.	Provide RICE therapy and supportive care.
Hematoma	Collection of blood within the tissue because of damaged blood vessels from injury, underlying fracture, or medications (such as warfarin). These may be small or very large, and patients may lose ≥1 L of blood. Symptoms may include pain and swelling.	Provide supportive care for small contusions (which often resolve spontaneously), RICE therapy, monitor for signs of continued bleeding.
Crush injury	External pressure may cause severe internal injuries, such as fractures and organ rupture.	Manage the patient's airway/ventilation/oxygen supplementation and shock as needed, control bleeding, and provide supportive care.

Bite wounds

Injury	Characteristics	Prehospital
Animal bites	Dog bites may cause any type of soft-tissue injury (lacerations, punctures, crush injury, avulsions) depending on the extent of the bite. Cat bites are often puncture bites with a high risk of infection. Pediatric and geriatric patients are most at risk of infection. Children are the most often victims of animal bites.	Check that the scene is safe and the animal is secured, control any bleeding, flush the wound with sterile NS or water, apply dressings, manage the patient's airway/ventilation/oxygen supplementation (especially with bites to the face/throat), and treat shock if needed. Check the rabies status of the animal involved if known. Report the bite according to legal requirements.
Human bites	If the bite is on the genitals, it indicates abuse. Most commonly bites are on the fingers from fist contact with someone's mouth. Human bites are prone to infection, especially if treatment is delayed.	Flush the wound with NS or water, apply a sterile dressing, and provide emotional support for victims of abuse. Document the patient's statement accurately in the event the bite becomes a legal matter.

Spider bites

Injury	Characteristics	Prehospital
Black widow	Initially there are two faint fang marks with a pale area surrounded by a red-blue ring. Muscle cramps, pain radiating to the upper chest (arm bites) or abdomen (leg bites) and weakness within 2 hours increasing to generalized pain, headache, itching chills, nausea, vomiting, dyspnea, hypertension, cardiac abnormalities, shock, and coma.	Provide supportive care and analgesia and benzodiazepine to relieve muscle spasms (per protocol). Take the spider in a sealed plastic bag to the receiving facility.
Brown recluse	Red, swollen bite site with severe pain and itching; "red, white, and blue" sign—a pale center with a central blister and reddish-blue peripheral discoloration with the blister becoming ischemic and necrotic—leaving an open ulcerated area that covers with black eschar and may expand in size. The following systemic reactions may occur within 6–12 hours in some patients: fever, vomiting, jaundice, hypotension, change in mental status, hemolytic anemia, disseminated intravascular coagulation, renal failure, seizures, coma, and death.	Provide supportive care and analgesia. If symptoms are severe, provide an IV access line and fluids.

Insect bites

Injury	Characteristics	Prehospital
Fire ants	Hives and blistering with severe itching, redness, pain, and burning. Some patients may develop systemic reactions and anaphylaxis.	Provide supportive care and cold compresses. Use the anaphylaxis protocol if necessary.
Wasps/bees	• Pain, itching, redness, and swelling (most common) • Severe allergic (hives) and/or anaphylactic (life-threatening) reactions	Wipe the area with gauze or scrape it with a sharp instrument to remove the stinger, wash with soap and water, apply ice, and elevate. Give antihistamines for an allergic response. Use the anaphylaxis protocol if necessary.
Scorpions	May cause local (burning, itching, pain, and redness) or severe neurologic and/or other systemic reaction, such as paresthesia, stroke, hypertension, tachycardia, respiratory distress, priapism, hemorrhage, nausea, and vomiting. Pregnant women may miscarry.	Immobilize the affected part below the level of the heart, apply cool compresses (the first 2 hours), monitor the patient's airway/ventilation/oxygen supplementation, start an IV access and give fluids if needed, and administer norepinephrine for severe hypotension.
Ticks	Pain may occur at the bite site. Ticks may carry numerous infections, including Lyme disease, so follow-up is essential.	Grasp the tick near the skin with tweezers and pull with steady upward pressure, disinfect the site, and save the tick in a plastic bag.

Classification of burns and rule of nines

Burn injuries may be chemical, electrical, or thermal and are assessed by the area affected, percentage of the body burned, and the depth of the burn, as follows:

- First-degree burns are superficial and affect the epidermis, causing erythema and pain.
- Second-degree burns extend through the dermis (partial thickness), resulting in blistering and sloughing of the epidermis.
- Third-degree burns affect the underlying tissue, including the vasculature, muscles, and nerves (full thickness).

Burns are classified according to the American Burn Association's criteria as follows:

- Minor: <10% body surface area (BSA) or 2% BSA with third-degree burns without serious risk to the face, hands, feet, or perineum.
- Moderate: 10%–20% BSA combined second- and third-degree burns in adults; age <10 years or ≤10% third-degree without serious risk to the face, hands, feet, or perineum.
- Major: 20% BSA; ≥10% third-degree burns; all burns are to the face, hands, feet, or perineum and will result in functional/cosmetic defect; or burns with inhalation or other major trauma.

The rule of nines estimates the BSA burned: Adults—head 9%, trunk (front) 18%, trunk (back) 18%, arm 9%, leg 18%, perineum 1%. Infants/Children—head 18%, trunk (front) 18%, trunk (back) 18%, arm 9%, leg 13.5%, perineum 1%.

Complications associated with burn injuries

Burn injuries begin with the skin but can affect all organs and body systems, especially with a major burn. Complications include the following:

- Cardiovascular: Cardiac output may fall by 50% as capillary permeability increases with vasodilation and fluid leaks from the tissues, resulting in hypovolemia and hypothermia. Vasoconstriction occurs as a compensatory mechanism, but it may impair circulation and result in further hypoxia.
- Pulmonary: Injury may result from smoke inhalation or (rarely) aspiration of hot liquid. Pulmonary injury is a leading cause of death from burns and is classified according to the degree of damage as follows:

First: Singed eyebrows and nasal hairs with possible soot in airways and slight edema, increasing hypoxia.
Second: Stridor, dyspnea, and tachypnea with edema and erythema of the upper airway, including the area of the vocal cords and epiglottis, resulting in severe hypoxia, sometimes with rapid onset.

- Infection: Open wounds are vulnerable to infection.
- Circumferential burns: Swelling beneath eschar can create a tourniquet effect, impairing distal circulation.

General management of chemical and electrical burns

Patients with severe burns may develop shock and impairment of all major body systems. If the burning process is ongoing, room-temperature water or NS should be applied to stop the burning and any smoldering clothes or jewelry should be removed, although if the clothing is adhered to the skin, it should be left in place. With facial or airway burns, the airway must be monitored constantly

- 152 -

with interventions as necessary and an IV access line should be provided for fluid replacement, based on the patient's weight and the extent of the burn (Parkland formula: 4 mL/kg/wt × BSA per 24 hours). The burned area should be covered with nonadherent dry clean dressings, and the patient should be kept warm for transport. Children experience greater fluid and heat loss because of their greater body surface relative to their size, and the paramedic should be alert to the possibility of child abuse. With **chemical burns**, any dry powder should be brushed off and wet chemicals should be flushed with copious amounts of water (by a paramedic wearing gloves and eye protection). With **electrical burns**, internal burns may be more severe than external burns, and the patient is at risk of cardiac arrest.

Dressings and Bandages

Dressing/Bandage	Characteristics
Sterile gauze	4×4 (sponge) or roller/wrapping gauze (Kerlix) used to protect skin or pack wounds to control bleeding. Roller gauze may be used to secure other dressings.
Nonadherent dressings	Designed not to stick to open wounds because of their special coating (Teflon, foam, petrolatum, hydrogel). Used on abrasions, burns, and lightly draining wounds.
Occlusive dressings	These have a waxy coating to make an air- and water-tight seal, but they are not as absorbent as gauze. Used for sucking chest wounds, abdominal eviscerations, and lacerations of the external jugular vein or carotid.
Trauma dressings	Dressings that often include a nonadherent pad, a clotting agent embedded in the dressing, and an elastic wrap in one piece so that they can be rapidly applied (e.g., an ACE bandage), include QuikClot Combat Gauze and Celox Rapid hemostatic gauze. Especially useful to control bleeding and to apply pressure to a wound.
Adhesive, roller bandages	May be elastic or nonelastic, and they are used to secure other dressing and/or apply compression.

High-pressure injection injury

High-pressure injection injury includes injection with oil, solvents, paint, water, grease, hydraulic fluids, air, or other substances. These types of injuries (most commonly on the hand or arm) are usually accidental, and the external injury may appear insignificant, often just a small puncture wound. However, internal injuries may be severe, especially with substances that are toxic to the body, and injuries to digits or limbs may require amputation (especially with paint) if not promptly treated with surgical intervention to wash the substance out and debride the tissue. Even nontoxic substances (such as air) may cause severe irritation and result in compartment syndrome. Only 100 psi are required to break the skin, but many types of high-pressure equipment have pressure up to 12,000 psi. Prehospital: Provide supportive care; control bleeding if necessary; monitor swelling, circulation, and sensation in the affected area; start an IV access line and give fluids if indicated; and provide rapid transport.

Head, scalp, and falcial injuries

Injury	Characteristics	Prehospital
Head	Open: Bleeding. Closed: Swelling and bruising, may have depression of the skull and underlying injury. Battle's sign (bruising over the mastoid process) and/or raccoon eyes (bruising about eyes) may indicate a basal skull fracture.	Apply direct pressure to control the bleeding; apply dry, sterile dressings. Monitor the patient's mental status. Be alert for signs of skull fracture.
Scalp	Copious bleeding may occur. May cause shock in infants and young children. Injuries above the ears increase the risk of brain injury.	As above. Manage the patient's airway/ventilation/oxygen supplementation if needed. Rapid transport is required with shock. Avoid closing the patient's mouth with bandages.
Facial	May include soft-tissue damage, facial bone fractures (nasal, orbital), eye injuries, and oral/dental injuries (tooth avulsions, mandibular/maxillary fractures). May have severe swelling, airway compromise, impaired vision, and bloody nose.	Maintain a patent airway, but avoid nasopharyngeal airways; suction as needed; take broken teeth to the hospital; examine the eyes; and control bleeding. Patch both eyes if one or both eyes are injured. Stabilize impaled objects in the eye(s), but remove impaled objects from the cheeks if any bleeding obstructs the patient's airway.

Brain and cervical spine injuries

Injury	Characteristics	Prehospital
Brain	Direct injury to brain tissue or damage from bleeding inside of the skull may occur. Altered mental status. Cerebrospinal fluid may leak from the nose/ears. Symptoms include the pupils being unequal, nausea and/or vomiting, bradycardia (slow heart rate), increased BP, and irregular breathing.	Immobilize spine; manage the patient's airway/ventilation/oxygen supplementation; provide shock prevention; control bleeding; and provide rapid transport.
Spine	Suspect with motor vehicle/pedestrian accidents; falls; hanging; blunt or penetrating trauma to the head, neck, or torso; diving accidents, and unresponsive trauma patients. May have tenderness in the area; pain on moving; numbness, tingling, or weakness; the inability to feel or move below the injury; difficulty breathing; and incontinence (bowel and/or bladder).	Responsive: Manually stabilize the head and neck in the position found until a cervical collar and backboard are in place. Question the patient's pain, sensations, and ability to move. Unresponsive: Stabilize the head and neck as above; manage the airway, ventilation, and oxygenation; question witnesses; and provide rapid transport.

Anatomy of the brain and spinal cord

The **brain** is protected by the skull and the meninges, the three layers of lining: the dura mater, arachnoid mater, and the pia mater. Brain tissue is comprised of gray matter (neurons [nerve cells]) and white matter (covered nerve pathways that conduct messages). The main part of the brain is the cerebrum, which is comprised of two hemispheres that contain the frontal parietal, temporal, and occipital lobes. The cerebrum controls higher brain functions, including thoughts, speech, vision, hearing, and actions. The cerebellum lies in the back of the brain below the cerebellum and controls the equilibrium and coordination. The brain stem controls involuntary functions, such as respirations, heart rate, temperature control, and nerve transmission. The brain stem is continuous with the **spinal cord**, which is also protected by the meninges and the vertebrae (cervical, thoracic, and lumbar). Cerebrospinal fluid circulates within the subarachnoid space of the brain and the spinal cord.

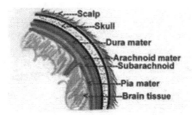

Concussions

Concussion is a brain injury in which structural damage is not apparent but neurological functioning is impaired. Patients may experience a brief loss of consciousness after a head injury and may experience confusion and even bizarre behavior (if the frontal lobe is affected). Other symptoms include severe headache, somnolence, dizziness, lack of coordination, confusion, disorientation, inappropriate emotional response, nausea, and vomiting. Symptoms are usually transient (lasting from minutes to hours), but up to 50% may have recurrent symptoms (such as difficulty concentrating, headaches, and dizziness) for months. The American Academy of Neurology classifies concussions as follows:

- Grade 1: Transient confusion without loss of consciousness with symptoms resolving in <15 minutes.
- Grade 2: Transient confusion without loss of consciousness with symptoms resolving in >15 minutes.
- Grade 3: Any loss of consciousness of any duration.

Prehospital: Provide supportive care and reassurance, monitor vital signs and neurological status for signs of increasing intracranial pressure that may indicate more severe injury,

and elevate the patient's head.

Signs of increasing intracranial pressure

Head trauma may result in **increased intracranial pressure** and cerebral edema. Patients often suffer initial hypertension, which increases intracranial pressure and decreases perfusion, and significant swelling, which also interferes with perfusion, causing hypoxia and hypercapnia (increased carbon dioxide), which trigger increased blood flow. This increased volume at a time when injury impairs autoregulation further increases cerebral edema, which, in turn, increases intracranial pressure and results in a further decrease in perfusion with resultant ischemia

- 155 -

(impaired circulation). If the pressure continues to rise, the brain may herniate. The mean arterial pressure must remain between 65 and 150 mm Hg for the brain to autoregulate intracranial pressure (the normal pressure is 2–12 mm Hg). Symptoms include Cushing's triad: wide pulse pressure, bradycardia, and irregular respirations. Initially: Decreased levels of consciousness, increased BP, and decreased pulse, Cheyne-Stokes (irregular) respirations, and pupils are reactive. Middle brain stem involvement: Wide pulse pressure, bradycardia, pupils sluggish or nonreactive, and hyperventilation. Lower brain stem: Pupil blown on the side of injury, irregular respirations, flaccid response to painful stimulation, and the BP and pulse decrease. Prehospital: Elevate the patient's head, manage the patient's airway/ventilation/oxygen supplementation, provide rapid transport, and start an IV access line.

Intracranial hematomas

Type	Characteristics	Prehospital
Epidural	Bleeding between the dura and the skull, pushing the brain downward and inward. The hemorrhage is usually caused by arterial tears, so bleeding is often rapid, leading to severe neurological deficits and respiratory arrest. The patient may be lucid and without symptoms for 2–6 hours after the injury.	Provide supportive care, keep the patient's head elevated to reduce intracranial pressure, note neurological status (movement, strength, mental status, pupils equal and reactive or unequal/fixed), and provide rapid transport. Provide an IV access line and fluids.
Subdural	Bleeding between the dura and the arachnoid mater, usually from tears in the cortical veins of the subdural space. It tends to develop more slowly than an epidural hemorrhage. If the bleeding is acute and develops within minutes or hours of injury, then the prognosis is poor. Subacute hematomas that develop more slowly cause varying degrees of injury.	
Intracerebral 	Bleeding into the substance of the brain from an artery. Sudden onset; it results in a hemorrhagic stroke with a lack of nutrients and oxygen to parts of the brain. May result from degenerative changes, hypertension, brain tumors, medications, or illicit drugs (crack, cocaine). Symptoms vary depending on the site, but they may include one-sided weakness, paralysis, difficult speaking, and severe headache, altered mental status.	Provide supportive care, keep the patient's head elevated to reduce intracranial pressure, note neurological status (movement, strength, mental status, pupils equal and reactive or unequal/fixed), provide rapid transport, start an IV access line, and give fluids.
Subarachnoid	Bleeding in the space between the meninges and brain and into the cerebrospinal fluid, usually resulting from aneurysm, arteriovenous malformation (AVM), or trauma. This type of hemorrhage compresses the brain tissue. The first presenting symptoms are severe headache, nausea and vomiting, nuchal rigidity, palsy related to cranial nerve compression, retinal hemorrhages, and papilledema.	

Nonspinal neck injuries and nasal fractures

Nonspinal neck injuries may result from blunt trauma or penetrating trauma, and they must be carefully assessed for underlying spinal cord injury. Open wounds may bleed profusely, especially if the carotid artery is breached, resulting in rapid exsanguination and death. The airway may be compromised. Difficulty swallowing indicates esophageal injury, whereas voice changes indicate laryngeal injury. Crackling on palpation indicates air in the tissues. Prehospital: Apply single-digit (gloved) pressure to control bleeding of the carotid artery or jugular veins; apply an occlusive dressing for an injury to the large vessels after the bleeding is controlled to prevent air from entering the bloodstream, which is life-threatening; and manage the patient's airway/ventilation/oxygen supplementation (advanced life support may be needed). Rapid or air medical transport may be needed. **Nasal fractures** (40% of facial fractures) may cause persistent bleeding and should be assessed for drainage of the cerebrospinal fluid and injury of the surrounding structures, including brain injury, skull fracture, and neck and cervical spine injury. Prehospital: Control any bleeding, elevate the patient's head, and manage the airway, but do not use a nasopharyngeal airway.

Unstable facial fractures

Unstable facial fractures are those of the midface, usually from blunt facial trauma and are often associated with other trauma because of the degree of force involved. Categories include:

- Le Fort I (low downward force): The hard palate and lower maxilla are separated from the rest of skull.
- Le Fort II (low or mid-maxilla force): The nasal bones and lower maxilla are separated from the facial skull and other cranial bones.
- Le Fort III (force to the bridge of the nose or the upper maxilla): The entire midface is separated from the cranium.

Symptoms may include malocclusion, open bite, apparent lengthening of the face, clear nasal discharge (cerebrospinal fluid), periorbital ecchymosis, pain, swelling, and epistaxis (nosebleed), vision disturbances, airway compromise. Prehospital: Suction if necessary, manage the patient's airway/ventilation/oxygen supplementation (usually with intubation; avoid a nasopharyngeal airway), control any bleeding, elevate the patient's head. (Cricothyroidotomy may be necessary if the airway is obstructed.) Patch both eyes if one or both are injured. Stabilize an impaled object in the eye, but remove an impaled object in the cheek; apply dry sterile dressings, but do not cover the mouth; provide rapid transport.

Orbital fractures and perforated tympanic membrane

Orbital fractures most often occur with blunt force against the globe causing a rupture through the floor of the orbital bone or a direct blow to the orbital rim, often related to an assault or sports injury. Injuries are most common in adolescents and young adults. Patients may be essentially asymptomatic, or they may exhibit ecchymosis and edema of the eyelid, infraorbital anesthesia from pressure or damage to the infraorbital nerve, decreased sensation of the cheek and upper gum on the injured side, diplopia (double vision), and enophthalmos (a sunken globe). Prehospital: Patch both eyes to prevent movement, provide supportive care, and use an ice compress to reduce edema. A **ruptured tympanic membrane** may result from pressure (diving, waterskiing), a direct blow to the ear, explosions, and a foreign object in the ear. Symptoms may include pain, hemorrhagic otorrhea (bloody drainage), and hearing impairment. Prehospital: Provide supportive care.

Mandibular fractures, laryngotracheal injuries, and non-CNS-associated spinal trauma

Mandibular fractures are most common in males 21 to 30 and result from a blow to the jaw from an assault, motor vehicle accident, or gunshot wound and are often associated with other injuries, such as head injury or midface fractures. Symptoms include malocclusion of teeth, pain, point tenderness, and ecchymosis of the floor of the mouth. Prehospital: Manage the patient's airway/ventilation/oxygen supplementation (avoid the nasal airway), use an ice pack to reduce edema, elevate the patient's head, and monitor him or her closely. **Laryngotracheal injuries** result from direct trauma and may result in swelling and hemorrhage. Symptoms include swelling, changes in voice, hemoptysis, subcutaneous emphysema (from open wounds), and structural irregularities. The patient must be assessed for associated injuries. Prehospital: Manage the patient's airway/ventilation/oxygen supplementation because airway obstruction is common, elevate the patient's head, and provide supportive care. May require a surgical airway. With **non-CNS-associated spinal trauma,** patients complain of pain and point tenderness, but neurological findings are intact. Provide sitting or standing spinal mobilization and supportive care; manage the patient's airway/ventilation/oxygen supplementation as needed.

Facial and dental injuries

Facial injuries may include soft-tissue injuries, fractures, and eye injuries. Facial fractures may result in airway obstruction, pain, swelling, bruising, deformation, and bleeding. Fractures of the maxilla and mandible (the upper and lower jaw) often result in damage to the teeth as well. **Dental fractures,** most commonly of the maxillary teeth, may occur in association with other oral and facial injuries and may be overlooked unless a careful dental examination is carried out. Fractures may range from chipping of the enamel to fracture of the tooth root. **Dental avulsions** are complete displacement of a tooth from its socket. The tooth may be reimplanted if done within 1–2 hours after displacement, although only permanent teeth are reimplanted, not primary teeth, so question the parents of children to determine if an avulsed tooth is permanent. Prehospital: Manage the patient's airway/ventilation/oxygen supplementation as needed, elevate the patient's head, and place the avulsed tooth in NS for transport.

Skull fractures

The skull is divided into eight cranial bones: one frontal bone (over the frontal lobe), two parietal bones (over the parietal lobes), two temporal bones (over the temporal lobes), one occipital bone (over the occipital lobe and cerebellum), one sphenoid bone (it forms part of the eye orbit), and one ethmoid bone (it separates the nasal cavity from the brain). **Skull fractures** include the following:

- Basilar: Occurs in the bones at the base of the brain and can cause severe brain stem damage.
- Comminuted: The skull fractures into small pieces.
- Compound: A surface laceration extends to a skull fracture, which may be overlooked because of heavy bleeding.
- Depressed: May be open and is often comminuted. Pieces of the skull are depressed inward on the brain tissue, often producing dural tears and underlying brain trauma.
- Linear/hairline: A skull fracture forms a thin line without any splintering, usually without underlying injury.
- Diastatic: Affects children younger than 3 years old, widening the skull sutures.

Spinal injuries and spinal cord injuries (SCIs)

Spinal injuries of the vertebrae include fractures, dislocations, open wounds, and flexion and extension injuries. Because the spinal cord lies within the vertebral column, injury to the vertebrae may cause **spinal cord injuries (SCIs)** and disrupt transmissions in nerves that connect the body and the brain. SCI may affect only a few nerves, or they may completely transect the spinal cord, resulting in permanent paralysis below the site of injury. SCIs should be suspected with head trauma, penetrating trauma, direct blunt trauma, falls, diving injuries, motor vehicle accidents, rapid deceleration accidents, and multisystem trauma. Assessment includes evaluating extremity movement, respiration control, sensation, reflexes, pain/tenderness, and vital signs. Prehospital: Logroll the patient to examine his or her back, immobilize the patient (seated or standing), apply a rigid cervical collar, lift and move him or her with care, and provide rapid transport. Elevate the torso of children 2–3 cm with padding so that the head is in a neutral position if using an adult immobilization device. Immobilize infants in their car seats, padding all the voids.

Spinal cord injuries (SCIs) may result from blunt trauma (such as automobile accidents), falls from a height, sports injuries, and penetrating trauma (such as a gunshot or knife wound). Damage results from mechanical injury and secondary responses resulting from hemorrhage, edema, and ischemia. The types of symptoms relate to the area and degree of injury, as below:

Injury	Characteristics
Anterior cord	This results from pressure/damage to the anterior spinal cord. The posterior column functions remain, so there are sensations of touch, vibration, and position remaining below the injury but with complete paralysis and loss of the sensations of pain and temperature. The prognosis is poor.
Brown-Séquard	The cord is hemisected from penetrating trauma, resulting in spastic paresis, loss of sense of position and vibration on the injured side, and loss of pain and temperature sensation on the other side. The prognosis is good.
Posterior cord	Motor function is preserved but without sensation.
Conus medullaris	Injury to the lower spine (lower lumbar and sacral nerves).
Cauda equina	Damage is below L1 with variable loss of motor ability, reflexes, and sensation in the groin area and bowel, bladder, and sexual dysfunction. Injury is to the peripheral nerves descending from the end of the spinal cord. These nerves can regenerate, so the prognosis is better than for other lesions of the spinal cord.
Central cord	This results from hyperextension or hyperflexion and ischemia or stenosis of the cervical spine, causing spinal contusion and quadriparesis (more severe in the upper extremities) with some loss of sensations of pain and temperature. Prognosis is good, but fine motor skills are often impaired in the upper extremities with paresis being more acute distally than proximally in the arms.
Spinal shock	Injury at T6 or above (usually a complete transection), results in flaccid paralysis below the lesion with loss of reflexes, sensations, and rectal tone, bradycardia, hypothermia, and hypotension (although not circulatory collapse). Some reflexes usually begin to return by day 2, followed by autonomic hyperreflexia. Symptoms may persist for 7–20 days.

- 159 -

Brain injuries, the coup/contrecoup pattern, and posturing

Primary brain injuries are those that result from the original trauma and include direct damage to brain tissue, such as may occur with a gunshot wound. **Secondary brain injuries** result from the effects of the primary injury, such as increasing intracranial pressure, ischemia (most common), hemorrhage, edema, and brain herniation. **Coup/Contrecoup** injuries are common in motor vehicle accidents and shaken baby syndrome. With acceleration/deceleration and contact injuries where the head hits a fixed object (such as a windshield) and snaps back from the impact, coup (on the side of impact) and contrecoup (on the opposite side) contusions may both occur. **Decerebrate (extension) posturing** (with the body stiff, legs straight, feet extended, arms straight, and the head/neck arched back) is associated with severe midbrain damage. **Decorticate (flexion) posturing** (with the body stiff, legs straight, and hands clenched on the chest) is associated with damage to the pathway connecting the brain and spinal cord and may include damage to the cerebral cortex, white matter, or basal ganglia.

Neurogenic shock

Neurogenic shock occurs with injury to the CNS above T6 (from trauma resulting in acute spinal cord injury and from blunt and penetrating injuries), neurological diseases, drugs, or anesthesia, impairs the ANS that controls the cardiovascular system. Symptoms include hypotension and warm, dry skin related to the lack of vascular tone that results in hypothermia from loss of cutaneous heat. Bradycardia is a common but not universal symptom. The severity of symptoms relates to the level of injury, with injuries above T1 capable of causing disruption of the entire SoNS and with lower injuries causing various degrees of disruption. Even incomplete SCIs can cause neurogenic shock. Prehospital: Monitor the patient's airway/ventilation/oxygen supplementation, start an IV access line with fluid resuscitation with crystalloid to keep mean arterial pressure at 85 to 90 mm Hg to maintain oxygen saturation >90%, perform spinal immobilization, administer norepinephrine or dopamine (per protocol) if hypotension persists and atropine for severe bradycardia, and provide rapid transport.

Trauma in pregnancy and pediatrics

Pregnancy trauma: The mother and fetus are each considered to be patients. Pregnant patients are susceptible to falls and domestic abuse. Pregnant women have an increased blood volume and heart rate, impaired venous return if in the supine (flat) position in third trimester, and an increased risk of vomiting and aspiration. Hypovolemia/shock lowers oxygen to the fetus, resulting in fetal stress. Vaginal bleeding may occur. Prehospital: Have suction available, monitor the patient's airway/ventilation/oxygen supplementation with 100% oxygen per nonrebreather mask and ventilation assistance if needed, transport on the left side (tilt the immobilization board if necessary), provide an IV access line and fluids if indicated and rapid transport.

Pediatric trauma: Assess the pediatric triangle (appearance, work of breathing, and circulation). The respiration rate varies with age, but the use of accessory muscles and sternal retraction indicate respiratory distress. Assess the brachial pulse in infants—a slow pulse indicates hypoxia. Prehospital: Manage hypovolemia/shock, prevent hypothermia, and manage the patient's airway/ventilation/oxygen supplementation as needed. Ventilate if he or she is bradycardic (BVM is preferred for children).

Trauma in geriatric patients and the cognitively impaired

Geriatric trauma: These patients are more susceptible to trauma because of aging processes, and they may be less able to maintain normal vital signs during hemorrhage. Polypharmacy is common, and medications may affect vital signs and blood clotting. The risk of cerebral bleeding is increased because of brain shrinkage. The cough reflex may be lessened. Fractures are common because of osteoporosis, especially hip fractures. Prehospital: splint fractures, monitor the patient's airway/ventilation/oxygen supplementation, monitor oxygenation with pulse oximetry, suction if necessary, and check the mouth for dentures (which may obstruct the airway). Spinal curvature may require padding of the spinal board.

Trauma in cognitively impaired patients: Disorders may include Alzheimer's or other forms of dementia, traumatic brain injuries, strokes, Down's syndrome, and autistic spectrum disorders. Patients may be more at risk of trauma, and assessment and history taking may be difficult. Perceptions of pain may be altered, and psychological reactions may vary. Prehospital: Remain supportive, reassure the patient, obtain information from the caregiver if necessary, and treat as indicated by the patient's condition.

Generalized hypothermia

Generalized hypothermia occurs when the body temperature falls to below-normal levels:

- Mild: 32°C –35°C (89.6°F–95°F).
- Moderate: 28°C–32°C (82.4°F–95°F).
- Severe: <32°C (<82.4°F).

Contributing factors include wet and cold environments, wind, age (geriatric/pediatric), medical conditions, substance abuse (alcohol, drugs), and poison. Up to 50% of trauma patients with severe injuries become hypothermic because of exposure, blood loss, shock, and standard procedures (such as administration of cold fluids and clothing removal). Indications of hypothermia include cold skin, shivering, decreased mental status (confusion, memory loss, lethargy, dizziness, mood changes, impaired judgment, difficulty speaking), decreased sensation of touch, decreased motor function (muscle rigidity, stiff posture, muscle/joint stiffness), and bradycardia. Prehospital: Remove the patient from the cold environment, remove any wet clothing, wrap in warm blankets, begin CPR if no pulse is obtained after 30–45 seconds of assessment, and use an AED if it indicates the need to defibrillate

Frostbite/Freezing

Frostbite is tissue damage from **freezing**, most often affecting the nose, ears, and distal extremities (hands/feet). The affected part feels numb and aches or throbs, becoming hard and insensate as the tissue freezes, resulting in circulatory impairment, necrosis of tissue, and gangrene. Degrees of frostbite/freezing are as follows:

1. Partial freezing with erythema and mild edema, stinging, burning, and throbbing pain.
2. Full-thickness freezing with increased edema in 3–4 hours and clear blisters in 6–24 hours; sloughing of skin with eschar formation, numbness, and then aching and throbbing pain.
3. Full-thickness freezing into the subdermal tissue with cyanosis, hemorrhagic blisters, skin necrosis, a "wooden" feeling, severe burning, throbbing, and shooting pains.
4. Freezing extends into the subcutaneous tissue (muscles, tendons, and bones) with a mottled appearance, nonblanching cyanosis, and eventually deep black eschar.

Prehospital: Remove the patient from the cold environment, handling him or her with care; remove wet clothing; cover the patient with a blanket; remove jewelry; manually stabilize the affected area; and transport rapidly. Do NOT break blisters, rub or massage the area, apply heat, rewarm if the area may refreeze, allow the patient to walk, or give him or her anything by mouth.

Heat-related illnesses

Condition	Characteristics	Prehospital
Heat stress	Increased temperature causes dehydration. Symptoms may include swelling of the hands and feet, flushing, itching, sunburn, dizziness, muscle cramps, and hyperventilation. The patient's temperature is normal.	Remove the patient from heat, give fluids to rehydrate, and give oxygen with a nonrebreather mask.
Heat exhaustion	Dehydration results in sodium depletion. Symptoms may include flu-like symptoms, headache, dizziness, fainting, nausea, vomiting, weakness, muscle cramping, rapid pulse, diaphoresis, and cold clammy skin. The patient's temperature is usually <106°F (41°C), and it may be normal.	Remove the patient from heat; use evaporative cooling techniques such as ice packs to the axilla, groin, and neck; rehydrate (one-half glass every 15 to 20 minutes). Give oxygen as above.
Heat stroke	There are two types, which may progress to multiorgan dysfunction syndrome with liver and kidney failure, and death. Exertional: Sudden onset after exertion. The patient's temperature varies because he or she is still sweating; there is diaphoresis, syncope, and loss of consciousness. Nonexertional: Sudden onset after heat exposure. The temperature is usually >106°F (41°C) rectally or >103°F (39.4°C) orally. There can be mild irritability, decorticate posturing, seizures, coma, and tachycardia.	Remove the patient from heat, apply evaporative cooling and ice packs as above; provide airway/ventilation/oxygenation support as needed, IV access line and fluids, and rapid transport.

Submersion/drowning

Submersion may cause aspiration (wet drowning) or trigger severe laryngospasm (dry drowning), although some people will be pulled from the water still breathing. **Drowning** is the leading cause of death in children younger than age 5, and it is the second leading cause of death in children younger than age 15. Most infant submersions are in bathtubs and result from intentional injury or lack of supervision. Adolescent/Adult submersions are often related to drugs, alcohol, or risk-taking behaviors. Submersion asphyxiation can cause profound damage to multiple organ systems, including the brain, heart, and lungs, from a lack of oxygen and aspiration. Hypothermia related to near drowning has some protective effect because blood is shunted to the brain and heart. Indications of submersion include coughing, vomiting, difficulty breathing, and respiratory and cardiac arrest. Prehospital: Initiate CPR if the patient is in arrest, manage the patient's airway/ventilation/oxygen supplementation with 100% oxygen (may need intubation), place him or her in the recovery position if he or she is unconscious or vomiting, provide suction as needed, start an IV access line, and provide rapid transport.

Snakebites

Pit vipers include rattlesnakes, copperheads, and cottonmouths. They have erectile fangs that fold until they are aroused; their venom is primarily hemotoxic and cytotoxic, but it may also have neurotoxic properties (affecting the blood, cells, and nerves at the bite site and systemically). Symptoms vary depending on the amount of venom that is injected (many bites are dry).

- Wounds usually show one or two fang marks.
- Swelling may begin immediately, or it may be delayed for up to 6 hours.
- Pain may be severe.
- There may be a wide range of symptoms, including hypotension and impairment of blood clotting that can lead to excessive blood loss, depending upon the type and amount of venom.
- Progressive weakness, vision problems, nausea and vomiting, altered consciousness, and seizures are expected.

Prehospital: Note the time elapsed from the time of the bite to the time of transport, reassure the patient, immobilize the extremity, cleanse the wound with soap and water, apply an ice pack to slow venous return and reduce swelling, transport immediately for further treatment such as with antivenom, and mark the extent of the swelling on the skin every 15 minutes.

Decompression sickness

Decompression sickness (dysbarism) occurs when a diver ascends too quickly and the body is unable to compensate for the pressure change. Because the pressure reduces too rapidly, dissolved gases in the blood, such as helium and nitrogen, form bubbles. These bubbles interfere with blood flow and can cause gas emboli, which can obstruct blood vessels and damage the alveoli in the lung. The gas emboli can affect all tissues with symptoms ranging from mild to severe with complete neurological and cardiovascular collapse. Typical mild to moderate symptoms include joint pain, numbness, tremors, amnesia, difficulty breathing, itch, tinnitus, vertigo, and localized swelling. Severe symptoms include pneumothorax, loss of consciousness, seizures, and weakness or paralysis of extremities. The onset of mild symptoms is gradual with more than 40% having symptoms within 1 hour, but the onset of severe symptoms may occur within minutes of surfacing. Prehospital: Rapid transport for recompression therapy is critical to survival (especially in severe cases); manage the patient's airway/ventilation/oxygen supplementation with 100% oxygen through a nonrebreather mask. Air transport must be below 1000 feet in altitude.

Electrical injuries

Low-voltage **electrical contact** most often causes a localized burn (first to third degree) to the hand or mouth (toddlers) with various degrees of tissue damage, although mouth contact may also result in cardiac or respiratory arrest. High-voltage electrical contact results in an entry and an exit wound with internal damage occurring between these wounds. Electrical current takes the shortest route to leave the body (flowing along blood vessels and nerves), so if the current passes from hand to hand, damage is usually more severe than if it passes from a hand to a foot. Severe injury may result in damage to bones, compartment syndrome, organ failure, and cardiac arrest from asystole or ventricular fibrillation. Vessels may be mildly or severely damaged. Abdominal organs may be damaged. Neurological damage with unconsciousness is common, especially if the current passes through the head. Peripheral nerve damage is also common, and damage to the spinal cord may occur. Prehospital: Manage the patient's airway/ventilation/oxygen supplementation, provide CPR/defibrillation as needed, provide rapid transport (with the head elevated if it was involved), start an IV access line, and give fluid resuscitation if needed.

Lightning injuries

Lightning injuries may occur with a direct strike (≤5%), side splash from a strike nearby, contact voltage when touching an item that has been struck, ground current (from a more distant strike), and blunt trauma from being too close to a strike (which often results in the patient being thrown). Symptoms may vary, but they can include external burns (Lichtenberg figures) in a fernlike pattern, acute pain, fixed and dilated pupils (temporary), eye injuries, confusion, headache, hearing loss, perforated eardrum, hypotension, paralysis/paresis, spinal cord injury, altered mental status, brain injury, fractures, and cardiac arrest. Patients may be responsive initially but lapse into unconsciousness as cerebral edema increases, resulting in secondary respiratory and/or cardiac arrest. Burns are usually mild because of the brief contact. Prehospital: Manage the patient's airway/ventilation/oxygen supplementation, provide CPR/defibrillation as needed, provide rapid transport (with the head elevated), start an IV access line, and give fluid resuscitation.

Multisystem trauma

Multisystem trauma (common) involves injury to more than one major system. Care includes the following points:

- Ensure the safety of the patient and all rescue personnel, and determine the need for additional resources.
- Consider the mechanism of injury and identify and manage life-threatening conditions.
- Manage the patient's airway/ventilation/oxygen supplementation (high concentration) as well as necessary spinal immobilization with him or her in a lying/sitting position, and make positioning decisions.
- Control hemorrhage, provide shock therapy, and maintain body temperature.
- Splint musculoskeletal injuries.
- Suspect additional injuries.
- Prioritize interventions and continue care en route rather than delaying transport.
- Evaluate the patient's condition by the injuries sustained (bleeding, difficulty breathing, lack of pulse) rather than by the patient's response (screaming, yelling).
- Complete the primary and secondary assessments, and obtain a medical history.
- Platinum ten—the first 10 minutes on the scene in which the patient should be extricated and stabilization efforts should be started.
- Golden hour—the first 60 minutes during which the patient should be stabilized and transported to the receiving facility.

Notify the receiving facility so that resources are prepared.

Blast injuries

Blast injuries may result from high-order explosives (TNT, nitroglycerin) or low-order explosives (pipe bombs, Molotov cocktails). Enclosed explosions usually cause more injury than do open-air blasts. Blast waves occur only with high-order explosives and result from high-pressure impulses.

Blast wind may occur with either type of explosives and involves superheated air. Ground shock may cause further injury. Immediate death may occur.

Injuries may include the following:

Type	Characteristics	Prehospital
Primary	Blast wave injury affects gas-filled organs/structures: lungs, eardrum, abdomen, eyes, and brain (20% of victims).	Be alert for a second explosive device or a device on a victim (who may be a perpetrator).
Secondary	Penetrating injuries from flying shrapnel affecting any part of the body along with abrasions, contusions, and lacerations. (Secondary injury is the most common cause of death.)	Carry out rapid triage. Control any bleeding, and manage shock. Manage the patient's airway/ventilation/oxygen supplementation. Provide CPR if necessary.
Tertiary	Injuries from being thrown by blast wind: fractures, spinal and brain injuries, and traumatic amputations.	Splint musculoskeletal injuries.
Quaternary	Other injuries and complications, such as difficulty breathing because of smoke inhalation, burns, and crush injuries.	Start an IV access and give fluid resuscitation. Provide rapid transport.

Special Patient Populations

Premonitory signs of labor

Lightening	As the fetal head engages and moves toward the birth canal, the fundal pressure on the diaphragm lessens, so the mother can breathe more easily, but pressure in the pelvic area increases, causing urinary frequency. The lower abdomen may protrude more than previously. Increased circulatory impairment may cause venous stasis and ankle edema as well as increased vaginal secretions as the vaginal mucous membranes become congested. Pressure on the nerves may result in leg cramps or increased pelvic and leg pain.
Braxton Hicks (BH)	BH contractions are short in duration, occur at irregular intervals in the lower abdomen, and do not change the cervix. They are often relieved by activity or mild analgesia. The intensity and frequency of BH contractions often increase immediately prior to the onset of true labor.
Cervical changes	The cervix ripens (softens) to allow for effacement (thinning) and dilation.
Bloody show	A mucous plug from pooled secretions forms at the opening of the cervical canal during pregnancy; when the cervix begins to efface, this mucous plug is expelled, exposing capillary vessels that bleed. The bloody show typically appears as pink mucus. Bloody show usually occurs within 24 to 48 hours of the onset of labor.
Ruptured membranes	Rupture of the membranes occurs in about 12% of women prior to the onset of labor, which usually then occurs within 24 hours. Before rupture, the membranes typically bulge through the dilating cervix; fluid comes in a gush, although it may come in smaller spurts in some cases. If the membranes rupture before engagement of the fetal head, the umbilical cord may prolapse with the fluid, increasing the risk to the fetus, so mothers should always seek medical attention after rupture. If the mother is at term and labor does not start within 24 hours of rupture, labor may be induced.

Stages of labor

First	Latent phase: The cervix begins to dilate; contractions are mild to moderate and occur every 3–30 minutes and are of short duration. Active phase: The cervix is dilated to 4–7 cm; contractions are every 1–5 minutes, lasting 20–40 seconds. Pain is increased. Transitional phase: The cervix is fully dilated (8–10 cm); contractions come every 1.5–2 minutes, lasting 60–90 seconds. There is increased pain, hyperventilation, crying, moaning, vomiting, and rectal pressure.
Second	From fully dilated cervix to delivery with contractions as in the transitional phase. The perineum begins to bulge, and the fetal head crowns as the mother begins to bear down and birth is imminent. Pressure on the rectum and anus may cause stool to be expelled. Birth occurs head first if it is a normal delivery, feet first if it is a breech delivery.
Third	Delivery of the placenta should occur 5–30 minutes after birth. Retained placenta occurs if more than 30 minutes elapse.
Fourth	The period of 1–4 hours after birth, which involves 250–400 mL blood loss, moderate hypotension (low BP), and tachycardia (rapid pulse).

Organs of pregnancy and vaginal bleeding

Organs of pregnancy include the uterus (womb). The placenta is attached to the walls of the uterus; it includes the umbilical cord, which provides blood, nutrients, and oxygen to the fetus. The fetus is inside an amniotic sac, which contains amniotic fluid that cushions the fetus. The opening to the uterus is the cervix, which thins and dilates for delivery. The vagina provides the birth canal.
Vaginal bleeding during the first trimester of pregnancy may indicate spontaneous abortion, ectopic pregnancy, or infection, although light occasional spotting may be normal. All vaginal bleeding during pregnancy should be assessed by a physician, and a large amount of bleeding may indicate a medical emergency. "Bloody show" near term may indicate that delivery is near. Prehospital: Use standard precautions, and position the patient on her left side. Place a sanitary pad over the vaginal opening, and save any soaked pads in a plastic bag so the physician can estimate the amount of blood loss. Manage the patient's airway/ventilation/oxygen supplementation, and provide emotional support. Provide an IV access line and fluids if indicated.

Spontaneous and elective abortion and ectopic pregnancy

Spontaneous abortion: Unplanned loss of pregnancy at or before 20 weeks. May result from trauma, fetal abnormality, or another cause. Indications include vaginal bleeding (mild to severe) and contractions. The patient may be very emotionally upset. Prehospital: Use the term "miscarriage" rather than "abortion," which has negative connotations for many; gather any products of conception in a plastic bag to take to the hospital; provide supportive care; place a sanitary pad over the vagina; and provide reassurance and emotional support.

Elective abortion: Planned loss of pregnancy at or before 20 weeks per surgical procedure or abortion pills (during the first 10 weeks). Patients may develop bleeding after surgery or as the fetus is expelled. Prehospital: Gather any products of conception in a plastic bag to take to the hospital, provide supportive care, place a sanitary pad over the vagina, and provide reassurance and emotional support.

Ectopic pregnancy: Pregnancy in which the egg fertilizes and attaches outside of the uterus (usually in the fallopian tubes), resulting in abdominal pain, absent menstrual periods, and vaginal bleeding. Prehospital: As above.

Delivery of a newborn

If the fetal head is obvious at the vaginal opening (crowning), **delivery** is imminent. Steps to delivery include the following:

- Wash hands and don PPE for standard precautions and obtain an OB kit and supplies.
- Position the patient on her back with hips elevated, knees bent, and legs apart.
- Position one person at the mother's head for support if possible while the other supports the baby's head during delivery.
- Provide oxygen to the mother.
- Provide an IV access line and NS, cardiac monitoring, and analgesia as needed.
- If the umbilical cord is around the baby's neck, attempt to slip it over the infant's head.
- Make note of the time of delivery.
- Lower the infant's head to facilitate the drainage of fluids and keep the mouth and nose suctioned with a bulb syringe.
- Clamp the cord or cut it if sterile equipment is available.

- Monitor the infant's airway, breathing, and circulation with the baby at the level of the birth canal.
- Monitor delivery of the placenta (afterbirth).
- If mother and infant are stable, allow the infant to nurse.
- Place a sanitary pad over the vaginal opening to contain any bleeding. Observe for hemorrhage.
- Massage the uterus in a circular motion to prevent excessive bleeding.

Complications of pregnancy and labor

Complication	Characteristic	Prehospital
Preterm labor	Labor between weeks 20 and 37; presents a risk to the fetus.	Provide supportive care in the left lateral position.
Premature rupture of membranes	Membranes rupture before the onset of labor; this may lead to preterm labor and risk to the fetus.	Manage the patient's airway/ ventilation/ oxygen supplementation (100%).
Substance abuse	May result in damage to the fetus and preterm labor. Many drugs restrict blood flow to the fetus, resulting in growth retardation and low oxygen. Some drugs, such as cocaine, affect the fetal nervous system. Sudden withdrawal of opiates may trigger preterm labor. Alcohol may result in fetal alcohol syndrome, characterized by facial abnormalities, growth retardation, and neurological defects.	Transport rapidly if there is severe bleeding or a risk of imminent preterm delivery. Start an IV access line and give NS for placental abruption.
Placental abruption	The placenta prematurely detaches, partially or completely, from the uterus. Related to maternal hypertension and the incidence increases with cocaine abuse. Partial detachment interferes with the functioning of the placenta, causing intrauterine growth retardation. Severe bleeding occurs with total detachment.	Provide supportive care in the left lateral position. Manage the patient's airway/ ventilation/ oxygen supplementation (100%). Transport rapidly if there is severe bleeding or a risk of imminent preterm delivery. Start an IV access line and give NS for placental abruption.
Placenta previa	The placenta implants over or near the internal cervical opening. Implantation may be complete (covering the entire opening), partial, or marginal (to the edge of the cervical opening). Results in increased incidences of hemorrhage in the third trimester. Symptoms include painless bleeding after the 20th week of gestation.	Provide supportive care in the left lateral position.

Pregnancy-induced hypertension/ Preeclampsia/ Eclampsia	Hypertension >140/90 associated with increased protein in the urine and edema (peripheral or generalized) or increase of ≥ 5 pounds of weight in one week after the 20th week of gestation. Severe preeclampsia is BP $\geq 160/110$. Symptoms include headache, abdominal pain, and visual disturbances. May progress to eclampsia (seizures) and death.	Manage the patient's airway/ventilation/oxygen supplementation (100%). IV access line and NS. Transport rapidly if there is severe bleeding, high BP $\geq 160/110$, seizures, or altered mental status. Provide ECG monitoring. Administer magnesium sulfate for preeclampsia/ eclampsia.
Cephalic (vertex) presentation	<u>Military:</u> Head straight, neck not flexed. <u>Brow:</u> Neck extended, brow presents first, can cause birth trauma, so episiotomy or cesarean section (C-section) is usually required. <u>Face:</u> Severely extended neck with face presentation, may prolong labor, increase swelling of the fetus, and cause neck trauma.	Provide supportive care. Manage the patient's airway/ ventilation/ oxygen supplementation (100%). Transport rapidly.
Breech presentation	Frank breech (buttocks presentation with legs extended upward) is the most common, but single- or double-footling breech (incomplete breech) or buttocks presentation with legs flexed (complete breech) can also occur. Breech presentation is most common with placenta previa, hydramnios, fetal anomalies, and multiple gestations. Cord prolapse is more likely. Head trauma may occur because molding does not occur, and the head can become entrapped.	

Prolapse of the umbilical cord

A **prolapse of the umbilical cord** occurs when the umbilical cord precedes the fetus in the birth canal and becomes entrapped by the descending fetus. With an <u>occult cord prolapse,</u> the umbilical cord is beside or just ahead of the fetal head. With a <u>nuchal cord prolapse,</u> the cord tightly wraps about the fetal neck. About half of prolapses occur in the second stage of labor and relate to premature delivery, multiple gestations, or other complications. As contractions occur and the head descends, pressure to the umbilical cord occludes the blood flow, causing hypoxia and bradycardia. The decrease in blood flow through the umbilical vessels can cause impaired gas exchange, and if pressure on the cord is not relieved, the fetus can suffer severe neurological damage or death. Prehospital: Elevate the presenting part off the cord, pull the cord off of the fetus's neck if possible, elevate the mother's knees to the chest to relieve pressure on the cord, provide 100% oxygen, and transport rapidly.

Hyperemesis gravidarum (HG) and Rh incompatibility

About 60–80% of pregnant woman suffer from nausea and vomiting (NV), especially during the first trimester, but only about 2% suffer **hyperemesis gravidarum** (HG). Symptoms of HG include severe (sometimes intractable) NV, weight loss, and dehydration. Prehospital: Provide intravenous fluids with 5% glucose in NS or Ringer's lactate; administer antiemetic drugs, including promethazine (Phenergan), prochlorperazine (Compazine), or chlorpromazine (Thorazine).

Rh incompatibility occurs if the mother is Rh– and the father is Rh+, putting their infant is at risk for hemolytic disease of the newborn (HDN). Sensitization can occur during abortion, placental abruption, amniocentesis, C-section, chorionic villus sampling, delivery, ectopic pregnancy, and toxemia. Women who are Rh– with an Rh+ mate receive the serum RhoGAM, containing anti-Rh+ antibodies in order to agglutinate any fetal red blood cells that pass over into the mother's circulatory system and thus prevent the mother from forming antibodies against them that will attack the infant and sensitize her for future pregnancies. ABO incompatibility is similar but is usually less severe.

Multiple gestations

In vitro fertilization and ovulation-inducing drugs have increased the incidence of high-order **multiple gestations** over the past 30 years. The trend of delayed childbearing has led to an increase in twin/multiple gestations. Infants born from multiple gestations are more likely to be born prematurely and with low birth weights. The incidence of premature birth and low birth weight is proportional to the number of fetuses. There may be growth restriction/growth discordance, oligohydramnios, and restriction of movement of one or more fetuses. Approximately 50% of twins and 90% of triplets are born premature, compared to 10% of singletons. With this increase in prematurity and proportion of infants born with low birth weight, there are increased morbidities, such as cerebral palsy and mental retardation. The risk for genetic disorders, such as neural tube defects and GI and cardiac abnormalities, is twice that of single gestations.

CHEAP TORCHES and TORCH panel

CHEAP TORCHES is the acronym used to recall common causes of congenital and neonatal infections. Many congenital infections are present for at least a month prior to birth and remain present at birth, such as the following:

> **C** = Chickenpox (varicella)
> **H** = Hepatitis (B, C, and E)
> **E** = Enterovirus (RNA viruses, including coxsackievirus, echovirus, and poliovirus)
> **A** = AIDS (HIV)
> **P** = Parvovirus (B19)
> **T** = Toxoplasmosis
> **O** = Other (group B streptococcus, Candida, Listeria, TB, lymphocytic choriomeningitis)
> **R** = Rubella (measles)
> **C** = Cytomegalovirus
> **H** = Herpes simplex virus
> **E** = Every other STD (chlamydia, gonorrhea, Ureaplasma, papillomavirus)
> **S** = Syphilis

Exposure to these pathogens in utero may cause a miscarriage or congenital defect, especially if the exposure was during the first trimester. Symptoms may include being small for gestational age, an enlarged liver and spleen, thrombocytopenia, skin rash, jaundice, seizures, or encephalitis. The

TORCH panel, which tests for toxoplasmosis, rubella, cytomegalovirus, and herpes simplex virus, is commonly used to screen pregnant women for infectious diseases.

Postpartum depression/psychosis

Postpartum depression occurs in >10% of mothers. Onset may occur any time within the first year, but it is most common around week 4 postpartum, before the onset of menses. The duration varies, but it is usually 3 to 14 months (half symptomatic at 6 months). Symptoms are typical of depression and include sadness, crying, insomnia or excess sleeping, difficulty concentrating or making decisions, phobias, anxiety, lack of interest in activities, and feeling of being out of control or helpless. The mother may be irritable and hostile, especially toward the child. She may also be suicidal. **Postpartum psychosis** may occur up to 3 months postpartum, but symptoms are usually evident within the first 3 weeks with sudden onset of psychotic symptoms, such as delusions, hallucinations, insomnia, anorexia, paranoia, and suicidal and/or homicidal ideation. In 4% of cases, mothers have committed infanticide. Prehospital: Ensure the safety of the infant, and provide supportive care.

Initial care of the newborn

Dr. Virginia Apgar developed the **APGAR assessment** in 1952. APGAR stands for **a**ppearance, **p**ulse, **g**rimace, **a**ctivity, and **r**espiration. The APGAR is the first test given to a newborn. It is used as a quick evaluation of a newborn's physical condition to determine if any emergency medical care is needed, and it is administered 1 minute and 5 minutes after birth. The test is administered more than once because the baby's condition may change rapidly. It may be administered for a third time 10 minutes after birth if needed. The baby is rated on the five subscales, and scores are added together. A total score of ≥7 is a sign of good health.

Sign	0	1	2
Appearance (skin color)	Cyanotic or pallor over entire body	Normal, except for the extremities	Entire body is normal.
Pulse (heart rate)	Absent	<100 bpm	>100 bpm.
Grimace (reflex irritability)	Unresponsive	Grimace	Infant sneezes, coughs, and recoils.
Activity (muscle tone)	Absent	Flexed limbs	The infant moves freely.
Respiration (breathing rate and effort)	Absent	Bradypnea, dyspnea	There is good breathing and crying.

Routine care of the newborn

Infants have poor temperature regulation ability, particularly preterm infants who lack brown fat, which is one of the body's tools to regulate body temperature, so **providing warmth** is critical as a component of resuscitation. An infant who is just seconds old and wet will need aggressive measures to keep him or her warm while any resuscitation efforts are being initiated. Infants lose heat through their heads, so one of the first steps should be to place a hat on the head or cover the head in some way. The infant should be vigorously dried with warmed blankets. Often, this stimulation, drying and warming, is all that is needed to establish a regular respiration pattern in the neonate. Preterm infants weighing <1500 grams should be placed in a plastic bag (made specifically for this purpose), if available, up to the height of the shoulders to prevent cold shock. A term infant with no distress can be placed on the mother's chest and covered with a warm blanket.

Establishing an airway

To **establish an airway**, the infant is placed supine with the head slightly extended in the sniffing position. A small neck roll may be placed under the shoulders to maintain this position in a very small premature infant. Once the proper position is established, the mouth and nose are suctioned (suction the mouth first to prevent reflex inspiration of secretions when the nose is suctioned) with a bulb syringe or catheter if necessary. The infant's head can be turned momentarily to the side to allow secretions to pool in the cheek where they can be more easily suctioned and removed to establish the airway. Stimulating the newborn is often all that is needed to initiate spontaneous respirations. This tactile stimulation can be accomplished by gently rubbing the back or trunk of the infant. Another technique that is used to provide stimulation is flicking or rubbing the soles of the feet. Slapping neonates as stimulation is no longer practiced and should NOT be used.

Managing airway and ventilation

Blow-by oxygen	Provide if the newborn is cyanotic and heart rate is >100 bpm and respiratory effort is adequate. Provide warm oxygen at 5 L/min. with a direct flow on the face. Avoid oral airways.
Bag-valve mask (BVM)	Provide if the newborn is apneic, the heart rate <100, and/or there is inadequate respiratory effort. Use an appropriate size and avoid excess pressure, which may cause pneumothorax, although initial ventilation requires higher pressure to expand the lungs. Disable the pop-off valve.
Intubation	Provide if other measures are ineffective and the heart rate is <60. Use a straight-blade laryngoscope size #1 for full term and size #0 for preterm with ETT 2.5 to 4.90 mm. Confirm placement through visualization, auscultation (lateral, superior chest wall, epigastric region), improvement in respirations, ETCO₂, and pulse oximetry. Secure the ETT. Provide PEEP as indicated at 5 cm H₂0. Gastric decompression may be necessary if the abdomen is distended. Provide CPR as needed.

ABCs of resuscitation of the neonate

The **ABC's of resuscitation** should begin immediately after delivery with assisted ventilation begun within 60 seconds if required.

A—**A**irway	An airway should be established as the very first thing tended to; if there is no airway, air cannot be moved during resuscitation attempts. This step includes clearing the mouth and nose of secretions and properly positioning the infant in the sniffing position.
B—**B**reathing	This step involves initiating breathing after the airway has been established; this can be done with stimulation, supplemental oxygen, or through artificial ventilation as indicated.
C—**C**irculation	Once an airway and breathing have been established, then the circulation is considered; chest compressions may be indicated here or the administration of IV epinephrine (if the heart rate is less than 60 bpm), and possible volume expanders (isotonic crystalloid at 10 mL/kg) can be used if the neonate is hypovolemic. Begin compressions to the lower third of the sternum with two thumbs or two fingers at a 3:1 ratio (90 compressions to 30 ventilations per minute). Increase oxygen to 100% during compressions.

Neonatal complications

Condition	Characteristics	Prehospital
Meconium in amniotic fluid	The infant is at risk for aspiration with complete obstruction (causing atelectasis and/or right-to-left shunt through the foramen ovale) or incomplete obstruction (causing pneumothorax or pneumonitis). The infant may be hypoxic, hypercapnic, and acidotic.	Avoid stimulating respirations. If there are no signs of distress, suction the mouth, nose, and throat. If there is respiratory distress, intubate and suction the trachea and ventilate with 100% oxygen.
Apnea	This is failure to breathe spontaneously or respiration pauses for >20 seconds. It usually results from hypothermia or hypoxia, but it may result from other causes, such as narcotics in the system.	Stimulate, ventilate, suction, and/or intubate as indicated.
Bradycardia	It usually results from hypoxia, so the airway must be assessed for obstruction.	Suction, BVM with 100% oxygen, intubation, chest compressions as indicated. Administer IV epinephrine.
Hypoglycemia	Blood glucose is <45 mg/dL. The infant exhibits twitching, limpness, lethargy, seizures, eye rolling, apnea, cyanosis, irregular respirations, and a high-pitched cry.	Manage the airway, ventilation, circulation. Administer dextrose 10% (D10).

Delivery of the preterm infant

A **preterm** infant is one born prior to 37 weeks' gestational age. In the United States, preterm birth is the most important factor influencing infant mortality, accounting for 75%–80% of all neonatal morbidity and mortality. Preterm birth is often associated with comorbidities. Findings may include the following:

- Respiratory distress syndrome because of inadequate surfactant production (hyaline membrane disease).
- Hypothermia because of inadequate subcutaneous fat, small amounts of brown fat, and large skin surface area to mass ratio.
- Hypoglycemia secondary to poor nutritional intake, poor nutritional stores, and increased glucose consumption associated with sepsis.
- Skin trauma or infection secondary to fragile, transparent, immature skin with less subcutaneous fat.
- Periods of apnea because of an immature respiratory center in the brain
- Intraventricular hemorrhage.
- Large trunk and short extremities.

The original cause of the preterm birth (such as maternal infection) may also play an integral role in the likely health problems associated with the infant's prematurity. Prehospital: Attempt resuscitation with signs of life, suction, ventilate/oxygenate, give compressions if indicated, administer epinephrine for bradycardia, and maintain body temperature.

Pediatric considerations

Pediatric patients have the following general considerations:

- Proportionately greater body surface area to body mass ratio, so they are at greater risk of fluid and heat loss, burns, and absorption of toxins.
- Higher respiratory rates and heart rates than adults, resulting in higher oxygen demand.
- Immature blood/brain barrier, resulting in more neurological symptoms.
- Immature immune system, resulting in a higher risk of infection.
- Narrower and shorter airway and smaller jaw, so the tongue may easily obstruct the airway.
- Soft tracheal cartilage that increases the risk of airway collapse, and a large epiglottis.
- More pliable ribs, which provide less protection for abdominal organs, which are more forward.
- Liver and spleen that are proportionately larger and at risk of injury.
- Bones that are softer with open growth plates: An open growth plate injury can impair growth.
- Less protection for the brain and spinal cord (increasing the risk of injury) and less subarachnoid space.
- Cerebral blood-flow needs twice that of adults, increasing the risk of hypoxia.
- Limited glucose stores and risk of hypothermia (especially in the first month).
- Anterior fontanel that closes by 12 months and posterior fontanel that closes by 3–4 months.

Pediatric seizures

Febrile seizure is a generalized seizure associated with fever (usually >38.8°C [101.8°F]) from any type of infection (upper respiratory, urinary tract) but without intracranial infection or other cause, occurring between 6 months and 5 years of age. Seizures usually last <15 minutes and are without subsequent neurological deficit. Prehospital: Provide fever control (acetaminophen OR ibuprofen) and a tepid-water bath. **Other types of seizures** may result from pathology, such as meningitis, cerebral edema, brain trauma, or brain tumors, but most seizures in children >3 are related to idiopathic epilepsy, which predisposes the child to recurrent seizures, usually of the same type. Seizures are characterized as focal (localized), focal with rapid generalization (spreading), and generalized (widespread). In most children, seizures become generalized with loss of consciousness. Seizure disorders with onset younger than 4 years of age usually cause more neurological damage than those with onset at older than 4 years of age. Prehospital: Place the patient on the floor or on a safe surface, loosen clothes, and protect him or her from injury during seizure. Afterward, place the patient in the recovery position, monitor the airway/ventilation, and provide oxygen supplementation (the patient may need assisted ventilation if he or she is cyanotic), and suction if needed.

Apparent life-threatening events (ALTEs) and sudden infant death syndrome (SIDS)

Infants with an **apparent life-threatening event (ALTE)** are those who are lifeless and without respirations but are successfully resuscitated or begin breathing spontaneously. With **sudden infant death syndrome (SIDS),** which is almost always related to respiratory arrest, the child cannot be resuscitated. There are numerous proposed causes for ALTE and SIDS, so a careful history, including familial history of SIDS, and physical examination or postmortem examination can provide important information, such as indications of child abuse or metabolic/infectious disorders. Prehospital: Continue resuscitative efforts (airway/ventilation/oxygen supplementation and compressions as indicated), and stabilize the infant if possible. The child with ALTE should be hospitalized for observation, further studies, and apnea monitoring because these children are at an increased risk for SIDS. For SIDS patients, the paramedic should provide support and information to the family. The protocol for reporting SIDS varies by state, but it usually involves notifying the coroner's office.

Growth and development of pediatric patients

Age	Characteristics
0–2 mos.	Sleeps up to 16 hours per day but should rouse easily. Cries for a reason; persistent crying may indicate illness. Limited head control. Gazes at faces.
2–6 mos.	Smiles voluntarily and makes eye contact, uses both hands, begins to hold his or her head up, rolls over, and sleeps through the night.
6–12 mos.	Sits, crawls, has pincer grasp, mouths objects (increasing risk of poisoning and aspiration), babbles, and speaks first words by 12 months. Exhibits separation anxiety from parents.
12–18 mos.	Begins to walk; imitates others; knows body parts and 4–6 words; lacks molars for grinding food, increasing the risk of aspiration; and has increased mobility.
18–24 mos.	Begins to run and climb, knows 100 words (24 months), clings to parents, attaches to special objects, labels objects, and begins to understand cause and effect.
2–5 years	Walks, runs, throws, catches, is toilet trained, has magical thinking and irrational fears, learns acceptable behavior, has temper tantrums, and develops modesty.

6–12 years	Loses baby teeth; thinks logically; becomes self-conscious; understand the finality of death; attaches importance to school, popularity, and peers.
12–20 years	Puberty begins, reasons (imperfectly), is self-conscious, seeks independence and peer approval, and takes risks.

Patients with special challenges

Condition	Issues	Prehospital considerations
Homeless/Indigent	Patients often are without medical care, increasing the risk of disease, and they may lack insurance. They may have mental health/substance abuse problems.	Know who will treat indigent patients and what resources are available in the community.
Bariatric	Increased risk of chronic disease. Patients pose handling/moving problems and require special bariatric equipment and multiple personnel to assist. Patients often have trouble breathing and must have their head elevated.	Recognize the need for bariatric equipment and know how/where to obtain it. Notify the receiving facility. Use properly sized equipment, such as BP cuffs.
Technology-/Device-assisted	Wide range of issues including ventilators, apnea monitors, vascular devices, dialysis shunts, colostomies, ileostomies, and feeding tubes. Patients may have special needs regarding care and transport.	Ask about the patient's equipment and needs. Avoid disturbing/damaging the devices if possible.

Geriatric considerations

Geriatric patients may have the following considerations:

- Decreased sensory input (hearing, vision, touch, pain); impaired depth perception and night vision; and decreased ability to differentiate colors.
- Hypertension, increasing the risk of heart attack and stroke.
- Decreased breathing capacity and decreased cough, increasing the risk of infection.
- Difficulty chewing and swallowing; digestive problems; and reflux when lying flat, increasing the risk of aspiration.
- Short-term memory deficit and slower reflexes.
- Decreased bone density, increasing the risk of breaks; loss of muscle tone.
- Increased risk of infection and less obvious symptoms of infection.
- Arthritis in the neck, interfering with airway assessment.
- Dentures that can obstruct the airway (leave them in place if possible during ventilation).
- Skin that is fragile and tears easily.
- Irregular pulse from underlying heart problems.
- Dementia (incidence increases with age), making history taking and treatment difficult.
- Atypical symptoms for illnesses, even if severely ill.
- Multiple comorbidities and multiple medications.
- Shock with BP greater than 100.

Delirium

Delirium is an acute sudden change in consciousness, characterized by reduced ability to focus or sustain attention, language and memory disturbance, disorientation, confusion, audiovisual hallucinations, sleep disturbance, and psychomotor activity disorder. Delirium differs from disorders with similar symptoms in that delirium fluctuates. Delirium occurs in 10%–40% of hospitalized older adults and about 80% of patients who are terminally ill. Delirium may result from drugs, such as anticholinergics, and numerous conditions, including infection, hypoxia, trauma, dementia, depression, vision and hearing loss, surgery, alcoholism, untreated pain, fluid/electrolyte imbalance, and malnutrition. Delirium increases the risks of morbidity and death, especially if untreated. Asking the patient to count backward from 20 to 1 and spell his or her first name backward can identify an attention deficit. Prehospital: Ensure the patient's safety, manage the patient's airway/ventilation/oxygen supplementation, and reorient the patient frequently. Haloperidol is the drug of choice, but it should be reserved for patients who are a risk to themselves or others.

Signs of neglect and lack of supervised care

Children and older or impaired adults may suffer from a profound **neglect or lack of supervision** that places them at risk. Indicators include the following:

- Appearing dirty and unkempt, sometimes with infestations of lice, and wearing ill-fitting or torn clothing and shoes.
- Being tired and sleepy during the daytime.
- Having excessive medical or dental problems, such as extensive dental caries.
- Missing doctor's appointments and not receiving proper immunizations.
- Being underweight for their current stage of development.
- Lacking assistive devices or misplaced hearing aids/eyeglasses.
- Left in soiled or urine-/feces-soiled clothing.
- Clothing is inadequate (such as lack of a coat/sweater during winter or dirty, torn, clothes).

Neglect can be difficult to assess, especially if the paramedic is serving a homeless or very disadvantaged population. Home visits may be needed to ascertain if there is adequate food, clothing, or supervision, and this is beyond the scope of care provided by the paramedic. Thus, suspicions should be reported to the appropriate authorities who can arrange a follow-up assessment of the home environment.

Elder abuse

Physical	Various types of assault related to hitting, kicking, pulling hair, shoving, and pushing. Patients may be forcibly confined, forced into seclusion, and/or force-fed to the point that they choke on food.
Psychological	Caregivers may threaten to hit the patient, brandish a weapon, and tell the person to commit suicide. Ongoing intimidation may make the patient terrified and anxious. Sometimes, caregivers threaten to injure pets or family members, increasing the patient's fear.
Sexual	Types of sexual abuse include the following: Physical: Fondling, kissing, and rape Emotional: Exhibitionism Verbal: Sexual harassment, using obscene language, and threatening

Financial	Financial abuse includes the following:

- Outright stealing of property or persuading patients to give away possessions
- Forcing patients to sign away property
- Emptying bank and savings accounts and using stolen credit cards
- Convincing the person to invest money in fraudulent schemes
- Taking money for home renovations that are not done

Child abuse

Children rarely admit to **abuse** (physical, sexual, or emotional) and often attempt to protect the abusing parent. Therefore, suspicion of abuse depends on other indicators, such as the following:

- **Behavioral:** The child may be overly compliant or fearful with obvious changes in demeanor when a parent/caregiver is present. Some children act out with aggression toward other children or animals. Children may become depressed or suicidal or present with sleeping or eating disorders. Behaviors may become increasingly self-destructive as the child ages, including inappropriate sexualized behavior.
- **Physical:** The type, location, and extent of injuries can raise the suspicion of abuse. Head and facial injuries and bruising are common, as are bite or burn marks and spiral fractures. There may be handprints or grab marks and unusual bruising, such as across the buttocks. Any bruising, swelling, or tearing of the genital area and the identification of sexually transmitted diseases are also causes for concern.

Suspected abuse must be reported to the appropriate authorities, according to protocol, with careful documentation of findings and statements by the child or caregivers.

Injuries consistent with domestic violence/abuse

Characteristic injuries	<ul><li>Ruptured eardrum</li><li>Rectal/genital injury—burns, bites, trauma</li><li>Scrapes and bruises about the neck, face, head, trunk, arms</li><li>Cuts, bruises, and fractures of the face</li><li>Spiral arm fractures (children)</li></ul>
Patterns of injuries	<ul><li>"Bathing suit" pattern—injuries on parts of the body that are usually covered with clothing because the perpetrator wants to hide the evidence of abuse</li><li>Head and neck injuries (50%)</li></ul>
Abusive injuries (rarely attributable to accidents)	<ul><li>Bites, bruises, rope and cigarette burns, and welts in the outline of weapons (belt marks)</li><li>Bilateral injuries of the arms/legs</li></ul>
Defensive injuries	<ul><li>Back-of-the-body injury from being attacked while crouched on the floor facedown</li><li>Located on the soles of the feet from kicking at a perpetrator</li><li>Located on the ulnar aspect of the hands or palm from blocking blows</li></ul>

Muscular dystrophy

Muscular dystrophies are genetic disorders with gradual degeneration of muscle fibers and progressive weakness and atrophy of skeletal muscles and loss of mobility. Pseudohypertrophic (Duchenne) muscular dystrophy is the most common form and is the most severe. Children typically have some delay in motor development, with difficulty walking and have evidence of muscle weakness by about age 3. Pseudohypertrophic refers to enlargement of muscles by fatty infiltration associated with muscular atrophy, which causes contractures and deformities of joints. Abnormal bone development results in spinal and other skeletal deformities. The disease progresses rapidly, and most children are wheelchair bound by about 12 years of age. As the disease progresses, it involves the muscles of the diaphragm and other muscles needed for respiration. Mild to frank mental deficiency is common. Cardiomegaly commonly occurs. Death most often relates to respiratory infection or cardiac failure by age 25. Treatment is supportive. Prehospital: Manage the patient's airway/ventilation/oxygen supplementation, and provide supportive care.

Cerebral palsy (CP)

Cerebral palsy (CP) is a nonprogressive motor dysfunction related to CNS damage associated with congenital, hypoxic, or traumatic injury before birth, during birth, or ≤2 years after birth. CP may include visual defects, speech impairment, seizures and mental retardation. There are four types of motor dysfunction, as follows:

1. Spastic: Constant hypertonia and rigidity lead to contractures and curvature of the spine.
2. Dyskinetic: Tremors and twisting with exaggerated posturing and impairment of voluntary muscle control.
3. Ataxic: Atonic muscles in infancy with lack of balance, instability of muscles, and poor gait later.
4. Mixed: Combinations of all three types with multiple areas of damage.

Characteristics of CP include athetosis (constant writhing motions), ataxia, weakness, or paralysis of all or some extremities. Some patients will remain dependent on others and require lifetime assistance with activities of daily living, but others will be able to function independently. Prehospital: Place in a position of comfort, secure but avoid constraints that prevent athetosis (if present), and allow the patient time to respond because his or her speech may be slow.

EMS Operations

Apparatus and equipment readiness

The paramedic should ensure that the ambulance is ready for use and that the tires are properly inflated, the gas tank is full, warning devices are working, and engine fluid levels are appropriate. All necessary safety equipment, such as PPE (masks, gowns, gloves, and goggles or face guards) and safety devices (safety vests, road flares, and signs) as well as seat belts and harnesses should be available and in proper working condition. All equipment in the cab, the compartments, and the rear of the ambulance should be in the proper place, labeled, and secured to prevent shifting during transportation. High-risk situations include going through intersections, inclement weather (especially with poor visibility), careless drivers, highway access, unpaved roads, and driver distractions (conversation, eating, drinking, mobile devices, music, GPS devices, and fatigue). During transportation, all personnel as well as patients should be properly secured with safety equipment.

Scene-of-incident safety considerations

The paramedic must do a 360° **assessment of the scene** of incident on arrival and determine safety considerations. The paramedic should make note of any gunshots heard, downed power lines, buildings in a state of collapse, leaking fuels/fluids, fire, smoke, broken glass, and other hazards. The paramedic may need to wait until the site is safe to proceed. The paramedic should assess the mechanism of injury (accidents) and the need for appropriate PPE (gloves, gown, mask, and face guard) and must keep the patient informed of all actions and prevent harm or further injury. The ambulance should be parked off of the roadway if possible or parked at a 45° angle (with the front wheels out) to shield the work area, making sure not to block access for other emergency vehicles. Parking uphill is safer than downhill and upwind rather than downwind. If flares are used to warn other drivers, they should extend at least 300 feet from a collision. Yellow warning lights are the scene are safest, but excessive lighting may blind other drivers at night.

Transferring a patient from the scene to an ambulance

Different types of **stretchers and transfer equipment** may be used for prehospital transfer, including the following:

- Wheeled: Stretcher that can be lowered and raised with a wheeled base allowing it to slide into the ambulance.
- Scoop: Two- to four-piece stretcher that can be connected and placed under a patient.
- Transfer sheet: A heavy plastic sheet can be used with patients up to 800 lb. to facilitate transfer.
- Flexible stretcher: Lightweight flexible (plastic, rubberized canvas) stretcher with webbing handles on both sides. Can be used to transfer patients around corners and up and down stairs where a wheeled stretcher cannot be used.
- Stair chair: Safety chair that can be used to transfer patients in tight spaces and up and down stairs.
- Lightweight stretcher: Folding stretcher made of lightweight materials.
- Basket stretcher (Stokes basket): Used primarily for rescues in the wilderness or from cliffs.

Patient positioning should be according to the possible or probable injury, with safety restraints always securing the patient to the gurney and the gurney to the vehicle.

- Left-side-lying: Pregnant patients should be placed in this position to increase circulation to the placenta, and unconscious patients should be placed in this position to prevent aspiration and choking if there is no indication of a spinal injury.
- Supine (flat on the back): Patient has a suspected pelvic fracture or neck injury (also requires a cervical collar).
- Supine (feet elevated above the heart): This is the position for patients in shock to increase circulation to the heart and brain as the BP falls.
- Trendelenburg (the entire stretcher is tilted so that the head is below the feet): Position for patients with a suspected spinal cord injury.
- Semi-Fowler's (30°–45° position): For patients with chest pain, stroke, and/or shortness of breath and no indication of a spinal cord injury.
- Fowler's (upright, 90° position): For patients with severe shortness of breath.

Environmental risk factors

When assessing a patient, it's important to consider that **environmental factors** may place the patient at an increased risk for harm or may be a factor in disease. There are a number of different types of environmental factors to consider.

Factors	Examples	Effects
Toxic chemicals	Lead, arsenic, muriatic acid, sulfuric acid, ammonia, lime	May result in poisoning (lead, arsenic) or burns (acids, ammonia, lime) through direct exposure or inhalation.
Physical objects	Guns, cars, knives, equipment	Accidents, gunshot wounds, stabbings, various injuries (blunt and penetrating).
Biological organisms	Bacteria, fungi, viruses	Infections.
Temperature variations	Heat, cold	Burns, dehydration, heat stroke, hyperthermia, hypothermia, frostbite.
Ambient noise	Sirens, loud music, traffic noise, work-related noise	Hearing loss/deafness, increased anxiety.
Psychosocial	Increased stress	Anxiety, hypertension, suicidal ideation.

Rescues in confined spaces

A **confined space** is one in which access is limited and the space is surrounded by walls or structures that are not suitable for habitation. A confined space may occur in a building (such as with a collapse), a silo, a motor vehicle (such as a large vehicle involved in a crash), a cistern or septic tank, or a well. A confined space may pose a risk to the patient and the paramedic because of difficulty moving about and accessing the patient as well as decreased ventilation that may result in the buildup of toxic gases and/or a lack of oxygen. Before entering a confined space, the paramedic should test the atmosphere and use the correct breathing equipment. This is especially important if the patient is nonresponsive, which is often an indication of poor air quality. The paramedic should also carefully assess his or her ability to access the patient and the best means of doing so.

Driving safety

The **ambulance driver** should stop briefly or slow significantly at intersections because other drivers may not hear or may ignore sirens. The driver should keep the brake covered with the left foot for fast braking and avoid excessive speeds because of the increased risk of accidents, especially on curves. The speed should be adjusted for road and weather conditions and should not be influenced by use of the siren (siren syndrome). Snow and ice should be cleared from the ambulance before driving it. At least one vehicle length should separate the ambulance from other vehicles for every 10 mph of speed. A spotter should always be used when backing up the ambulance because of poor visibility. All personnel in the ambulance should be seated and secured with seat belts or safety harnesses before the ambulance moves. Studies have shown that CPR is most effective if done from a sitting position in an ambulance rather than standing despite common practice. Patients and gurneys should also be secured.

Lights and sirens

Lights and sirens should be used together, and they are indicated when going to a scene and when transporting a patient in a serious emergent situation. There are four types of warning lights used on emergency vehicles such as ambulances: rotating lights (resulting in a flashing sensation), fixed flashes (usually red or blue), strobe lights, and LED lights. Red (the most common) and blue lights are generally used to indicate emergency vehicles and can be used to obtain the right-of-way or to block the right-of-way. These colors may be interchangeable, although in some states the color blue is restricted to law enforcement vehicles. Amber lights are warning lights and can be used by all vehicles, but they do not require others to stop. Some emergency vehicle lights change to amber when the vehicle is parked. White warning lights cannot be used on the rear of an emergency vehicle. Green lights are sometimes used to indicate a mobile incident command post, but in some states, green lights may also indicate private security vehicles or volunteer firefighters.

Incident management

FEMA IS-700.A outlines the **National Incident Management System (NIMS)**, which, under the direction of the Federal Emergency Management Agency (FEMA), an agency of the U.S. Department of Homeland Security, provides the foundation for collaboration among different governmental and nongovernmental agencies, jurisdictions, and specialties/disciplines in handling large-scale incidents that threaten life, property, and/or the environment. Components of FEMA IS-700.A include the following:

- Preparedness: Focuses on planning, procedures and protocols, training and exercises, personnel qualifications/certifications, and equipment certification, and it includes the National Response Framework, which ensures that local jurisdictions retain control but use a unified approach and establish protocols.
- Communications and information management: Systems must be interoperable, reliable, portable, scalable, resilient, and redundant.
- Resource management: Includes personnel, equipment, supplies, and facilities, which must be inventoried and categorized using a standardized approach.
- Command and management: Includes the Incident Command System (this standardized approach outlines the responsibilities of the incident commander, area command, command staff, and general staff), multiagency coordination systems, and public information.
- Management and maintenance: The National Integration Center is responsible for management.

- Flexibility: Components are scalable and adaptable to all types of incidents.
- Standardization: The NIC develops standards in cooperation with standards development organizations.

ICS-100.B, the Incident Command System course, meets NIMS requirements for operational personnel and outlines a standardized approach to incident management. ICS is used for any type of major event, planned or otherwise, and large- or small-scale incidents, including natural (disasters), technological (hazmat release), and human-caused (civil disturbance) hazards. ICS outlines the chain of command (the incident command in control and the orders going through supervisors). Every incident requires an incident action plan, resource management, and processes for reimbursement. The incident commander establishes an incident command post and staging areas (gathering places) as well a base (coordination area for logistic and administrative functions), camps (for sleeping, eating, and sanitary services), helibases, and helispots. Primary features of ICS include common terminology, establishment/transfer of command, chain of command/unity of command, management of objects, incident action planning, modular organization, manageable span of control, comprehensive resource management, incident facilities and locations, integrated communications, information and intelligence management, accountability, and dispatch/deployment.

Chain of command/Unity of command/Unified command

Each organization must establish the **chain of command** for its incident command system. Although these may vary somewhat, an incident commander is ultimately in charge with individuals being assigned as incident managers in different areas, such as triage, treatment, transport, security, and liaison. **Unity of command** means that each incident commander should have control over personnel assigned to his or her area, and each individual within the chain of command should have a clear understanding of whom to report to at the scene so that communication is efficient and timely. **Unified command** means that when multiple agencies are involved from multiple jurisdictions, the chain of command that has been established is recognized and respected even though each agency retains its own authority and accountability and is responsible for carrying out its own duties. A unified command system prevents duplication of effort as well as neglect of important functions.

Incident action plan

The purpose of the **incident action plan** is to outline control objectives, resources, and strategies for dealing with an incident. Incident action plans should be updated frequently. Incident action plans may be designed for various types of incidents and modified as needed to include:

- Goals and objectives, including expected outcomes.
- Strategies and tactics for responding and accomplishing the goals and objectives.
- An outline of the chain of command for the incident command system, including the span of control (the number of people reporting to an individual).
- Tasks assigned to each level in the chain of command.
- Safety/Health plan for responders to prevent injury/illness and to treat as needed.
- Communications plan outlining how information will be exchanged, including alternative methods of command if, for example, cell phone towers are out of commission.
- Logistics plan regarding the acquisition and use of resources, such as supplies, personnel, and equipment.
- Maps and demographic information.

Incident commander

When a multiple-casualty or mass-casualty event occurs, the first lead emergency medical responder on the scene generally assumes the role of **incident commander** and carries out a rapid assessment of the scene and begins to call for additional resources as indicated while another medical responder begins triage. The incident commander should begin to establish a command center in an area that is safe and out of the way of emergency vehicles while awaiting assistance. This first incident commander will relinquish the role when the staffed and/or assigned incident commander arrives to take command, and he or she should then report to the person who is assuming the role of staging officer. The incident commander's duties include establishing command, assessing needs, developing a plan, coordinating all activities, delegating responsibilities, ensuring the safety of all personnel and patients, liaising with other agencies, and communicating information.

Primary triage and resource management

Primary triage is a rapid method (30–60 seconds) of prioritizing patients based on the severity of their condition and is carried out at the scene of multiple casualty incidents. All patients are triaged and tagged according to the following international color-coding priority (P) guidelines on the foot or wrist (not on the clothing):

- P1—Red: Immediate care is needed for urgent systemic life-threatening conditions, such as airway/breathing problems, severe bleeding, severe burns (especially with breathing problems), decreased mental status, shock, and severe medical problems, or a Glasgow Coma Scale score ≤13.
- P2—Yellow: Delayed care and able to wait 45–60 minutes for treatment. Conditions include burns (without breathing problems), multiple bone/joint injuries, back and/or spinal cord injuries (unless the patient is in respiratory distress).
- P3—Green: Hold, able to wait hours for treatment of minor injuries.
- P4—Black: Deceased.

Resource management involves identifying a triage officer, who remains at the scene during the event, and identifying the need for additional personnel and equipment and providing those to the patients with the highest priority.

Secondary triage/retriage

During a mass-casualty incident, triage is done quickly, and patients may be scattered over a wide area with many patients being red-tagged for emergency care. Patients coded black are left in place, but those with other-color tags should be moved and segregated in separate sections of a holding area to await treatment and/or transport. The patients should be **retriaged** as they are moved into the holding area to determine if the tagging color is still appropriate. Additionally, **secondary triage** may be carried out in the separate sections, especially if some must be airlifted, to determine which patients have the best chance of survival and should receive priority for transfer and treatment. Secondary triage may also help to determine which trauma center (based on location or level of care) or hospital is most appropriate for the patient considering the patient's condition, transport time, and the surge capacity of the healthcare institutions.

Centers for Disease Control and Prevention's guidelines for field triage of injured patients

The **CDC's guidelines for field triage** of injured patients is a four-step algorithm that is used to identify the most seriously ill patients and transport them to an appropriate treatment center.

Step	Assess	Findings requiring priority treatment	Plan
1	Vital signs/Level of consciousness	Glasgow Coma Scale score of ≤13, systolic BP <90 mm Hg, respiratory rate <10 or >29 per minutes (<20 in an infant <1 year), or need of ventilatory support.	Highest level trauma center
2	Anatomy of injury	Penetrating injuries, flail chest, ≥ two or more long-bone fractures, crushed/mangled/pulseless extremity, amputations, pelvic fractures, open/depressed skull fracture, or paralysis.	Highest level trauma center
3	Mechanism of injury/High-energy impact	Falls—adults >20 feet and children >10 feet or 2–3 times their height. High-risk auto crash with intrusions, partial or complete ejection, or there is a death in the same passenger compartment. Auto vs. pedestrian/bicycle with victim thrown, run over, or sustaining a significant impact. Motorcycle crash >20 mph.	Trauma center
4	Special patient/system considerations	Older adults, children, pregnancy >30 weeks, burns, patients on anticoagulants or with bleeding disorders (based on the paramedic's best judgment).	Trauma center/ hospital

START method of triage

With the **START method of triage**, the paramedic starts triage with the first victim encountered, tags the patient, and then moves on to the next patient, assessing in order: (1) respirations, (2) perfusion, and (3) mental status (RPM) and using the standard red-yellow-green-black color-coding system. Walking wounded are tagged as green.

Respirations	Present.	Red tag if >30. Continue to perfusion assessment if <30.
	Not present—position the airway.	Red tag if respirations recur or black code (death) if none.
Perfusion	Radial pulse absent or capillary refill of greater than 2 seconds.	Control bleeding and red tag.
	Radial pulse present and capillary refill of less than 2 seconds.	Continue to mental status assessment.
Mental status	Cannot follow simple directions.	Red tag.
	Can follow simple directions.	Yellow tag.

JumpSTART method of triage for pediatric patients

JumpSTART is a pediatric triage method developed only for use in multiple-casualty incidents.

Able to walk	No	Continue to breathing assessment.
	Yes	Green tag. Carry out secondary triage.
Breathing	No	Step 1: Position the upper airway and red tag if breathing. Step 2: Give five rescue breaths and red tag if breathing. Black tag if breathing does not recur.
	Yes	Respiratory rate <15 or >45, red tag. Respiratory rate 15 to 45, continue to pulse assessment.
Palpable pulse	No	Red tag.
	Yes	Continue to AVPU assessment
Alert, voice, pain, unresponsive (AVPU) assessment	Inappropriate pain, posturing, or unresponsive	Red tag.
	A, V, or P is appropriate	Yellow tag.

Critical incident stress management (CISM)

Critical incident stress management (CISM) is a procedure to help people cope with stressful events, such as disasters, in order to reduce the incidence of post-traumatic stress syndrome (PTSS).

- Defusing sessions usually occur very early, sometimes during or immediately after a stressful event, and they are used to educate personnel who are actively involved about what to expect over the next few days and to provide guidance in handling their feelings and stress levels.
- Debriefing sessions usually follow in one to three days and may be repeated periodically as needed. These sessions may include people who were directly involved as well as those who were indirectly involved. People are encouraged to express their emotions about the event. Critiquing the event or attempting to place blame is not productive as part of the CISM process.
- Follow-up is done at the end of the process, usually after about week, but this time frame can vary.

Air medical transport

Air medical transport is indicated when the patient is in need of a high level of care that may be available on an aircraft but not an ambulance, when the patient's condition and need for treatment are time critical, when the patient is located in a remote area where access by ambulance is difficult or would be delayed (helicopter), or when local medical services have exceeded their capacity. Helipads are often available at large hospitals, so the patient can be treated immediately after arrival. Some disadvantages include inclement weather (which may interfere with flight plans) as well as altitude and airspeed limitations. Depending on the aircraft, the cabin size may be inadequate for the patient, personnel, and equipment. Difficult terrain, such as forested or hilly areas may not provide an adequate landing site. Cost is the biggest difference between ground and air transport with air transport often costing tens of thousands of dollars with only part, or in some cases none, of the costs being covered by insurance.

The pilot in command (PIC) of rotorcraft and fixed-wing aircraft is responsible for the **safety** of the aircraft, crew, emergency medical personnel, and the patient. As with all takeoffs and landings, the medical staff and crew must be seated and secured by seat belts. Helmets should be in place and secure. Patients who are violent, confused, or combative should be physically restrained for transport and may also require chemical restraints to ensure their own personal safety as well as the safety of the medical and flight crew. Patients should be offloaded ONLY when a crew member signals the receiving medical personnel to approach the aircraft. With high-altitude fixed-wing air transports, cabins are pressurized but only to the equivalent of 6000–8000 feet, not to sea level. Rotorcraft are usually used to transfer a patient from the scene of an incident to a primary care facility or from the primary care facility to another type of facility, whereas a fixed-wing aircraft is usually used from one facility to another over longer distances.

A **communication specialist** should coordinate all air medical services, including communications within an agency and between agencies regarding all aspects of transport. The communication specialist should have radio communication skills and knowledge of medical terminology, including knowledge of how to obtain information about a patient, navigation, map usage, customer service, weather, aircraft emergencies, as well as FAA and Federal Communications Commission (FCC) regulations that relate to air medical transport. The communication specialist should be familiar with the radio frequencies utilized by emergency medical services. The dispatcher determines whether an aircraft should take off. The communication center may be located in a medical facility, airport, or other space, but it should be free of distractions and have emergency backup electrical power. All air medical transport team members should have knowledge of the radio communication system. Some systems include radio or radio-phone communication, and some systems require team members to carry pagers, such as two-way satellite pagers. All incoming and outgoing communication should be recorded.

Helicopters have the advantage over fixed-wing aircraft of being able to load a patient at or near the scene rather than having to transport the patient by ambulance to an airport. A paved surface is not necessary for a helicopter landing site, but level grassy or paved sites are preferred, ideally with 100 × 100 feet of clear space, but a minimum area of 60 × 60 feet may be used. Additionally, the area should be free of debris that may be disrupted by the rotor blades and should be clear of structures that may interfere with the aircraft, such as power poles, tall trees, power lines, cables, and antennas. A rotor aircraft does not require that people approach in a crouching position, but people should avoid holding anything over their heads and should generally approach from the front of the aircraft and avoid the rear of the aircraft and the rear rotors.

State statutes require that aircraft used for air ambulance service must be licensed to provide that service, and the service must ensure that all required medical equipment is available. Although statutes may vary slightly from one state to another, most require that the service be able to provide basic and advanced life support and should provide patients with a description of services and costs. Additionally, the aircraft and crew must comply with Federal Aviation Administration (FAA) regulations and carry insurance to cover injuries that may occur in transport. The FAA carries out periodic inspections of aircraft and issues resource documents regarding safety and operations. Federal regulations establish weather guidelines for safe flying. The U.S. Department of Transportation provides guidelines regarding standards of care. The Commission on Accreditation of Medical Transport Systems establishes voluntary accreditation standards, but air medical services associated with hospitals must meet hospital accreditation standards, typically those of the Joint Commission.

Scene management at the site of a vehicle extrication

Scene management at the site of an accident that requires vehicle extrication incudes initial evaluation of any hazards at the site (360° evaluation), such as oncoming traffic, fallen wires, spilled fuel, and fire/explosion risk or presence. The scene must be secured (45° parking, police security, flares, and cones) and EMS should don protective equipment as necessary and access the patient to provide life-saving care. The patient must be disentangled from the motor vehicle as much as can be done safely. The patient is prepared for extrication (such as by applying pressure to bleeding sites and placing a cervical collar), removed from the vehicle, and then prepared for ground or air transport and provided emergent treatment. For extrications in difficult terrain, assess the following:

- <u>Terrain</u>: Forests, desert, cliff, water, snow.
- <u>Obstacles</u>: Trees, rocks, light, unavailability of landing sites.
- <u>Methods to be used:</u> Helicopter extrication, overland carry, type of extrication.
- <u>Alternative solutions:</u> Abort; contact search and rescue.
- <u>Safety issues:</u> Review all safety concerns.

Motor vehicle extrication (car, truck)

For **vehicle extrication,** the vehicle must be stabilized before EMS personnel attempt to enter the vehicle or administer aid to the patient, especially if the vehicle may slide or is on its side and rescue personnel must access the vehicle from the top because the vehicle may shift and further endanger the patient as well as EMS personnel. EMS personnel can access the vehicle through a window (breaking it if necessary) or a door if one is operable (the patient may be able to assist in opening a window or door). EMS personnel should carry an airway (in case the patient requires ventilation), dressings (to apply pressure if the patient is bleeding), and a rigid cervical collar (to protect against spinal injury or further spinal damage), and they should do rapid triage on access to the patient. Oxygen is usually not administered until after the patient is extracted because of the danger of fire, especially if the patient is saturated with fuel, and CPR is not done until the patient is in the supine position on a solid surface. If patients are apneic and pulseless, they must be removed as quickly as possible even with only manual protection of the spine being provided.

For **vehicle extrication**, once EMS personnel have gained access to the motor, they should unlock its doors if possible to allow others to more easily gain access. EMS personnel should ensure that the engine is turned off, the parking brake is set, and the transmission is set to park. If possible, an emergency response person should disconnect the battery to decrease the risk of fire and explosion. If the patient can be removed, a short backboard should be applied before moving the patient. If the patient is wedged between the seat and the steering wheel, the seat may be slid back manually while rescuers support the patient. If the seat has become dislodged from the track, then the patient should be completely immobilized because this type of mechanical damage can result in severe physical injury. If the patient's legs are trapped, lifting the steering wheel away may also lift the dashboard and help to release the patient.

If a patient must be **cut from a vehicle** (such as when the vehicle is on its side and access must be through a U-shaped flap in the roof), he or she should be warned of the noise and should be covered with a safety blanket (heavy aluminized). In some accidents, **air bags** may not deploy, but movement of the patient or vehicle may cause them to deploy, resulting in danger to the patient and

EMS personnel. If the air bags have not deployed, then the battery cables should be disconnected or cut (negative side first) to prevent deployment and personnel should avoid being in front of the path of deployment. EMS personnel

should check for side air bags as well as front. The air bags should be deactivated before the steering column is moved (keeping in mind that deactivation can take up to 30 minutes), and care should be taken to avoid cutting or drilling into an air bag.

Since the 1990s, vehicles have been equipped with **seat belt pretensioners** on three-point (shoulder harness) systems in the front and often also in the back. The purpose of seat belt pretensioners is to tighten any slack in the belts in an accident, pulling the person back into the seat and in the proper position for deployment of the air bag. Evidence of pretensioners is not always visible, although an accordion sleeve near the buckle end may be an indication. This sleeve compresses if the pretensioner fires. Although an undeployed pretensioner poses less threat to EMS personnel than an undeployed air bag, it can increase the risk of injury to the patient or EMS personnel, so the seat belt should be disconnected or cut immediately on access to the patient. If the patient was not wearing the seat belt on impact and the pretensioner fired, the seat belt will be tightly vertical along pillar B. If the seat belt pretensioner fired while being worn, it will be extended and will not be retractable.

Although large and heavy pieces of equipment, such as hydraulic rescue tools (including the Jaws of Life, cutters, spreaders, truck jacks, and rams), pneumatic tools, and come-along tools, are often used in vehicle extrication, a tool kit with **simple hand tools** should also be readily available. Hand tools may also be needed to access and safely remove a patient from a vehicle. Tools that may be needed for disassembly include adjustable wrenches, screwdrivers (flat and Phillips), flashlight, penlight, medical scissors, headlamp, pliers, bolt cutters, hammers, axes, crowbars, rescue knives (specially designed to cut through seat belts and clothing), and tin snips. Combination rescue tools are available that can be used for a variety of purposes, such as shutting off gas valves, prying open windows, and cutting through battery cables. Tool belt pouches are available to hold small tools that may be needed during an extrication.

Cribbing and chocking are used to raise a vehicle and prevent it from rolling, such as when a patient is caught beneath a vehicle. Cribbing consists of 2×4 blocks and wedges and 4×4 blocks and wedges that are used to create crib boxes to hold an air bag. Cribs are usually made of Douglas fir or southern yellow pine, which can hold 500 psi and crushes slowly. The cribbing is stacked with a 4-inch overhang (to allow for compression), and it should not exceed 48 inches in height. The crib box is put in place with the air bag on top. Chocks are large stepped wedges that are placed in front of or behind the wheels to keep them from rolling when the air bag is inflated. As the air bag is slowly inflated, capture cribbing stacks are placed on both sides behind it to hold the vehicle when the air bag is deflated. Once the vehicle is elevated and secured, the air bag is deflated and the crib box is removed to allow room for extrication of the patient.

Some vehicles are powered by **alternative fuels**, such as compressed natural gas (CNG) or liquefied natural gas (LNG), so EMS personnel should look for CNG/LNG logos, often on the right rear or near the refueling port or the right rear of the cab (semitruck). A "natural gas vehicle" warning may be located near the bottom of the rear doors. CNG tanks may be located behind cabs in semitractors, and some may have additional saddle tanks. The power should be turned off and the 12-volt battery positive and negative cables should be cut. The emergency shut-off valve should be located and turned off, although each tank can also be turned off manually. Electric vehicles pose the risk of stranded energy. Batteries should always be considered energized with a potential for high-voltage injury. Damaged lithium ion batteries that are leaking or sparking are at risk for thermal runaway (fire). The car battery should be shut down immediately. If the battery is damaged, the vehicle must be relocated at least 50 feet from any combustible material.

Bus extrication

Before accessing patients involved in a **bus crash,** the bus must be stabilized, especially if it is on its side or if it is upside down. If the engine is still running, a stop button is often located on the left side of the front panel. Access to the bus may be through the front door if possible. Access may also be through the front windshield (which can be removed through removal of the rubber locking strip that surrounds the window), side windows, the emergency exit door or window, the bathroom window, or an opening cut into the top of the vehicle. Removal of injured patients (usually on stretchers) from inside the vehicle often requires rapid triage and assistance of multiple EMS personnel. If the vehicle remains upright but patients are completely or partially beneath the vehicle, they should be removed quickly because they may be crushed if the air suspension system deflates.

Aircraft extrication

Communication is essential if EMS personnel are responding to an **aircraft crash site** because the paramedics need to know when the crash occurred, the type and size of the aircraft, the number of passengers and crew, reports of fire or explosion, and whether the aircraft is private, commercial, or military as well as the status (fire, collapse) of any structure(s) that the aircraft may have impacted. For a small plane with the cabin still reasonably intact, extrication may be similar to a motor vehicle, but severe crashes in which the cabin is destroyed and large airplane crashes pose significantly different problems because passengers may have been thrown about inside or outside of the aircraft and seats and belongings and body parts may block access. Victims may lie in the roadway, so emergency vehicles must proceed with caution. Fire and explosions may be a severe risk, and rescuers may need to wait for fire suppression. Triage may begin outside of the aircraft while the aircraft (or the remains of the aircraft) is secured.

Extrication considerations

Part of the stabilization of the scene is ensuring that it is secure. An **outer perimeter** is established to block public and media access, and an **inner perimeter** is established immediately around the scene of the rescue and the working crew. Three **control zones** are established as follows:

- Hot (coded red): This encompasses the inner perimeter and the crew as well as any area that is dangerous, such as an area contaminated by hazardous material or one in danger of release of toxins.
- Warm (coded orange): Area for trained personnel in support of those in the hot zone. Decontamination of patients, crew, and equipment is carried out in this zone.
- Cold (coded yellow): This is the staging area and the command post (if necessary for the emergent situation). No members of the public or media should be allowed in the cold zone.

Zones are usually established by placement of police cars and fire-line tape.

The **path of least resistance** is an important concept to understand for rescues, especially if they involve fire and any products of combustion (smoke, heat, gas). Fire's path of least resistance is usually vertical and upward, although fire also spreads horizontally, especially if a vertical path is not available. It's for this reason that if there is a fire on the top floor of a building, the roof is breached to prevent horizontal spread. External factors, such as gusts of wind, can affect the path of least resistance. Water, on the other hand, also flows vertically, but downward and then horizontally if the downward flow is blocked. If the paramedic is rescuing patients from a building, they will often be found near the path of least resistance, such as a near a door or window. Patients should also be transported according to the path of least resistance, that is, the route that is the easiest and safest.

Multistep rescue process

The **multistep rescue process** includes the following 10 steps:

1. Preparation: Training, readying equipment, and preparing for different types of rescues.
2. Response: Using protocols for dispatch; contacting others, such as utility companies, which may have the necessary knowledge or equipment.
3. Situation size-up: 360° site survey to identify hazards and determine the need for additional personnel or equipment. Determine if the situation is rescuer/equipment intensive.
4. Stabilization: Establishing perimeters and control zones, monitoring hazardous atmosphere, carrying out lockout/tagout of industrial equipment.
5. Access: Gaining access to the patient and providing emergent care.
6. Disentanglement: Freeing the patient.
7. Removal: Continuing critical and life support while assisting the patient to move or carrying the immobilized patient. Rapid extraction if his or her condition is life threatening.
8. Transport: Transporting by various means with decontamination done as needed.
9. Scene security: Police or others providing protection of the scene, crew, and patients.

Postevent analysis: Reviewing procedures performed and the problems encountered.

Occupational Safety and Health Administration (OSHA)

The **Occupational Safety and Health Administration** (OSHA) is part of the U.S. Department of Labor, and it is charged with ensuring safe, healthful working conditions and setting and enforcing workplace standards. OSHA covers most employers in the private sector, but state and federal safety regulations also generally conform to OSHA standards. Employers must provide safety training, inform workers of chemical hazards, and provide required PPE. OSHA must be notified of a workplace-related death within 8 hour and a workplace-related injury that results in hospitalization, the loss of an eye, or amputation within 24 hours. Workers may file a complaint about workplace conditions with OSHA and request an inspection. OSHA's Whistleblower Protection Program prohibits retaliation by the employer. OSHA provides Hazardous Waste Operations and Emergency Response Standard (HAZWOPER) training courses (8-hour, 24-hour, 40-hour, and refresher) for first responders. OSHA has established regulations and guidelines that are industry specific. For example, OSHA has regulations regarding EMS. OSHA requires that hazardous material be color coded, with red indicating danger; yellow, caution; orange, warning; and fluorescent orange/orange-red, biological hazard.

Hazardous materials and waste

Hazardous materials are any that may cause harm (health or physical hazard) to humans or animals by themselves or through interaction with something else. Hazardous materials may be any of the following:

- Chemical: These include blister agents, blood agents, choking agents, nerve agents, asphyxiants, and irritants. These can enter the body through inhalation, absorption, ingestion, and injection.

- 191 -

- Radiological: Nuclear material and radioactive substances (alpha/beta particles).
- Physical/Biological: Infectious wastes, blood and other body fluids, and biotoxins.

Almost any material or substance can be classified as hazardous depending on various factors, such as its location, amount, and interactions. Exposure occurs when a person/animal comes in contact with the hazardous material, and contamination is the residue resulting from exposure. Absorption is the method by which hazardous material enters the bloodstream. Exposure and contamination may result in an immediate response (blistering, itching, and pain) or a delayed response (nausea, vomiting, cancer, and lung disease).

The Environmental Protection Agency (EPA) classifies **hazardous wastes** according to the following characteristics:

- Ignitable: Liquids and nonliquids that can ignite and cause fires with flash points of <60°C/140°F).
- Corrosive: Based on pH (<2 or >12.5) or the ability to corrode steel.
- Reactive: Wastes that are unstable, may react with water, or that may result in toxic gases. They may also explode.
- Toxic: Heavy metal compounds that are harmful if ingested or absorbed.

Wastes may also be classified as listed wastes. These include wastes from manufacturing and industrial processes. Hazardous wastes are often produced in manufacturing, nuclear power plants (nuclear wastes), and healthcare facilities (needles and materials contaminated with body fluids). Nuclear wastes are classified as mixed waste because they contain a radioactive component as well as a hazardous component. Hazardous wastes can result in disease (such as from needle punctures), injury (from fire and explosions), and death (from toxic exposure and disease).

The purpose of **hazardous waste site characterization** is to identify hazards and select the appropriate PPE. The team leader is responsible for the assessment, but he or she may request assistance from outside experts, such as chemists. The three steps to site characterization include:

- Offsite characterization: Gather information/data before personnel enter the site, including the location, a description of the activities, the duration of the event, terrain information (photographs, maps), habitation/population data, accessibility, paths of least resistance, and properties of any hazardous materials/substances. Conduct the needed interviews and review of records. Perimeter reconnaissance is done with observations, air sampling, and development of a preliminary site map.
- Onsite survey: Verify the information gathered from perimeter reconnaissance, survey the area and situation, note potential exposure to hazardous materials (dust, liquid, dead animals, gas) and safety hazards (obstacles, terrain, poisonous plants), and develop a site safety plan. The entry team should have at least four members: two to enter and two for outside support who can enter the site in an emergency.
- Ongoing monitoring: Monitoring should be continuous.

Types of **chemical hazardous waste materials** include the following:

- <u>Blister agents:</u> Include sulfur mustard (mustard gas) and nitrogen mustard, which are both highly toxic. Exposure by inhalation, contact, or ingestion results in skin irritation (erythema and blistering) and eye irritation and injury to the respiratory system as well as bone marrow suppression and gastrointestinal and neurological damage. The patient should be decontaminated within 1 to 2 minutes by flushing the eyes with water for up to 20 minutes and removing clothing and showering with soap (if available) and water for 20 minutes. Rescuers should use a self-contained breathing apparatus (SCBA), PPE (including eye protection), and chemical-protective gloves.
- <u>Asphyxiants:</u> Gas exposure (such as by butane, helium, and propane) lowers oxygen levels and results in suffocation. Patients require oxygen administration and may need CPR. This is especially a risk in confined spaces. Rescuers should use an SCBA.
- <u>Blood agents:</u> These include cyanide chloride, hydrogen cyanide, and arsine. Exposure by inhalation or ingestion. They prevent oxygen transfer from blood to cells. The patient may need oxygen and an antidote. Rescuers should use an SCBA.
- <u>Carcinogens:</u> Agents such as asbestos, nickel compounds, and ionizing radiation that result in genetic mutation and cancer. There are various types of exposure. Patients must be removed from exposure. The rescuer must wear adequate PPE, and in some cases, he or she should use a mask or SCBA.
- <u>Choking agents:</u> Often, a chemical weapon is used (ammonia, chlorine) that is designed to inhibit breathing and incapacitate the person. Exposure is by inhalation, contact, or ingestion (rare). They may be corrosive to the skin and result in fluid in the lungs, leading to suffocation. Patients require supportive treatment and oxygen. Rescuers should use PPE and SCBA for most agents.
- <u>Convulsants/Nerve agents:</u> These include hydrazine and strychnine. Exposure may be by inhalation, contact, and ingestion. The severity of convulsion and nervous system impairment is dose related. Patients require supportive treatment. Rescuers need SCBA and protective suits (according to the exposure level of the agent).

Safety data sheets (SDSs)

Safety data sheets (SDSs), formerly known as material safety data sheets (MSDSs), explain how to handle caustic substances in the event of an accident or injury and provide pertinent information on the composition and toxic effects of the chemicals in a lab. SDSs outline the proper storage of chemicals, procedures for cleanup and dumping of caustic substances, procedures in the event of a chemical spill or injury, and proper locations in the facility for cleanup. The SDS should also contain information indicating which substances may cause allergic effects or asthma from contact or inhalation. Emergency rescue services should obtain SDSs for common chemicals and products. Manufacturers and suppliers should have SDSs on file and can be contacted for copies. The OSHA/Environmental Protection Agency (EPA) Occupational Chemical Database provides links for SDSs for some products. SDSs are available from various other sources, including the Toxicology Data Network (TOXNET) and poison control centers. There are also pathogen safety data sheets for biological hazards.

Multiple-casualty incidents versus mass-casualty incidents

Multiple-casualty incident

- Involves more than one person, but different jurisdictions may quantify the total number of persons differently. Usually refers to an incident involving at least three patients.
- Usually involves only one jurisdiction and only one to three agencies (ambulance, fire department, and police).
- Requires triage, but generally only primary.
- Standards of care are maintained, and all patients not coded black (deceased) are transported for care.

Mass-casualty incident

- Also involves more than one person but may involve much larger numbers—dozens, hundreds, to thousands.
- Often involves multiple jurisdictions and agencies.
- Requires triage but may also involve separate waiting areas for color-coded individuals and secondary triage.
- Standards of care may be modified and patients coded black (expectant) and not expected to live may be left in the field and/or receive delayed care if they are still living after red- and yellow-coded individuals are transported.

Role of the transportation officer in a mass-casualty incident

During a mass-casualty event, the **transportation officer** must maintain constant communication with hospitals and trauma centers, triage officers, police, ground ambulance services, and air medical transport services. The transportation officer controls the flow of patients for treatment and must determine where to route patients in order to prevent a backlog at the receiving facility and must coordinate incoming and outgoing ambulances in the transportation staging area. The transportation officer must obtain information about each facility's surge capacity and the number and types of patients that the facility is prepared to care for. The transportation officer must also coordinate air medical transport flights and determine, with the triage officer, which patient to transport by air according to the severity of their injuries, availability of treatment options, and appropriate levels of care. The speed of transportation and care is often critical in a mass-casualty incident because delays often result in increased death rates.

Role of triage in a mass-casualty incident related to terrorism or a disaster

In a mass-casualty incident related to terrorism or a disaster, **rapid triage** and tagging must occur and patients must be sorted according to priority for transportation or field treatment. Because of the large numbers of casualties, triage should begin with the first patient encountered, proceeding from one to another. According to some plans, patients who are alive but expected to die are coded red, but this can result in overtriage, with too many red-coded individuals having to be transported and/or treated, resulting in patients dying during the wait. With other plans, patients expected to die are black-coded as "expectant" and left in the field or left aside until red- and yellow-coded individuals are transported and/or treated. If patients are undertriaged (such as patients who should be coded red being coded yellow instead) this can also result in increased deaths while other patients are waiting for transport and/or treatment.

Mass casualty shooting and improvised explosive device (IED) incidents

Terrorist or other attacks that involve active shooters or improvised explosive devices (IEDs) often result in injuries similar to those encountered in combat situations in which the most common

- 194 -

causes of death are extremity hemorrhage, tension pneumothorax, and airway obstruction. The **THREAT acronym** provides guidance for dealing with these situations in the following ways:

- <u>Threat suppression:</u> Use of police protection, ballistic vests, concealment, cover, and situational awareness. One concern is that most of the protective gear available to emergency medical personnel is for ballistics rather than explosive devices.
- <u>Hemorrhage control:</u> Use of tourniquets (military style) and hemostatic dressings (QuikClot) to control bleeding.
- <u>Rapid extrication to safety:</u> Move patients and personnel out of the danger zone to prevent further injuries.
- <u>Assessment by medical providers:</u> Includes provision of a nasopharyngeal airway or upright seating and leaning forward for airway compromise and spinal precautions.
- <u>Transport to definitive care:</u> Medical treatment should continue during transport.

Safety issues associated with active shooter and terrorist bomb attacks

With **active shooters,** standard protocol has been for emergency response services to wait until the police have removed the threat and secured the area before moving in to care for victims; however, this delay in treatment may result in death, so some authorities are now recommending that emergency response personnel enter the scene with police while wearing appropriate protective equipment although this does pose some risk, especially with additional shooters or secondary attack.

With a **terrorist bombing** and improvised explosive devices (IEDs), situational awareness is critical because multiple explosive devices (some undetonated) may be at the scene. IEDs may be inside backpacks, suitcases, and packages left unattended, but in emergency situations, innocent people often drop backpacks and packages and run away. Additionally, attackers wearing suicide vests or belts may mix in with other victims or people escaping the blast area.

Bomb threat standoff recommendations

Threat	Explosive capacity (lb)	Mandatory evacuation distance (ft)	Preferred evacuation distance (ft)	Shelter-in-place zone (ft)
Pipe bomb	5	70	1200+	71–1199
Suicide bomber	20	110	1700+	111–1699
Suitcase/ Briefcase	50	150	1850+	151–1849
Automobile	500	320	1900+	321–1899
SUV/Van	1000	400	2400+	401–2399
Small truck	4000	640	3800+	641–3799
Container truck	10,000	860	5100+	861–5099
Semitrailer	60,000	1570	9300+	1571–9299

Source: U.S. Department of Homeland Security.

B-NICE hazardous material (hazmat) incidents associated with terrorist attacks

Category	Response
B—Biological (bacteria, viruses, fungi, and toxins)	Inhalation type—evacuate for 80 feet, shut down air-handling systems, wear appropriate PPE and SCBA, and avoid contamination. Visible agent—decontaminate with soap and water. Symptoms may vary but are usually delayed.
N—Nuclear/Radiological	Inhalation type (most common)—Isolate/Secure the area, avoid smoke/fumes, stay upwind, and use PPE and SCBA. Isolate victims and decontaminate as appropriate. Symptoms are usually delayed.
I—Incendiary	Be on alert for multiple devices and sabotaged fire suppression equipment. Symptoms include burns, pain, and trauma.
C—Chemical	Isolate/Secure the area, decontaminate victims with soap and water, and be on alert for chemical dispersal devices. Approach toward uphill and upwind. Isolate symptomatic patients from others. Symptoms vary but may include burns, blistering, vomiting, breathing difficulty, and neurological damage.
E—Explosives	Be alert for secondary devices, undetonated devices, and secondary hazards (unstable buildings and debris). Remove victims from the area, secure the perimeter, and stage away from the incident area. Decontaminate as necessary. Symptoms include burns, amputations, cuts, and penetrating and blunt trauma.

"All-hazards" safety approach to mass-casualty incidents

The **"all-hazards" safety approach** to mass-casualty incidents aims to provide plans that can be used to deal with all types of hazards (natural disasters, terrorist attacks, and mass-casualty incidents) as well as encompassing the four components of emergency management: mitigation, preparedness, response, and recovery. Organizations in an area coordinate to develop joint action plans that can be activated in response to incidents with the chain of command clearly outlined. This approach lowers costs to individual organizations and provides for faster and more effective response. However, although the basic structure may be the same for responding to all hazards, there are inevitable differences between (for example) a terrorist attack with active shooters and a natural disaster, such as a hurricane, which can be anticipated and mitigated to some degree. For this reason, modifying existing incident action plans to meet the needs of a situation is essential.

Treating terrorists and criminals

In mass-casualty incidents, **terrorists and criminals** involved in the incident may be injured and require treatment, and EMS personnel may feel conflicted about providing treatment when others have been injured or killed, but it's important to provide treatment to terrorists and criminals the same as any other individuals because (1) they are in need of help and (2) their survival may be critical to identifying coconspirators and to providing reasons for the attack. However, these individuals may pose risks to emergency medical personnel, so they should be examined while under police guard. The individual's hands should be examined first to check for weapons and detonators and secured (with handcuffs, if possible). Clothes should be examined and removed very carefully in case the person is wearing a suicide device of some type. Emergency medical personnel should also be aware that the individuals may be feigning injury or unconsciousness.

Paramedic Practice Test

1. Which of the following statements regarding allergies is **FALSE**?

    a. A type I allergic reaction can be life-threatening
    b. Immunity can be natural or acquired
    c. Anaphylactoid reactions are mediated by an antigen-antibody reaction
    d. Immunity can be artificially induced

2. All of the following patients are at high risk of latex allergy **except**

    a. Tollbooth operators
    b. Asthmatics
    c. Hairdressers
    d. Patients with allergic rhinitis

3. You are called by the husband of a 25-year-old woman who has developed a severe allergic reaction to shellfish. On arrival, the woman's face is swollen, and hives appear on her arms and legs. She complains of tightness in her neck and has difficulty breathing. The first step in treating this patient is to

    a. Administer IV epinephrine
    b. Transport the patient to the hospital
    c. Administer high-concentration oxygen
    d. Administer IV saline solution

4. All of the following drugs may be given safely in addition to epinephrine **except**

    a. Beta agonists
    b. Beta-blockers
    c. Antihistamines
    d. Corticosteroids

5. Which of the following is **NOT** a typical sign of an allergic reaction?

    a. Urticaria
    b. Diarrhea
    c. Bronchoconstriction
    d. Altered mental status

6. In performing defibrillation, the paddles should be placed

    a. Over the sternum
    b. Over the pacemaker
    c. To the right of the upper sternum and to the left of the left nipple
    d. To the left of the upper sternum and to the right of the right nipple

7. In performing defibrillation, the following may be used to decrease paddle-skin interface resistance

    a. Creams used in ECG monitoring
    b. Pads soaked in alcohol
    c. Pads soaked in water
    d. Pads soaked in saline

8. In performing defibrillation, you should

    a. Remove nitroglycerin patches before defibrillation
    b. Place the paddles together before firing the defibrillator
    c. Alternate cardiopulmonary resuscitation with defibrillation
    d. Perform open air discharge of the defibrillator to remove an unwanted charge

9. Which of the following statements regarding asynchronous cardiac pacing is **FALSE**

    a. Asynchronous pacing is typically used in asystole
    b. Asynchronous pacing may be used to control dysrhythmia
    c. Asynchronous pacemakers are used more frequently than demand pacemakers
    d. The asynchronous mode may be used to determine heartbeat in cases of electrocardiogram interference

10. Transcutaneous cardiac pacing should be used in

    a. Patients with open wounds
    b. Bradycardia
    c. Cardiac arrest
    d. Pulseless electrical activity

11. According to American Hospital Association guidelines, in which of the following cases is resuscitation appropriate?

    a. Presence of a DNAR order
    b. Septic shock
    c. Asystole
    d. Drug overdose

12. Which of the following statements regarding biphasic defibrillation is **FALSE**?

    a. Biphasic defibrillation of 115 J is equivalent to 200 J monophasic defibrillation
    b. Initial defibrillation should be 4 J/kg for a pediatric patient
    c. Initial defibrillation should be at 360 J monophasic energy
    d. The optimal current for ventricular defibrillation is 30 to 40 A

13. You are called to the home of an 88-year-old woman suffering from an acute pulmonary episode. The patient complains of extreme dyspnea. She is sitting upright but leaning forward and breathing through pursed lips; wheezing and rhonchi are evident. Initial assessment of this patient indicates that she is suffering from

    a. COPD
    b. Asthma
    c. ARDS
    d. Pneumonia

14. The signs and symptoms in the patient described above are indicative of

    a. Pneumonia
    b. Bronchitis
    c. Emphysema
    d. Asthma

15. Typical signs and symptoms of chronic bronchitis include

a. Nonproductive cough
b. Pink or red complexion
c. Chronic cyanosis
d. Pursed-lip breathing

16. All of the following are indicated in treatment of a patient in respiratory distress **except**

a. Establishing an IV line
b. Applying a cardiac monitor
c. Pulse oximetry
d. Withholding oxygen

17. Which of the following letters in the acronym OPQRST used in obtaining a history of a patient in respiratory distress is **INCORRECT**?

a. O = onset
b. S = sensitivity
c. P = provocation
d. Q = quality

18. Which of the following is indicative of a perfusion problem?

a. Asthma
b. Atherosclerosis
c. Shock
d. Carbon monoxide poisoning

19. Which of the following statements regarding obstructive airway disease is **TRUE**?

a. A patient can manifest COPD and asthma at the same time
b. Patients with emphysema are referred to as "blue bloaters"
c. Patients with chronic bronchitis are referred to as "pink puffers"
d. Childhood asthma usually persists throughout adulthood

20. The wife of a 50-year-old man calls for assistance for her husband, who is having a severe asthma attack. On arrival, the patient is in respiratory distress, with loud and rapid respirations and audible wheezing. The patient's wife states that he has recently discontinued corticosteroid therapy. After administering oxygen, the next step should be to

a. Administer CPAP
b. Administer albuterol
c. Administer BiPAP
d. Administer ketamine

21. Inspiratory wheezing in the patient described above may indicate

a. Upper airway occlusion
b. Respiratory failure
c. Secretions in the large airways
d. Pneumonia

22. A PEFR test is most often used

    a. In patients in severe respiratory distress
    b. In children less than 5 years of age
    c. Before drug administration
    d. In patients with ARDS

23. The sister of an 85-year-old woman calls for assistance, stating that she thinks her sister is having a stroke. On arrival, the patient is conscious but slightly confused and her speech is slurred. Her sister states that a few moments ago, the patient appeared disoriented and did not seem to recognize her own name; she also has a history of hypertension. The patient states that she feels better and does not want to go to the hospital. Proper initial treatment for this patient should include

    a. Managing hypertension
    b. Establishing time of symptom onset and transporting
    c. Administering anticoagulant therapy
    d. Performing a CT scan

24. All of the following are useful in the diagnosis of stroke **except**

    a. CPSS
    b. LAPSS
    c. Medical history
    d. 50% Dextrose

25. The following statements regarding TIAs are true **except**

    a. The signs and symptoms of a TIA are the same as those of stroke
    b. A TIA is the most important predictor of a brain infarction
    c. TIAs are associated with permanent neurological damage
    d. Initial assessment of a patient with a TIA is the same as that of a stroke victim

26. You are called to the home of a 40-year-old woman complaining of severe "gas pains" and cramps in her stomach. On arrival, the patient is lying on the couch, holding her lower abdomen. She states that she was experiencing severe cramping in her lower abdomen, with profuse sweating and nausea; the pain progressed in severity but has now subsided. The first step in caring for this patient is to

    a. Conduct an initial scene survey
    b. Offer pain medication
    c. Transport to the hospital
    d. Perform a complete physical examination

27. In using the mnemonic OPQRST to obtain a history of abdominal pain, the letter P stands for

    a. Pain onset
    b. Pain severity
    c. Past medical history
    d. Provocation

28. Which of the following would NOT be considered in obtaining a SAMPLE history for the patient described above?

    a. Change in bowel habits
    b. Regularity of menstrual periods
    c. Pain location
    d. Last meal or oral intake

29. An example of a condition associated with visceral pain is

    a. Cholecystitis
    b. Peritonitis
    c. Ulcer
    d. Morphine addiction

30. After obtaining a thorough patient history from the patient described in Question 26, you find that she has had 2 or 3 previous episodes of cramping pain, increasing in intensity, then quickly subsiding. Pain radiates to the right upper quadrant and usually occurs at night, especially after consuming fried or fatty foods. This patient is probably suffering from

    a. Pancreatitis
    b. Cholecystitis
    c. Crohn's disease
    d. Bowel obstruction

31. Which of the following statements regarding nasogastric intubation is **FALSE**?

    a. Nasogastric intubation is indicated in cases of abdominal distention
    b. Nasogastric intubation may be associated with gastrointestinal bleeding
    c. Nasogastric intubation is not indicated in unconscious patients
    d. Nasogastric intubation is indicated only under medical direction

32. All of the following statements regarding dialysis are true **except**

    a. Dialysis patients with chronic renal failure cannot tolerate increased potassium levels
    b. Dialysis may be associated with dysrhythmias
    c. Dialysis patients are at increased risk of hemorrhage
    d. Peritoneal dialysis is slower than hemodialysis

33. In treating graft occlusion associated with thrombosis in a patient with acute or chronic renal failure, you should

    a. Irrigate the graft
    b. Clear the graft by aspiration
    c. Obtain the blood pressure in the extremity with an arteriovenous graft
    d. Administer fluids intravenously in an alternative site

34. In the case of poisoning, gastric lavage is indicated

    a. Before tracheal intubation
    b. After tracheal intubation
    c. In adults only
    d. 2 to 3 hours after ingestion

35. Which of the following statements regarding gastric lavage is **FALSE**?

    a. Gastric lavage is contraindicated in the case of gasoline ingestion
    b. Gastric lavage is contraindicated in the case of ingestion of caustic agents
    c. Only water should be used for gastric lavage in pediatric patients
    d. Only normal saline should be used for gastric lavage in pediatric patients

36. All of the following statements regarding use of syrup of ipecac are true **except**

    a. Syrup of ipecac is suitable for routine use in the out-of-hospital setting only
    b. Syrup of ipecac is contraindicated in patients with altered consciousness
    c. Syrup of ipecac is contraindicated in pregnancy
    d. Syrup of ipecac is commonly found in patients' homes

37. The antidote for calcium channel blockers is

    a. Bicarbonate
    b. Ethanol
    c. Calcium
    d. Glucagon

38. The mother of a 2-year-old boy calls to report her son has ingested most of a small bottle of baby oil. On arrival, the child is crying, with a loud hacking cough. His mother states that he spontaneously vomited after swallowing the contents of the bottle. The first line of treatment for this child is to

    a. Decontaminate the stomach
    b. Administer activated charcoal
    c. Administer syrup of ipecac
    d. Provide a patent airway

39. An example of a hydrocarbon associated with significant toxicity is

    a. Asphalt
    b. Baby oil
    c. Tar
    d. Grease

40. Which of the following symptoms is associated with methanol poisoning?

    a. Cyanosis
    b. Hemolytic anemia
    c. Bacterial pneumonia
    d. Blindness

41. Which of the following plants is **NOT** poisonous?

    a. Mistletoe
    b. Buttercups
    c. Marigold
    d. Daffodil

42. Which of the following is **NOT** indicated in treatment of cyanide poisoning associated with smoke inhalation?

    a. Cyanide antidote kit
    b. Amyl nitrate
    c. Hydroxocobalamin
    d. Oxygen

43. The principal treatment for tick bite is

    a. Nail polish
    b. Isopropanol
    c. Burning match
    d. Tick removal

44. Benzodiazepines are used to treat overdose of

    a. Tricyclic antidepressants
    b. Heroin
    c. Cocaine
    d. PCP

45. Diazepam is **NOT** indicated in overdose of

    a. Antipsychotics
    b. Opioids
    c. Cocaine
    d. Lysergic acid diethylamide or LSD

46. Which of the following statements regarding treatment of drug-induced cardiovascular emergencies is **FALSE**?

    a. Naloxone is used in treating meperidine-induced seizures
    b. Benzodiazepines are used in treating acute coronary syndrome
    c. Benzodiazepines are used in treating acute anticholinergic syndrome
    d. Naloxone is used in treating opioid poisoning

47. Treatment of drug-induced ventricular fibrillation may include

    a. High-dose epinephrine
    b. Propranolol
    c. Electrical defibrillation
    d. Calcium

48. Which of the following is NOT a major mechanism of heat loss?

    a. Convection
    b. Absorption
    c. Radiation
    d. Conduction

49. The manager of a golf course calls to report that a 65-year-old man has collapsed after playing golf for several hours in 100º F heat. The patient did not seem to be aware of his surroundings and began talking to himself shortly before collapsing. On arrival, the patient is conscious but suffering from convulsions; his skin is flushed and his core body temperature (CBT) is increased. After initiation of BLS and ALS measures, proper treatment for this patient should be to

    a. Submerge the patient in ice water
    b. Administer large quantities of fluids
    c. Remove the patient's clothing
    d. Cover the patient with blankets and transport

50. A common symptom of heat stroke is

    a. Profuse sweating
    b. Absence of sweating
    c. Electrocardiogram changes
    d. Increased muscle tone

51. All of the following are indicated in the treatment of hypothermia **except**

    a. Passive rewarming
    b. Removing the patient's clothing
    c. Active internal rewarming
    d. Active external rewarming

52. Which of the following is a clinically significant factor in the care of a drowning victim?

    a. Aspiration of contaminants
    b. Dry drowning
    c. Wet drowning
    d. Duration of submersion

53. Which of the following is **NOT** significant in pressure-related diving emergencies?

    a. Henry's law
    b. Newton's law
    c. Dalton's law
    d. Boyle's law

54. Acute mountain sickness may result in

    a. Coma
    b. Cough with frothy sputum
    c. Altered consciousness
    d. Impaired memory

55. According to Centers for Disease Control (CDC) guidelines, in the absence of blood, universal precautions for prevention of HIV transmission do **NOT** apply to exposure to

    a. Semen
    b. Amniotic fluid
    c. Vomitus
    d. Synovial fluid

56. Which of the following statements regarding HCV infection is **FALSE**?

    a. HCV is often transmitted through sexual contact
    b. HCV infection most often results from needle-stick injury
    c. No vaccine has been developed for HCV
    d. Most patients with HCV are asymptomatic

57. You are called to a homeless shelter to assist a 42-year-old man whose severe coughing is "disrupting" the other residents. On arrival, an emaciated man is coughing violently and wiping his mouth with a handkerchief. He complains of fatigue and states that he has been coughing up blood. He admits to being HIV-positive, but states that he has never had any type of lung disease. This patient is most likely suffering from

    a. HCV
    b. TB
    c. Pneumonia
    d. HBV

58. Which of the following statements regarding TB infection is **FALSE**?

    a. TB is more prevalent in patients with HIV infection
    b. Residents of homeless shelters are at high risk of TB
    c. TB can be transmitted by coughing or sneezing
    d. The most common form of TB transmission is through the skin or mucous membranes

59. To prevent the transmission of TB to the paramedic, all of the following are required by the National Institute for Occupational Safety and Health (NIOSH) **except**

    a. Surgical mask
    b. N-type respirator
    c. HEPA filter
    d. Respiratory protection program

Questions 60 and 61 refer to the following scenario:

> The mother of a 4-year-old boy calls you, stating that her son has been projectile vomiting and has a "bad rash" on his foot. On arrival, the boy says he has a "bad headache" and a "stiff neck." He has a low-grade fever, and a petechial rash is visible.

60. The most likely diagnosis in this patient is

    a. Rubella
    b. Measles
    c. Tetanus
    d. Meningitis

61. Treatment of the patient should include all of the following **except**

    a. BSI precautions
    b. Placement of a surgical mask
    c. Antibiotics
    d. Analgesics

62. Which of the following statements regarding rabies infection is **FALSE**?

  a. An animal suspected of carrying rabies should be killed
  b. Rabies vaccine is given by a series of injections in the stomach
  c. Rabies infection may result in eye and facial muscle paralysis
  d. Tetanus prophylaxis may be indicated for rabies

63. Which of the following statements regarding SARS is **TRUE**?

  a. The majority of SARS cases improve spontaneously
  b. Quarantine is no longer required for SARS patients
  c. SARS is usually transmitted via close contact with family members or coworkers
  d. SARS may be transmitted via blood transfusion

64. Which of the following statements regarding bird flu is **FALSE**?

  a. Bird flu may be transmitted by pigs
  b. Bird flu may be transmitted among humans
  c. Bird flu may be transmitted among different bird species
  d. Antiviral therapy is not indicated for bird flu prophylaxis

65. Which of the following is **NOT** part of the recommended procedure for transport of SARS patients?

  a. Used needles should be collected in sharps containers
  b. Non-patient areas of the vehicle should also be cleaned
  c. Paramedics who may have been exposed to SARS after patient transport may continue working
  d. Compressed air may be used to clean the vehicle and any reusable equipment

Questions 66 and 67 refer to the following scenario:

> The brother of a 30-year-old man calls to request assistance because his brother is "completely out of control." On arrival, the patient is pacing around the room and shouting obscenities. His brother states that the patient had been throwing objects around the room and had threatened to "kill somebody." He also states that the patient had been treated in the past for "manic-depression" but discontinued taking his medication because he had been sick with the flu. You observe a bottle of vodka on the table.

66. In assessing this patient, you should first

  a. Conduct a brief physical examination
  b. Restrain the patient and transport to the hospital
  c. Interview the patient
  d. Contact the police for assistance

67. While interviewing the patient, he suddenly accuses you of "interrogating" him and begins throwing objects around the room. To manage this situation, you should first

  a. Offer the patient a last chance to cooperate
  b. Call the police and leave the scene
  c. Apply chemical restraint
  d. Restrain the patient using wrist restraints

- 206 -

68. All of the following agents are useful in chemical restraint **except**

    a. Haloperidol
    b. Diazepam
    c. Lithium
    d. Diphenhydramine

69. In caring for a victim of sexual assault, which should be done first?

    a. Examine the patient's genitalia
    b. Obtain a sexual history
    c. Move the patient to a separate room
    d. Remove and bag the patient's clothing for law enforcement

70. You are called to the scene of a severe traffic accident involving a 25-year-old pregnant woman. The woman is 6 months pregnant and has sustained significant head trauma. Your first priority in managing this patient is to

    a. Assess fetal heart rate
    b. Administer high-concentration oxygen
    c. Transport the patient in the supine position
    d. Apply a pneumatic antishock garment

71. Treatment of third-trimester bleeding should include all of the following **except**

    a. IV fluid therapy
    b. Measurement of fundal height
    c. Vaginal examination
    d. Administration of high-concentration oxygen

72. Which of the following should **NOT** be used to determine the need for resuscitation of a baby just born?

    a. Apgar score
    b. Muscle tone
    c. Crying
    d. Amniotic fluid

73. All of the following should be used to stimulate uterine contraction following delivery **except**

    a. Administering oxytocin
    b. Packing the vagina to control bleeding
    c. Massaging the uterus
    d. Encouraging breastfeeding

74. Which of the following is an example of safe ambulance operation?

    a. Using high beams to increase visibility
    b. Using a police escort in response to an emergency call
    c. Using lights and sirens to provide absolute right of way
    d. Using warning devices during transport of a patient with life-threatening injury

75. The 2-second rule should be applied in gauging braking distance for

 a. Larger emergency vehicles
 b. Poor roadway conditions
 c. Type III emergency vehicles
 d. Heavy vehicle weight

76. Which of the following statements regarding air medical services is **FALSE**?

 a. Ground ambulances are faster than air ambulances within a 30-mile range in urban areas
 b. Fewer crashes occur with air than with ground ambulances
 c. Fewer individuals survive helicopter crashes
 d. Air ambulances can accommodate more patients and equipment

77. You arrive at the scene of a crash of a small chartered plane. Two of the passengers are conscious and have sustained minor injuries; one has broken his arm in several places. A third passenger is unconscious, with a carotid pulse but not a radial pulse. The pilot has suffered significant head trauma with severe hemorrhage and has a respiratory rate of less than 10 breaths per minute. The primary line of treatment for these patients is to

 a. Administer epinephrine
 b. Set any broken limbs
 c. Reposition the airway and control hemorrhage
 d. Treat for hypovolemia

78. The START technique is used for

 a. Assessing the airway
 b. Primary triage
 c. Critical incident stress management
 d. Secondary triage

79. Proper treatment for the passenger with the broken arm described above would be to

 a. Direct the patient to remain at the scene for further assistance
 b. Assess the patient's respiratory rate
 c. Evaluate the patient's mental status
 d. Check the patient's pulse rate

80. In the case of the passenger described above with a carotid pulse but no radial pulse, you should

 a. Assess mental status
 b. Classify as delayed
 c. Classify as critical
 d. Classify as dying

81. During a blizzard, a commuter plane crashes into a river, submerging all of the passengers; the water temperature is 35ºF. All of the following rescue techniques are valid **except**

 a. Lifting victims onto a back board
 b. Directing multiple passengers to huddle together
 c. Directing a single passenger to assume the fetal position
 d. Putting on a PFD before rescue

82. Which of the following statements regarding hypothermia is **FALSE**?

    a. Rapid hypothermia can improve brain viability
    b. The effectiveness of the cold protective response depends on age
    c. Resuscitation should not be attempted after prolonged submersion in extremely cold water
    d. Sudden exposure to extremely cold water can lead to laryngospasm

83. In the case of a confined-space emergency,

    a. Use the SCBA as an air supply
    b. Obtain a copy of the OSHA permit
    c. Shoring is required for all cave-ins
    d. Approach the lip of the cave-in to assess the scene

84. During a severe thunderstorm, a car is hit by downed electrical wires, trapping the two passengers inside. Proper management of this situation should include

    a. Securing the downed wires
    b. Extricating the passengers from the vehicle
    c. Instructing the passengers to remain inside the vehicle
    d. Instructing the passengers to climb out the back window

85. In rescuing an accident victim in an airbag-equipped car, you should

    a. Disconnect the car battery if the airbag is deployed
    b. Maintain a safe distance of 20 inches for passenger-side airbags
    c. Turn on the ignition to test whether the battery is disconnected
    d. Place a hard board between the passenger and the airbag

86. During a high-angle rescue attempt, which of the following is mandatory?

    a. ALS
    b. Endotracheal intubation
    c. Supplemental oxygen
    d. IV line

87. Tactics for paramedic safety in the course of a potentially violent situation include all of the following **except**

    a. Avoidance
    b. Tactical retreat
    c. Confrontation
    d. Concealment

88. A bulletproof vest is **NOT** effective against

    a. Knives
    b. Ice picks
    c. Handgun bullets
    d. Airgun pellets

89. Which of the following is useful for protection against hazardous materials?

    a. SCBA
    b. Air-purifying respirator
    c. Level C clothing
    d. Level D clothing

90. You are called to the scene of a hazardous chemical spill caused by an overturned truck. On arrival, the truck driver has suffered severe leg trauma; the drivers and passengers of nearby vehicles were not seriously injured. Proper emergency treatment of the truck driver should include

    a. Wound debridement
    b. Removal from the hot zone
    c. IV therapy
    d. Spinal immobilization

91. Following a hazardous materials or "hazmat" incident, proper procedure should include all of the following **except**

    a. Showering to remove potential contaminants
    b. Leave the incident immediately and continue to the next emergency
    c. Hazmat establishment of a decontamination corridor
    d. Debriefing of rescue personnel

92. Which of the following statements regarding pediatric anatomy is **FALSE**?

    a. Children have a larger body surface area-to-body mass ratio
    b. A child in shock may maintain a normal blood pressure
    c. The liver and spleen are less often injured in children
    d. In children, the muscles provide the primary means of support for the chest wall

93. In assessing a 5-year-old girl who is not acutely ill, the paramedic should

    a. Monitor vital signs every 5 minutes
    b. Allow the child to play with the stethoscope
    c. Conduct a physical exam from toe to head
    d. Obtain an electrocardiogram reading

94. The mother of a 4-year-old boy calls at 2 AM to report that her son has awakened with "a terrible cough and trouble breathing." On arrival, the child is sitting upright in bed and coughing; nasal flaring and slight cyanosis are present. The mother states that the child has had a "bad cold" over the last 2 weeks and is running a low fever. This child is likely suffering from

    a. Croup
    b. Epiglottitis
    c. Pneumonia
    d. Airway obstruction

95. Proper management of the child described above should include

    a. Intubation
    b. Parenteral antibiotics
    c. Bronchodilators
    d. Cool humidified air

96. Treatment of status epilepticus in a child may include all of the following **except**

    a. Diazepam
    b. Glucagon
    c. Intubation
    d. Cardiac monitoring

97. Which of the following is **NOT** indicated in the emergency treatment of a child with hyperglycemia?

    a. IV fluid therapy
    b. Insulin
    c. Glucose testing
    d. Dextrose

98. A possible cause of SIDS is

    a. Suffocation
    b. Regurgitation
    c. Allergies
    d. Upper airway obstruction

99. You are called to the apartment of an 85-year-old woman complaining of shortness of breath, pain in her right calf, and a "racing heart." The patient states that she has a history of CHF. On examination, tachycardia and tachypnea are present, as well as mild edema of the right calf. This patient is most likely suffering from

    a. Bacterial pneumonia
    b. Pulmonary embolism
    c. Myocardial infarction
    d. Heart failure

100. Aggressive airway management, including supplementary oxygenation and IV bronchodilator therapy, is indicated in

    a. COPD
    b. Cerebral vascular disease
    c. Pulmonary embolism
    d. Bacterial pneumonia

101. Sudden disorientation, with incoherent speech, mental confusion, and excitement, is associated with

    a. Alzheimer's disease
    b. Dementia
    c. Delirium
    d. Senility

102. Which of the following statements regarding trauma management of elderly patients is **FALSE**?

    a. PaO_2 decreases with age
    b. Rapid fluid IV administration is indicated in elderly patients
    c. Elderly patients may require higher arterial pressures for perfusion
    d. Adjustment of stroke volume may be decreased in response to hypovolemia

103. The rule of nines is useful for

    a. Infants
    b. Irregularly shaped burns
    c. Burns over a large area of the body
    d. Children over 10 years of age

104. A moderate burn may be classified as

    a. A full-thickness burn covering greater than 10% of body surface area
    b. A partial-thickness burn covering 15% of body surface area
    c. A burn from contact with a caustic chemical
    d. A burn from contact with high-voltage electricity

105. In managing a burn victim, the paramedic should

    a. Apply ointment to the burn
    b. Remove blisters already formed
    c. Cover the patient with a sterile blanket
    d. Place an ice pack on the burn

106. The sister of a 20-year-old woman calls to report that she has found her sister in the family car with the windows rolled up and the heat on. The young woman is semi-conscious and has been in the car for about 3 hours. Her sister states that the young woman has been depressed because of the break-up of a serious relationship. Proper treatment of this patient may include all of the following **except**

    a. High-concentration oxygen
    b. Pulse oximeter
    c. Sodium thiosulfate
    d. Hyperbaric oxygen

107. In the patient described above, the most appropriate line of action following medical care is to

    a. Transport the patient immediately
    b. Question the patient's sister about the patient's medical history
    c. Ask the patient directly about suicidal intent
    d. Call law enforcement

108. A carbon monoxide blood level of 10% produces

    a. No symptoms
    b. Electrocardiogram abnormalities
    c. Coma
    d. Nausea and vomiting

109. Increasing intracranial pressure may be controlled by

    a. IV fluid therapy
    b. The Valsalva maneuver
    c. Blood replacement therapy
    d. Osmotic diuretics and steroids

110. All of the following may be used to determine left ventricular function **except**

    a. PCWP
    b. RAP
    c. LAP
    d. PAP

111. Which of the following drugs increases respiration?

   a. Diazepam
   b. Aspirin
   c. Epinephrine
   d. Morphine

112. The following drug may be safely given to a pregnant woman:

   a. Morphine
   b. Aspirin
   c. Diazepam
   d. Oxytocin

113. Drugs that are given during pregnancy only if the potential benefit justifies the risk to the fetus are classified as

   a. Category X
   b. Category B
   c. Category C
   d. Category D

114. The nasal cannula is typically used in patients with

   a. Apnea
   b. Chest pain
   c. Hypoxia
   d. Respiratory insufficiency

115. Which of the following devices may be used in patients with apnea?

   a. Bag-mask device
   b. Nasal cannula
   c. Partial nonbreather mask
   d. Nonbreather mask

116. Which of the following statements regarding rescue breathing is **FALSE**?

   a. The jaw-thrust technique is used in patients with suspected spinal injury
   b. Use of an oropharyngeal or nasopharyngeal airway is contraindicated in an unconscious patient
   c. Mouth-to-stoma ventilation is more sanitary than the mouth-to-mouth technique
   d. The mouth-to-nose technique requires the patient's mouth to be closed

117. The bag-mask device should **NOT** be used to

   a. Provide supplemental oxygen to a spontaneously breathing child
   b. Provide ventilation to a child in respiratory arrest
   c. Provide ventilation under extreme environmental temperatures
   d. Provide ventilation to a patient who has not been intubated

118. Nasal airways may be used in all of the following cases **except**

   a. Unconsciousness
   b. Cervical spine injuries
   c. Seizures
   d. Fractured skull

- 213 -

119. Cuffed endotracheal tubes may be indicated for

    a. Infants
    b. Children 8 to 10 years old or older
    c. Children less than 8 years old
    d. Adults only

120. Which of the following statements regarding blind intubation is **FALSE**?

    a. Blind intubation may be necessary in disaster situations involving many victims
    b. Blind intubation is indicated when the airway cannot be visualized
    c. Nasotracheal intubation is a blind procedure
    d. Blind intubation is indicated in patients with spinal fractures

121. An inaccurate pulse oximeter reading may result from

    a. Cyanosis
    b. Spinal injury
    c. Nail polish
    d. Hypertension

122. In-line stabilization is required for intubation of

    a. Infants
    b. Children under the age of 10
    c. Patients with hypertension
    d. Patients with spinal injuries

123. Use of the LMA is contraindicated in

    a. Unconscious patients
    b. Patients with an intact gag reflex
    c. Patients with an unstable neck injury
    d. Patients who cannot be positioned for tracheal intubation

124. Paralytic agents may **NOT** be used in the emergency intubation of

    a. Patients with facial hair
    b. Agitated trauma patients
    c. Combative patients
    d. Pediatric patients

125. All of the following are useful in RSI **except**

    a. Mallampati score
    b. Lidocaine
    c. Cricothyrotomy
    d. Preoxygenation

126. Air bags are most effective in

    a. Rear-impact collisions
    b. Frontal collisions
    c. Multiple collisions
    d. Rollover impacts

127. Which of the following statements regarding transport of a child in the ambulance is **FALSE**?

    a. Infants and young children can be transported in a child safety seat
    b. A child safety seat can be secured to a stretcher
    c. Older children can be secured to a stretcher
    d. The parent and child can be secured to a stretcher together

128. Hypovolemia may be associated with all of the following **except**

    a. Septic shock
    b. Hemorrhage
    c. Fainting
    d. Cardiogenic shock

129. Which of the following is a sign of uncompensated shock?

    a. Hypotension
    b. Unconsciousness
    c. Coma
    d. Combativeness

130. Jugular vein distention is associated with

    a. Anaphylactic shock
    b. Septic shock
    c. Cardiogenic shock
    d. Distributive shock

131. Which of the following wounds requires closure?

    a. Ring finger injury
    b. Abrasion from a motorcycle crash
    c. Contusion from a car accident
    d. Puncture wound from an animal bite

132. The wife of a 44-year-old man calls to report that her husband has suffered a deep wound to his forearm as the result of a broken power saw. On arrival, the wound is bleeding profusely. The first step in controlling hemorrhage should be to

    a. Apply a tourniquet
    b. Apply direct pressure
    c. Apply a splint
    d. Apply a pneumatic pressure device

133. Prehospital care of an open wound may involve all of the following **except**

    a. Applying antibacterial ointment
    b. Irrigating the wound with water
    c. Debridement of the wound
    d. Dressing the wound

134. After a building collapse, a construction worker is trapped beneath a steel beam for several hours. His right leg has been crushed under the beam and his left has been amputated. Initial treatment of this patient should include

a. Aggressive hydration with 5% dextrose in water and 0.45% normal saline
b. Fasciotomy of the right leg
c. Administration of calcium chloride
d. Administration of furosemide

135. Management of the patient's left leg should include

a. Applying a tourniquet to the remaining portion of the left leg
b. Searching for the amputated limb
c. If found, treating the amputated limb in the same manner as avulsed tissue
d. Fasciotomy to the remaining portion of the left leg

136. You are called to the scene of a car accident in which a 35-year-old man has hit a pole; damage to the vehicle is minimal, and no other cars were involved. The victim does not appear to be injured and claims he was not hurt; however, he admits to have been drinking before the accident and is clearly intoxicated. The MOI in this case is

a. Positive
b. Negative
c. Uncertain
d. Distraction

137. Which of the following statements regarding spinal injury is **FALSE**?

a. Spinal injury can occur without SCI
b. SCI only occurs with spinal injury
c. SCI may occur without spinal injury
d. SCI without spinal injury is more common in children

138. Which of the following statements regarding spinal immobilization is **FALSE**?

a. A rigid cervical collar does not provide adequate spinal immobilization
b. In immobilization to a long spine board, the torso should be immobilized before the head
c. Short spine boards should be used for immobilization of patients in a confined space
d. Short spine boards should be used for patients requiring immediate resuscitation

139. A 10-year-old boy has been ejected from an all-terrain recreational vehicle and has suffered potential spinal trauma. The boy is wearing a full-face helmet. Proper prehospital care for this patient should include all of the following **except**

a. Removal of the helmet
b. Manual in-line immobilization
c. Immobilization on a short spine board
d. Immobilization on a long spine board

140. A 45-year-old woman loses control of her vehicle on an icy road and rams into a tree. The patient complains that she has lost all feeling in her right leg and that she has "wet herself." Hypotension and vasodilation are present. This patient may be suffering from

a. Neurogenic hypotension
b. Spinal shock
c. Autonomic hyperreflexia
d. Spondylosis

141. Distended neck veins are usually associated with

a. Open pneumothorax
b. Closed pneumothorax
c. Tension pneumothorax
d. Flail chest

142. Which of the following statements regarding tension pneumothorax is **FALSE**?

a. Tension pneumothorax may result from sealing an open pneumothorax with occlusive dressing
b. Tension pneumothorax may be fatal
c. Tension pneumothorax may be relieved by thoracic decompression
d. Tension pneumothorax is primarily identified by chest percussion

143. Management of abdominal trauma should include all of the following **except**

a. Scene assessment
b. Fluid replacement
c. Replacement of eviscerated organs
d. Use of a PASG

144. Traction splints may be used for

a. Pelvic fracture
b. Hip injury
c. Knee injury
d. Femoral fracture

145. Which of the following statements regarding treatment of fractures and dislocations is **FALSE**?

a. Knee realignment is indicated by a "popping" into the joint
b. A dislocated elbow can be realigned at the scene
c. Fractures and dislocated joints should be immobilized in the direction of injury
d. Hip realignment is indicated by a "popping" into the joint

146. An extra heart sound may be indicative of

a. Congestive heart failure
b. Ventricular systole
c. Ventricular diastole
d. Myocardial infarction

147. The ECG lead aV$_F$ is an example of a

    a. Bipolar limb lead
    b. Unipolar limb lead
    c. Unipolar chest lead
    d. Bipolar chest lead

148. In an ECG reading, the QRS complex follows the

    a. Q-T interval
    b. T wave
    c. ST segment
    d. P wave

149. Which of the following methods may be used to calculate heart rate when the heart rhythm is irregular?

    a. Triplicate method
    b. Six-second count method
    c. R-R method
    d. Heart rate calculator ruler

150. All of the following may be used to treat paroxysmal supraventricular tachycardia **except**

    a. Adenosine
    b. Vagal maneuvers
    c. Magnesium
    d. Valsalva maneuver

Answer Key and Explanations

1. C: An anaphylactoid reaction is the most severe form of allergic reaction and is not mediated by an antigen-antibody reaction. A type I allergic reaction may lead to life-threatening anaphylaxis. Immunity can be natural or can be artificially induced through immunization.

2. D: Individuals in occupations that may involve prolonged exposure to latex, such as hairdressers, food handlers, healthcare workers, and tollbooth operators, are at high risk of latex allergy. Patients with asthma or with a genetic predisposition to allergies may also be at high risk; however, patients with allergic rhinitis are at no particular risk of latex allergy.

3. C: The first step in managing a patient with an anaphylactic reaction is to provide adequate airway support; the patient should be placed in a comfortable position and high-concentration oxygen should be administered. Intramuscular epinephrine may be given to patients with clinical signs of shock; however, intravenous epinephrine should only be given in rare instances and with authorization from medical direction. Saline is given only in the presence of hypotension or when the patient does not respond to epinephrine.

4. B: Beta-blockers can increase the severity of anaphylaxis and induce a severe reaction to epinephrine; however, beta agonists, antihistamines, corticosteroids, antiarrhythmics, and vasopressors may be given as additional drug therapy.

5. D: Signs of a mild allergic reaction include urticaria or hives, cramping or diarrhea, and bronchoconstriction; however, altered mental status, as indicated by a sense of impending doom, confusion, and agitation, is typically associated with anaphylaxis.

6. C: In performing defibrillation, paddles should not be placed over the sternum or over the generator of an implanted automatic defibrillator or pacemaker. Place one paddle to the right of the upper sternum below the clavicle and the other to the left of the left nipple immediately over the apex of the heart.

7. D: Various gels, creams, and pastes are useful in decreasing paddle-skin interface resistance; however, use only those made specifically for defibrillation and not for electrocardiogram monitoring. Pads soaked in saline are safe but those soaked in alcohol may ignite.

8. A: Nitroglycerin patches should be removed before defibrillation; placing paddles together can cause pitting, which may burn the patient. Alternating cardiopulmonary resuscitation with defibrillation may transfer gel from the patient's chest to the paddle handles. To remove an unwanted charge, simply turn off the defibrillator.

9. C: Asynchronous pacing is used less often than demand pacing, usually as only a last resort. Asynchronous pacing may be used in cases of asystole, to control tachydysrhythmia such as torsades de pointes, and in cases when artifact on the electrocardiogram interferes with its ability to read the actual heartbeat.

10. B: Transcutaneous cardiac pacing is primarily used in cases of symptomatic bradycardia, heart block associated with reduced cardiac output, or pacemaker failure. Cardiac pacing is usually ineffective in cardiac arrest or pulseless electrical activity and is not recommended in patients with open wounds or burns.

11. D: Resuscitation should not be attempted in patients with a valid Do Not Attempt Resuscitation (DNAR) order, in cases when vital functions have deteriorated, such as in patients with septic or cardiogenic shock, or in patients with asystole; however, resuscitation may be indicated in special cases, such as in young children or in those with hypothermia, electrolyte abnormalities, toxin exposure, or drug overdose.

12. B: Initial defibrillation should be attempted at 360 J monophasic energy; initial defibrillation for pediatric patients is 2 J/kg, followed by 4 J/kg if necessary. Biphasic defibrillation of 115 J is as effective as monophasic defibrillation of 200 J; the optimal current for ventricular defibrillation is 30 to 40 A.

13. A: Patients with chronic obstructive pulmonary disease (COPD) typically have an acute episode of worsening dyspnea and may be leaning forward to aid breathing. These patients may use accessory muscles as well as pursed-lip breathing to aid in respiration.

14. C: The thin, barrel-chest appearance of this patient, as well as the presence of wheezing, rhonchi, and pursed-lip breathing, are indicative of emphysema.

15. C: Typical signs and symptoms of chronic bronchitis include chronic cyanosis, productive cough, and resistance on inspiration; pink or red complexion, nonproductive cough, and pursed-lip breathing are indicative of emphysema.

16. D: In all patients in respiratory distress, the paramedic should establish an IV line and apply a cardiac monitor. Pulse oximetry and administration of high-concentration oxygen are also indicated; however, oxygen should not be withheld to avoid reduction of the hypoxic drive.

17. B: In the acronym OPQRST, used in obtaining a focused history in patients with respiratory distress, O = onset, P = provocation, Q = quality, R = region and radiation, S = severity, and T = time.

18. C: Conditions indicative of a perfusion problem include shock, anemia, pulmonary embolism, and trauma; asthma is indicative of a ventilation problem and atherosclerosis and carbon dioxide poisoning of diffusion problems.

19. A: Patients with chronic bronchitis and emphysema, known together as chronic obstructive pulmonary disease (COPD), may have both COPD and asthma at the same time but in varying degrees of severity. Patients with emphysema are referred to as "pink puffers" due to increased production of red blood cells; those with bronchitis are referred to as "blue bloaters" because they often appear cyanotic. In contrast to adult-onset asthma, childhood asthma usually improves or resolves with age.

20. B: The primary goal in managing an acute asthma attack is to ensure an adequate airway and reverse the bronchospasm. After administering high-concentration oxygen and consulting medical direction, the next step is usually to administer a fast-acting bronchodilator such as albuterol. Continuous positive airway pressure (CPAP) and biphasic positive airway pressure (BiPAP) should only be used if the patient has adequate spontaneous respirations; ketamine is used to sedate a patient before endotracheal intubation.

21. C: Inspiratory wheezing may indicate the presence of secretions in the large airways but does not necessarily indicate upper airway occlusion.

22. C: Peak expiratory flow rate (PEFR) tests are used in patients experiencing an acute asthma attack to determine baseline airflow before drug administration. PEFR tests are not useful in

children less than 5 years of age or in patients in severe respiratory distress. Positive end-expiratory pressure (PEEP) is often used in patients with adult respiratory distress syndrome (ARDS).

23. B: Initial management of a stroke patient should include providing life support, confirming signs and symptoms, and establishing the time of stroke onset to determine whether fibrinolytic therapy should be administered; the patient should then be transported to the hospital as soon as possible for definitive care. Management of hypertension is not indicated in the initial treatment of stroke.

24. D: Both the Cincinnati Prehospital Stroke Scale (CPSS) and the Los Angeles Prehospital Stroke Screen (LAPSS) are useful in diagnosing stroke; if the patient is conscious, obtaining a medical history may also be useful. 50% dextrose is administered during glucose analysis only when indicated.

25. C: Transient ischemic attacks (TIAs) present with the same signs and symptoms as those of stroke; thus, assessment of a patient with a TIA is the same as that for a patient with stroke. TIAs are important predictors of brain infarction; however, they are not associated with permanent neurological deficits.

26. A: The first step in treating a patient with abdominal pain is to survey the scene to determine whether the patient's condition is due to trauma or a medical condition; the area should be inspected for signs of alcohol or drug use, such as medication bottles. Pain medication should not be given to a patient with abdominal pain because it may mask critical signs and symptoms. Following the initial survey, a physical examination should be performed to identify any abdominal injuries. Transport should be provided only if abdominal pain persists for 6 or more hours.

27. D: In the mnemonic OPQRST, the letter P stands for provocative or palliative. The patient should be asked what improves or worsens pain; for example, whether sitting or lying down affects pain. The letter O stands for onset and S severity; past medical history is part of the SAMPLE history.

28. C: Pain location is included as part of the OPQRST evaluation (R or region); women of childbearing age should be asked about menstrual and/or pregnancy history. Changes in bowel habits and last meal or oral intake are key elements of the SAMPLE history in patients with abdominal pain.

29. A: Conditions associated with visceral or organ pain include cholecystitis, pancreatitis, and intestinal obstruction. Peritonitis and ulcer are associated with somatic pain, or constant pain localized to a specific area; morphine addiction is associated with dehydration, obstruction, and decreased intestinal motility.

30. B: Cholecystitis is often associated with cramping abdominal pain radiating to the upper right quadrant; pain increases in intensity, then subsides, and usually occurs at night, often after consuming fried or fatty foods. Cholecystitis is more common in women. Pancreatitis is associated with severe epigastric pain, often accompanied by abdominal distention; bowel obstruction usually results from fecal impaction or tumor. Crohn's disease is a chronic condition marked by diarrhea, anorexia, and weight loss.

31. C: Nasogastric intubation is indicated only in unusual circumstances and only under medical direction; nasogastric intubation is indicated in conscious patients with an intact gag reflex but may be attempted in unconscious patients with a protected airway. Complications associated with nasogastric intubation include gastrointestinal bleeding, nasal hemorrhage, and perforation of the esophagus.

32. A: Dialysis patients with chronic renal failure can tolerate increased potassium levels better than patients with normal kidney function; however, dialysis patients are at increased risk of hemorrhage and may suffer dysrhythmias resulting from myocardial ischemia. Peritoneal dialysis is slower than hemodialysis but is just as effective over time.

33. D: In the case of graft occlusion resulting from thrombus formation, attempting to clear the graft by irrigation or aspiration or obtaining blood pressure measurements in an extremity with an arteriovenous graft is not recommended; intravenous infusion of fluids should be initiated in an alternative site.

34. B: Gastric lavage should only be performed in patients who have ingested a lethal amount of poison within the last hour; in intubated or comatose patients, gastric lavage should be performed after tracheal intubation to prevent aspiration pneumonia. Gastric lavage can be safely performed in both adults and children.

35. C: Only normal saline should be used for gastric lavage in pediatric patients to prevent water absorption. Gastric lavage is contraindicated in the case of ingestion of low-viscosity hydrocarbons such as gasoline or caustic agents due to the increased risk of aspiration.

36. A: Syrup of ipecac is no longer the drug of choice in cases of poisoning and is not recommended for routine use; however, it is still commonly found in patients' homes. Syrup of ipecac is contraindicated in pregnant patients and in patients in a state of altered consciousness.

37. C: The antidote for calcium channel blocker ingestion is calcium; bicarbonate is indicated for cyclic antidepressants, ethanol for methanol, and glucagon for beta-blockers.

38. D: Baby oil is a hydrocarbon and ingestion is particularly dangerous; thus, the first step in treating hydrocarbon ingestion is to provide adequate ventilatory and circulatory support. Decontamination of the stomach or administration of activated charcoal or syrup of ipecac is not recommended for hydrocarbon ingestion.

39. B: Baby oil is a particularly dangerous hydrocarbon because of the risk of aspiration; asphalt, tar, and grease are not aspirated or absorbed in the gastrointestinal tract and thus do not have significant toxicity.

40. D: Ingestion of as little as 4 mL of methanol can cause blindness; cyanosis, hemolytic or aplastic anemia, and bacterial pneumonia are associated with hydrocarbon ingestion.

41. C: Ingestion of the marigold plant is not dangerous; however, ingestion of mistletoe, buttercups, or daffodils may be toxic.

42. A: Use of the cyanide antidote kit in patients with cyanide poisoning due to smoke inhalation may reduce the amount of hemoglobin needed for oxygen transport, resulting in anoxia and death. Inhalation of amyl nitrite followed by supplemental oxygen and administration of hydroxocobalamin may be useful in detoxification.

43. D: Removal of the tick with forceps, tweezers, or protected fingers is the principal treatment for tick bite; use of nail polish, isopropanol, or a burning match head are ineffective and may cause the tick to salivate or regurgitate into the bite wound.

44. C: Benzodiazepines are the primary treatment for cocaine overdose; alkalinization and anticonvulsant therapy may be useful in treating overdose of tricyclic antidepressants. Naloxone is

effective in treating overdose of heroin and other opioids. Phencyclidine (PCP) overdose may result in violent or unpredictable behavior; thus, these patients are usually rapidly transported for physician evaluation.

45. B: Naloxone is indicated for treatment of overdose of opioids such as heroin, morphine, or codeine; diazepam may be used in treating cocaine, antipsychotic, or lysergic acid diethylamide (LSD) overdose.

46. A: Naloxone is used in treating opioid poisoning but is not indicated for treatment of meperidine-induced seizures; benzodiazepines may be used in the treatment of acute coronary and anticholinergic syndrome.

47. C: Electrical defibrillation or cardioversion may be used in treatment of drug-induced ventricular tachycardia or fibrillation. High-dose epinephrine and propranolol are contraindicated in sympathomimetic poisoning associated with refractory ventricular fibrillation; calcium is indicated in drug-induced cardiogenic shock.

48. B: The major mechanisms of heat loss are radiation, conduction, convection, and evaporation.

49. C: In a case of suspected heat stroke, the top priority following BLS and ALS measures is to initiate rapid cooling; however, submerging the patient in ice water or cold water can induce peripheral vasoconstriction and convulsions. The patient should be moved to a cool environment and his or her clothing should be removed; administration of too much fluid can result in pulmonary edema. Patients suffering from hypothermia should be covered with warm blankets and transported.

50. B: Sweating is usually absent in cases of heat stroke; changes in electrocardiogram and increased muscle tone are symptoms associated with hypothermia.

51. C: Active internal rewarming techniques, including peritoneal or pleural lavage, extracorporeal circulation, and use of esophageal warming tubes, are invasive and are not recommended for out-of-hospital care. Replacing wet with dry clothing can help retain body heat; passive rewarming techniques, such as removing wet clothing and wrapping the patient in blankets, and active external rewarming through the use of radiant heat, forced hot air, or warmed IV fluids, are useful in managing hypothermia.

52. D: The most significant clinical factors in prehospital care of a drowning victim are duration of submersion and duration and severity of hypoxia. Aspiration of contaminants or amount of aspirated fluid do not affect outcome.

53. B: Henry's law, Dalton's law, and Boyle's law outline the properties of gases and are thus significant in pressure-related diving emergencies; Newton's law is relevant in the study of physics.

54. D: Acute mountain sickness can result in headache, anorexia, vomiting, and impaired memory; high-altitude pulmonary edema is characterized by cough with or without frothy sputum, and high-altitude cerebral edema may result in altered consciousness or coma.

55. C: According to the CDC guidelines regarding universal precautions for prevention of transmission of HIV, hepatitis B, or other blood-borne pathogens, exposure to vomitus in the absence of blood is not subject to universal precautions; however, universal precautions must apply to exposure to semen, vaginal secretions, tissue, and fluids such as synovial or amniotic fluid.

56. A: HCV is transmitted in the same manner as other forms of hepatitis and most often results from needle-stick injury; however, HCV is not often transmitted through sexual contact. Most patients with HCV infection are asymptomatic; no vaccine has yet been developed for HCV.

57. B: Tuberculosis (TB) should be suspected in HIV-positive patients with undiagnosed lung disease; typical signs and symptoms of TB include coughing, hemoptysis, fever, and fatigue. Pneumonia is an acute infection of the bronchioles and alveoli of the lungs marked by tachypnea, high-grade fever, and cough with yellow-green phlegm. Symptoms of hepatitis C virus (HCV) usually develop within 2 to 3 months of infection and include anorexia, nausea and vomiting, and generalized rashes; hepatitis B virus (HBV) is marked by an influenza-like illness that lasts less than 6 months and may lead to cirrhosis or other liver disease.

58. D: TB is most prevalent in homeless shelters, nursing homes, and other facilities and in patients with HIV infection. TB is most commonly transmitted by the coughing or sneezing of bacteria into the air and less often through the skin or mucous membranes.

59. A: A surgical mask is ineffective in preventing inhalation of TB bacteria; however, it should be placed on the patient before transport. NIOSH recommends use of an N-type respirator and an ambulance ventilation system including a high-efficiency particulate air (HEPA) filter to prevent paramedic exposure to TB while transporting the patient; a complete respiratory protection program should be implemented whenever respirators are required.

60. D: Nuchal rigidity, projectile vomiting, headache, and petechial rash are classic signs of meningitis. Tetanus is marked by stiffness of the jaw and rubella by a diffuse macular rash; measles is characterized by a blotchy red rash.

61. D: In treating a patient with signs and symptoms of meningitis, universal and body substance isolation (BSI) precautions should be taken, including placement of a surgical mask on the patient. Antibiotics are key in the treatment of meningitis and are usually given 30 to 60 minutes after arriving at the emergency department; analgesics are effective in the management of pneumonia.

62. B: Rabies vaccine is given by injection over a period of several weeks; however, injections are no longer given in the stomach. Tetanus prophylaxis may be indicated for treatment of the bite wound. If left untreated, rabies infection can result in eye and facial muscle paralysis. An animal suspected of being rabid should be killed by the proper authorities and examined for rabies antibodies.

63. A: More than 80% of severe acute respiratory syndrome (SARS) cases improve spontaneously; strict quarantine is the most effective mode of treatment. SARS is seldom transmitted via contact with family members or coworkers and is not transmitted through blood transfusion.

64. B: Bird flu is transmitted among birds and occasionally pigs but cannot be transmitted among humans; antiviral therapy is not indicated for bird flu prophylaxis due to reduce risk of developing a resistant strain of the virus.

65. D: Compressed air may allow infectious material to become airborne and should not be used to clean a vehicle or equipment used in transporting a severe acute respiratory syndrome (SARS) patient; used needles and scalpel blades should be collected in sharps containers and disposed of in accordance with hospital requirements and all non-patient areas of the vehicle should also be cleaned. Paramedics with suspected SARS exposure who are asymptomatic may continue working during the 10-day period following exposure.

66. C: In assessing a patient with a behavioral emergency, the first step should be to establish rapport by providing a limited and supportive interview; the paramedic should listen to the patient's account of events, showing support and empathy. The patient's personal space should be respected, and physical touch should be limited. Calling the police or using restraints is unnecessary if the patient is cooperative.

67. A: In managing a violent patient, the paramedic should offer him or her a final chance to cooperate before applying physical restraint; physical restraint is only warranted after all techniques to calm the patient have been exhausted. A single paramedic should not be left alone with a violent patient; at least four individuals should be present to help restrain the patient. If the patient is armed, the paramedic should move other individuals out of range, call law enforcement, then leave the scene. Chemical restraint should not be attempted without approval from medical direction.

68. C: Lithium is used in the treatment of bipolar disorder; diazepam is a benzodiazepine and haloperidol an antipsychotic used for chemical restraint. Diphenhydramine is used to reverse extrapyramidal side effects associated with antipsychotic drugs.

69. C: Before obtaining a patient history or examining the patient, the patient should be moved to a private area; obtaining a sexual history is irrelevant to patient care and may upset the patient. The patient's genitalia should be examined only if severe injury is suspected; the patient's clothing should be disturbed as little as possible to avoid damaging any evidence.

70. B: A pregnant trauma victim should be treated in the same manner as a nonpregnant victim; all pregnant women should be given high-concentration oxygen and transported. Transport should not be delayed to assess fetal heart rate. Women beyond 4 months' gestation should not be transported in the supine position to avoid hypotension; the left lateral recumbent position is preferred. The pneumatic antishock garment is rarely used and only under medical direction.

71. C: In managing a patient with third-trimester bleeding, vaginal examination may increase bleeding and/or induce labor and thus should not be attempted. Airway, ventilatory, and circulatory support should be provided as needed and IV fluid therapy initiated; fundal height should be documented for baseline measurement.

72. A: The Apgar score (appearance, pulse, grimace, activity, respiration) should not be used to determine the need for resuscitation of a baby just born. Presence or absence of crying and/or breathing and appearance of muscle tone should be used to assess the infant; the amniotic fluid should be clear and without signs of infection.

73. B: Packing the vagina should not be attempted to control postpartum hemorrhage; oxytocin and uterine massage may aid in stimulating uterine contraction. Placing the infant close to the mother's breast facilitates breastfeeding and may promote uterine contraction.

74. D: Warning devices are generally used only during transport of patient with life- or limb-threatening injury; lights and sirens should never be used to provide absolute right of way. Police escorts may result in collision as a result of motorist confusion and should not be used in responding to a routine emergency call; low beams should be used during all responses regardless of weather conditions to increase visibility.

75. C: The 2-second rule is useful for gauging braking distance for conventional type I, II, or III emergency vehicles under normal road and weather conditions; braking distance should be increased for larger or heavier vehicles and under poor roadway or weather conditions.

76. D: Air ambulances have specific space and weight restrictions that may limit the number of patients, emergency and flight personnel, and equipment that can be carried. In the urban setting, ground ambulances are faster that air ambulances within a 30-mile range. Although fewer crashes occur with air than with ground ambulances, helicopter crashes have fewer survivors.

77. C: In this case, primary triage should be used to classify accident victims according to treatment priority; the only treatment given during primary triage is to ensure an airway or control severe hemorrhage.

78. B: The START, or simple triage and rapid treatment technique, is used to classify a patient's status in primary triage according to ability to walk, breathing, pulse/perfusion, and mental status; in secondary triage, the patient is reassessed and labeled with a tag indicating priority of care. Critical incident stress management is used to assist distressed rescue personnel after a large-scale incident.

79. A: According to the START technique of primary triage (simple triage and rapid treatment), patients who can walk and understand basic commands are classified as delayed or walking wounded; these patients should be advised to remain at the site for further assistance or to walk to another treatment site. If the patient is unable to walk, the respiratory rate should be assessed.

80. C: A patient with a carotid pulse but no radial pulse should be classified as critical; if both the carotid and radial pulses are present, mental status should be assessed before triage classification. Conscious patients who are able to walk are classified as delayed; if no pulse is present, the patient should be classified as dying.

81. A: Submerged victims should not be lifted onto a back board; rather, the board should be allowed to float up to the patient. Before attempting a water rescue, the paramedic should put on a personal flotation device (PFD); multiple victims submerged in the water should be directed to huddle together to conserve body heat, while a single victim should be told to assume the fetal or heat escape-lessening position (HELP).

82. C: Resuscitation should be attempted in all victims of prolonged exposure to extremely cold water unless death is obvious; rapid hypothermia can actually improve brain viability. Sudden exposure to extremely cold water can cause laryngospasm, resulting in aspiration, hypoxia, and unconsciousness. The effectiveness of the cold protective response depends on the patient's age, lung volume, position in the water, and water temperature.

83. B: On arrival at the site of a confined-space emergency, a copy of the Occupational Safety & Health Administration (OSHA) permit should be obtained to properly assess the scene; in the case of a cave-in or trench collapse, the paramedic should not approach the lip, as the risk of a second collapse is high. Shoring or a trench box is required for cave-ins 5 feet deep or greater; the self-contained breathing apparatus (SCBA) provides only a limited supply of air, may cause entrapment, or may have to be removed to reach the victim, and thus should not be used for confined-space rescue.

84. C: In the case of downed electrical wires, paramedics should not attempt to replace the wires or approach patients until the scene is safe; passengers inside a vehicle entrapped by downed wires should be directed to remain inside to avoid the risk of electrical injury.

85. B: In the case of both deployed and undeployed airbags, the 5-, 10-, 20 rule should be used to determine a safe distance during rescue: a distance of 5 inches should be used for side impact airbags, 10 inches for driver-side airbags, and 20 inches for passenger-side airbags. The car battery

should be disconnected when a passenger is trapped behind an undeployed airbag; to verify that the battery has been disconnected, turn on the lights rather than the ignition. Do not place a hard board or other device between the passenger and the airbag.

86. C: During a rescue attempt, basic life support (BLS) techniques are mandatory, including airway control with supplemental oxygen. Advanced life support (ALS) techniques should only be provided if necessary; endotracheal intubation, IV lines, and ECG leads may complicate the rescue attempt.

87. C: In the case of a potentially violent situation, avoidance, tactical retreat, cover and concealment, and distraction and evasive maneuvers are useful tactics to ensure paramedic safety; confrontation should be avoided.

88. B: A bulletproof vest is effective against most handgun bullets and knives; however, it may not protect against thin or dual-edged weapons such as an ice pick.

89. A: The self-contained breathing apparatus (SCBA) provides the highest level of respiratory protection against hazardous materials; because an air-purifying respirator requires constant monitoring and must be fitted to the wearer, it is not recommended for protection against hazardous materials. Level C clothing is used for transport of contaminated patients; level D clothing provides only minimal protection.

90. D: Patient care in the hot zone should be limited to airway management, spinal immobilization, and hemorrhage control; removal of the patient from the hot zone is usually performed by trained personnel, such as firefighters and/or hazmat teams. IV therapy should only be given under the direction of a physician; invasive procedures such as wound debridement should not be performed to prevent hazardous materials from entering the patient's body.

91. B: Following a hazmat incident, the hazmat team will establish a decontamination corridor; rescue personnel should shower twice to remove any potential contaminants and should be debriefed as to the nature of the hazardous substances, signs or symptoms of exposure, and any acute or chronic health issues that may arise.

92. C: Compared with adults, a child's liver and spleen are larger and more vascular and are thus more easily injured; children also have a larger body surface area-to-body mass ratio, increasing the risk of hypothermia, hyperthermia, and dehydration. Because children are able to use vasoconstriction to decrease the size of blood vessels, they are able to maintain blood pressure longer than adults; for this reason, a child in shock may have a normal blood pressure. In children, the muscles rather than the bones provide the primary means of support for the chest wall.

93. B: In assessing a child who is not acutely ill, the paramedic should allow the child to become more familiar with the paramedic team and medical equipment by conversing with the child and allowing him or her to play with the stethoscope; this "transition stage" may be helpful in putting the child at ease. In a seriously ill or injured child, vital signs should be monitored every 5 minutes and continuous electrocardiogram monitoring should be performed; the physical exam should be conducted from toe to head in children younger than 2 years and from head to toe in older children.

94. A: Barking cough, nasal flaring, cyanosis, and low-grade fever are indicative of croup; croup typically occurs in children 6 months to 4 years of age with a history of recent upper respiratory infection. Patients usually present at night with signs of respiratory distress and may be sitting upright to facilitate breathing. Croup is sometimes confused with epiglottitis, a bacterial infection in children 3 to 7 years of age characterized by swelling of the epiglottis and supraglottic structures; however, unlike croup, epiglottitis is of rapid onset and marked by high fever, drooling, and

Copyright © Mometrix Media. You have been licensed one copy of this document for personal use only. Any other reproduction or redistribution is strictly prohibited. All rights reserved.

inspiratory stridor. Pneumonia is an acute infection of the lower airway and lungs marked by chest pain, rales, rhonchi, and tachypnea.

95. D: Symptoms of croup may be dramatically improved by exposure to cool humidified air; intubation and parenteral antibiotic therapy are indicated in a child with epiglottitis and bronchodilators in a child with severe pneumonia.

96. C: Intubation is usually not indicated in children with status epilepticus unless the child does not respond to initial treatment. Diazepam is effective in treating seizures in the majority of cases; glucagon may be used to treat hypoglycemia. Cardiac monitoring is used to detect cardiac rhythm or conduction abnormalities.

97. B: Insulin is usually not given in the prehospital setting in a child with suspected hyperglycemia; glucose testing should be performed following airway, ventilatory, and circulatory support. IV fluid therapy may be given if the child is dehydrated; if hyperglycemia cannot be confirmed with glucose testing, dextrose may be given to rule out hypoglycemia.

98. D: Possible causes of sudden infant death syndrome (SIDS) include immaturity of the central nervous system, upper airway obstruction, brainstem abnormalities, and cardiac conduction disorders; suffocation, regurgitation or aspiration of vomitus, and allergies are not associated with SIDS.

99. B: The presence of sudden tachycardia and tachypnea, as well as mild discomfort and edema of the calf, is indicative of pulmonary embolism; in the elderly, pulmonary embolism may be associated with congestive heart failure (CHF). Because the signs and symptoms of pulmonary embolism are similar to those of bacterial pneumonia, the two conditions are often mistaken for each other. Dyspnea is commonly seen in elderly patients with bacterial pneumonia, pulmonary embolism, myocardial infarction, and other conditions, making diagnosis difficult. Signs and symptoms of heart failure include dry, hacking productive cough, nocturia, and anorexia.

100. A: Aggressive airway management is indicated in chronic obstructive pulmonary disease (COPD) to treat acidosis and hypoxia, which may be life-threatening. Emergency care for patients with pulmonary embolism and bacterial pneumonia should provide adequate airway, ventilatory, and circulatory support; in patients with cerebral vascular disease, the primary goal of treatment is to identify stroke and transport the patient for immediate care.

101. C: Delirium is characterized by rapid onset of disorientation to time and place and may result from physical illness; dementia and Alzheimer's disease are marked by slow, progressive loss of awareness.

102. B: Rapid fluid IV administration may cause volume overload in the elderly; thus, the paramedic must be careful not to overhydrate an older patient. Partial pressure of oxygen in arterial blood (PaO_2) decreases with age; elderly patients may require higher arterial pressures for perfusion of vital organs as a result of atherosclerotic peripheral vascular disease. Adjustment of heart rate and stroke volume may be decreased in the elderly in response to hypovolemia.

103. D: The rule of nines is used to estimate burn injury size for adults and children over 10 years of age; it may be difficult to apply to irregularly shaped burns or burns scattered over a large area of the body.

104. B: Moderate burns may be classified as partial-thickness burns covering 15% to 25% of body surface area (BSA) in adults and 10% to 20% of BSA in children or the elderly and full-thickness

burns covering less than 10% of BSA; burns from contact with caustic chemicals or high-voltage electricity may be classified as major burns.

105. C: Covering the patient with a sterile blanket will preserve body heat and prevent too much heat loss. Applying ointment or ice to a burn may increase the severity of the injury and/or cause shock. Removal of blisters is at the discretion of the hospital burn-unit and not the concern of the paramedic.

106. B: In patients with carbon monoxide poisoning, the proper line of treatment is to ensure a patent airway, provide ventilation, and administer high-concentration oxygen; sodium thiosulfate and hyperbaric oxygen may also be given. The pulse oximeter is not a reliable indicator of effective oxygenation in cases of carbon monoxide poisoning.

107. C: Contrary to popular belief, asking a patient directly about his or her suicidal intentions does not encourage the patient to commit suicide; following medical care, establishing rapport with the patient and providing emotional support are essential. Law enforcement should only be consulted when the patient is armed.

108. A: A carbon monoxide level of 10% is commonly seen in smokers, truck drivers, traffic police, and others who are chronically exposed to carbon monoxide and is asymptomatic. A carbon monoxide level of 20% may cause nausea and vomiting, 30% may cause electrocardiogram abnormalities, and 40% to 60% may cause coma.

109. D: Administering osmotic diuretics and/or steroids to a patient with increasing intracranial pressure may reduce cerebral edema and inflammation. IV fluid therapy should be restricted in such patients; the Valsalva maneuver may increase intraabdominal pressure. Blood replacement therapy is used in patients with acute blood loss.

110. B: Pulmonary capillary wedge pressure (PCWP), pulmonary artery pressure (PAP) monitoring, and left atrial pressure (LAP) monitoring provide an accurate measure of left ventricular function; right atrial pressure (RAP) monitoring directly measures pressure in the right atrium and indirectly measures right ventricular pressure.

111. C: Epinephrine stimulates respiration and ventilation. Diazepam and morphine may decrease respiration; however, aspirin does not significantly affect respiratory function.

112. A: Morphine is considered a Pregnancy Category B drug and may be given to a pregnant woman in low doses for a short period of time; aspirin and diazepam are Category D drugs and should not be given during pregnancy except in the case of life-threatening disease. Oxytocin is administered after delivery to control postpartum bleeding.

113. C: Category C drugs may be given in pregnancy only if the potential benefit justifies the fetal risk; Category X drugs carry significant fetal risk and are contraindicated in pregnancy. Category B drugs have not been confirmed to provide a risk to pregnant women; Category D drugs are only indicated in the case of life-threatening disease.

114. B: The nasal cannula delivers only low-concentration oxygen and thus should be reserved for patients with chest pain or chronic pulmonary disease; it should not be used in patients with severe hypoxia, apnea, or respiratory insufficiency.

115. A: The bag-mask device may be used in patients with respiratory insufficiency or with a variety of pathological conditions; the nasal cannula and partial nonbreather and nonbreather masks should not be used in patients with apnea or respiratory insufficiency.

116. B: Use of the oropharyngeal or nasopharyngeal airway is indicated in an unconscious patient; the jaw-thrust position without the head-tilt technique should be used in those with suspected spinal injury. In the mouth-to-nose technique, the paramedic should keep one hand on the patient's forehead and use the other to close the patient's mouth. The mouth-to-stoma ventilation method is bacteriologically safer than the mouth-to-mouth technique.

117. A: The bag-mask device is primarily used for pediatric patients in respiratory arrest and should not be used to provide supplemental oxygen to a spontaneously breathing child; it may be used with a mask in patients who have not been intubated and is effective in extreme environmental temperatures.

118. D: The nasal airway may be used in unconscious patients and in those with cervical spine injury or seizures; however, it is contraindicated in patients with fractures of the basal skull or facial bones.

119. B: Cuffed endotracheal tubes are not indicated for infants or children under 8 years of age because narrowing of the cricoid cartilage acts as a natural cuff and prevents air leakage; they may, however, be used in older children.

120. D: Blind intubation is not an accepted prehospital procedure and should only be performed when the airway cannot be visualized due to the presence of blood or other secretions, in the case of patient entrapment, or in disaster situations with many victims and limited equipment. Nasotracheal intubation is a blind procedure and is only indicated in patients with spontaneous respirations, when laryngoscopy cannot be performed, or when movement of the cervical spine is limited; blind intubation is not indicated in patients with spinal injury.

121. C: Inaccurate pulse oximeter readings may result from a variety of factors, including hypotension, jaundice, hypothermia/vasoconstriction, and patient use of nail polish.

122. D: Manual in-line stabilization is required for intubation of patients with suspected spinal injuries; intubation of these patients is dangerous and must be authorized by medical direction.

123. B: The laryngeal mask airway (LMA) may be used in patients with an unstable neck injury, when conventional endotracheal intubation is unsuccessful, or when the patient cannot be positioned for tracheal intubation; patients must be unresponsive and without an intact gag reflex.

124. A: Paralytic agents are indicated in agitated or combative patients who require emergency intubation, such as those with a head injury or other trauma, and are acceptable for use in children; however, these agents should not be used in patients in whom ventilation or intubation may be difficult, such as those with facial hair, short necks, or obstructions.

125. C: Rapid sequence intubation (RSI) is used to rapidly bring a patient to an unconscious state through complete neuromuscular paralysis. The Mallampati score is used to assess the difficulty of intubation; preoxygenation with 100% oxygen is then accomplished, followed by pretreatment with lidocaine to prevent an increase in intracranial pressure and/or laryngospasm. Cricothyrotomy should only be performed if RSI is unsuccessful.

126. B: Airbags are most effective in frontal or near-frontal collisions.

127. D: A parent and child should never be secured to a stretcher together; however, a child safety seat can be safely secured to a stretcher using two belts placed at a 90º angle to each other. Infants and young children can be transported safely in a conventional child safety seat; older children can be secured to a stretcher.

128. C: Hypovolemia is associated with a variety of conditions and injuries such as hemorrhage, dehydration, burns, endocrine disorders, and tissue injury. Hypovolemia may occur in septic shock, and elements of cardiogenic shock may occur in hypovolemia; fainting is associated with vasogenic shock, a mild, reversible form of shock.

129. B: Unconsciousness, delayed capillary refill, and decreased systolic and diastolic blood pressure are signs of uncompensated shock. Hypotension and coma are signs of irreversible shock; patients in compensated shock may be confused or combative.

130. C: Patients in cardiogenic shock may show signs of congestive heart failure such as jugular vein distention. Anaphylactic shock and septic shock are types of distributive shock, which may result from vasodilation; signs of distributive shock include warm, flushed skin.

131. A: Wounds that require closure include ring finger injuries, wounds to the face, lips, or eyebrows, wounds over joints, and degloving injuries; abrasions are partial-thickness skin injuries resulting from the scraping or rubbing away of layers of skin. Contusions result from blood vessel disruption below the epidermis and may cause bruising; puncture wounds such as those caused by an animal bite are generally small but may result in severe injury to underlying tissue.

132. B: The first step in controlling hemorrhage should be to apply direct pressure over the injury; a pressure dressing may then be applied over the wound and secured with an elastic bandage. Splinting alone is not effective as a means to control bleeding; a pneumatic pressure device should be used only after other methods have been tried to control bleeding. A tourniquet is not indicated as a means to control hemorrhage and should be used only as a last resort.

133. C: Prehospital care of an open wound usually involves cleansing the wound with sterile water, applying an antibacterial ointment if the patient is not allergic, and dressing the wound; debridement of the wound should not be attempted.

134. A: Crush syndrome may result from prolonged immobilization or compression such as in a building collapse or other catastrophic event when patient rescue has been delayed for several hours. Treatment of potential crush syndrome should include administration of high concentration oxygen, aggressive hydration with 5% dextrose in water and 0.45% normal saline, and alkalinization of the urine; calcium chloride is not indicated unless the patient is at risk of hyperkalemia. Furosemide may acidify the urine and should not be given; fasciotomy of a crushed limb is not recommended in the prehospital setting because of the risk of infection and must be authorized by medical direction.

135. C: Transport should not be delayed to search for an amputated limb; however, if the amputated limb is found, it should be treated in the same manner as avulsed tissue. Direct pressure and elevation should be used to control hemorrhage the remaining portion of the left leg; fasciotomy or application of a tourniquet is not recommended.

136. C: The mechanism of injury (MOI) must be assessed to determine the need for spinal immobilization. Spinal immobilization is necessary in the case of a positive MOI, such as a high-speed motor vehicle accident, a fall from greater than 3 times the patient's height, or a blunt or penetrating injury near the patient's spine, but is not required when the MOI is negative, as in the

case of a twisted ankle, an object dropped on the foot, or an isolated soft-tissue injury. When the MOI is uncertain, as in the case of a low-speed motor vehicle crash, the paramedic must assess the reliability of the patient to determine the need for spinal immobilization; patients who are intoxicated, in an abnormal mental state, or who have distracting injuries are not considered reliable.

137. B: Spinal injury can occur with or without spinal cord injury (SCI); likewise, SCI can occur without spinal injury. SCI without radiological evidence of spinal injury is more commonly seen in children.

138. D: Short spine boards are primarily used for spinal immobilization of patients in a sitting position or in a confined space; a rigid collar alone is insufficient for spinal immobilization and should be used in conjunction with a short or long spine board. Long spine boards should be used for spinal immobilization of unstable patients with life-threatening injuries, patients requiring immediate resuscitation, or in situations where the time required to apply the device would put the patient's life in jeopardy. Immobilization of the torso to a long spine board should be performed before immobilizing the head.

139. C: A short spine board should be used for patients in a sitting position or in a confined space. Prehospital care of a pediatric patient with suspected spinal injury should include manual in-line immobilization, placement of a rigid cervical collar, and immobilization on a long spine board; an adult long spine board may be used if a pediatric device is not available. Full-face helmets should be removed to assess the patient's airway and ventilatory function.

140. B: Signs and symptoms of spinal shock include paralysis distal to the injury site, hypotension, vasodilation, and loss of bowel and bladder control; neurogenic hypotension is a rare condition and is not usually a cause of hypotension in patients with suspected spine injury. Autonomic hyperreflexia is marked by paroxysmal hypertension, bradycardia, and distended bladder or rectum; spondylosis is a structural defect of the spine and may result in stress fracture.

141. C: Tension pneumothorax is a life-threatening condition and must be managed immediately in the prehospital setting; signs and symptoms of tension pneumothorax include distended neck veins, diminished or absent breath sounds, increasing dyspnea, and hypotension. Open pneumothorax results from exposure of the pleural space to atmospheric pressure due to chest injury and is characterized by a sucking or gurgling sound through the open chest wound; closed pneumothorax occurs in patients with penetrating chest trauma and is marked by chest pain, dyspnea, and tachypnea. Flail chest occurs when three or more ribs are fractured in two or more places and is characterized by paradoxical movement of the injured section of the chest wall during breathing.

142. D: Tension pneumothorax is an often fatal condition that occurs when air in the thoracic cavity is trapped in the pleural space; the condition may result from sealing an open pneumothorax with an occlusive dressing. Chest percussion alone is not reliable in identifying tension pneumothorax; thoracic decompression may be used to relieve tension pneumothorax in patients with closed chest trauma.

143. C: Management of an abdominal injury should be limited to stabilizing the patient and rapidly transporting him or her for surgical care; eviscerated organs should not be replaced into the peritoneal cavity because of the risk of infection. A thorough on-scene survey should be performed to identify the cause of the abdominal injury; airway maintenance, ventilatory support, and fluid

replacement should be provided, and use of a pneumatic antishock garment (PASG) may be indicated depending on local protocol.

144. D: Traction splints should be used only for midshaft femoral fractures and should not be used for injuries of the hip or knee or fractures of the pelvis.

145. B: A severe fracture or dislocated joint (with exception of elbow) can be safely realigned and should be immobilized in the direction of the injury; successful realignment of the knee or hip is indicated by a "popping" into the joint. Realignment of a dislocated elbow should never be attempted in the prehospital setting.

146. A: An extra heart sound may be heard before S_1 or after S_2 and may be indicative of congestive heart failure. The first heart sign occurs during ventricular systole and the second during ventricular diastole; heart sounds are not indicative of myocardial infarction.

147. B: The augmented limb lead aV_F is an example of a unipolar electrocardiogram (ECG) lead; limb leads I, II, and II are bipolar limb leads and V_1 to V_6 unipolar chest leads.

148. D: The QRS complex follows the P wave; the ST segment immediately follows the QRS complex. The T wave is the first deviation from the ST segment and ends with the return of the T wave to baseline. The Q-T interval is measured from the beginning of the QRS complex to the end of the T wave.

149. B: The triplicate and R-R methods are useful in determining heart rate only when the heart rhythm is regular; when used alone, the heart rate calculator ruler is not a reliable method of calculating heart rate and is accurate only when the rhythm is regular. Although the 6-second count method is the least accurate means of determining heart rate, it is useful in estimating heart rate in the presence of an irregular rhythm.

150. C: Vagal maneuvers and adenosine should be used as first-line treatment of paroxysmal supraventricular tachycardia; the Valsalva maneuver may successfully terminate tachycardia. Magnesium is used in the treatment of atrial fibrillation or flutter.

How to Overcome Test Anxiety

Just the thought of taking a test is enough to make most people a little nervous. A test is an important event that can have a long-term impact on your future, so it's important to take it seriously and it's natural to feel anxious about performing well. But just because anxiety is normal, that doesn't mean that it's helpful in test taking, or that you should simply accept it as part of your life. Anxiety can have a variety of effects. These effects can be mild, like making you feel slightly nervous, or severe, like blocking your ability to focus or remember even a simple detail.

If you experience test anxiety—whether severe or mild—it's important to know how to beat it. To discover this, first you need to understand what causes test anxiety.

Causes of Test Anxiety

While we often think of anxiety as an uncontrollable emotional state, it can actually be caused by simple, practical things. One of the most common causes of test anxiety is that a person does not feel adequately prepared for their test. This feeling can be the result of many different issues such as poor study habits or lack of organization, but the most common culprit is time management. Starting to study too late, failing to organize your study time to cover all of the material, or being distracted while you study will mean that you're not well prepared for the test. This may lead to cramming the night before, which will cause you to be physically and mentally exhausted for the test. Poor time management also contributes to feelings of stress, fear, and hopelessness as you realize you are not well prepared but don't know what to do about it.

Other times, test anxiety is not related to your preparation for the test but comes from unresolved fear. This may be a past failure on a test, or poor performance on tests in general. It may come from comparing yourself to others who seem to be performing better or from the stress of living up to expectations. Anxiety may be driven by fears of the future—how failure on this test would affect your educational and career goals. These fears are often completely irrational, but they can still negatively impact your test performance.

> **Review Video:** 3 Reasons You Have Test Anxiety
> Visit mometrix.com/academy and enter code: 428468

Elements of Test Anxiety

As mentioned earlier, test anxiety is considered to be an emotional state, but it has physical and mental components as well. Sometimes you may not even realize that you are suffering from test anxiety until you notice the physical symptoms. These can include trembling hands, rapid heartbeat, sweating, nausea, and tense muscles. Extreme anxiety may lead to fainting or vomiting. Obviously, any of these symptoms can have a negative impact on testing. It is important to recognize them as soon as they begin to occur so that you can address the problem before it damages your performance.

> **Review Video:** 3 Ways to Tell You Have Test Anxiety
> Visit mometrix.com/academy and enter code: 927847

The mental components of test anxiety include trouble focusing and inability to remember learned information. During a test, your mind is on high alert, which can help you recall information and stay focused for an extended period of time. However, anxiety interferes with your mind's natural processes, causing you to blank out, even on the questions you know well. The strain of testing during anxiety makes it difficult to stay focused, especially on a test that may take several hours. Extreme anxiety can take a huge mental toll, making it difficult not only to recall test information but even to understand the test questions or pull your thoughts together.

> **Review Video:** How Test Anxiety Affects Memory
> Visit mometrix.com/academy and enter code: 609003

Effects of Test Anxiety

Test anxiety is like a disease—if left untreated, it will get progressively worse. Anxiety leads to poor performance, and this reinforces the feelings of fear and failure, which in turn lead to poor performances on subsequent tests. It can grow from a mild nervousness to a crippling condition. If allowed to progress, test anxiety can have a big impact on your schooling, and consequently on your future.

Test anxiety can spread to other parts of your life. Anxiety on tests can become anxiety in any stressful situation, and blanking on a test can turn into panicking in a job situation. But fortunately, you don't have to let anxiety rule your testing and determine your grades. There are a number of relatively simple steps you can take to move past anxiety and function normally on a test and in the rest of life.

> **Review Video:** How Test Anxiety Impacts Your Grades
> Visit mometrix.com/academy and enter code: 939819

Physical Steps for Beating Test Anxiety

While test anxiety is a serious problem, the good news is that it can be overcome. It doesn't have to control your ability to think and remember information. While it may take time, you can begin taking steps today to beat anxiety.

Just as your first hint that you may be struggling with anxiety comes from the physical symptoms, the first step to treating it is also physical. Rest is crucial for having a clear, strong mind. If you are tired, it is much easier to give in to anxiety. But if you establish good sleep habits, your body and mind will be ready to perform optimally, without the strain of exhaustion. Additionally, sleeping well helps you to retain information better, so you're more likely to recall the answers when you see the test questions.

Getting good sleep means more than going to bed on time. It's important to allow your brain time to relax. Take study breaks from time to time so it doesn't get overworked, and don't study right before bed. Take time to rest your mind before trying to rest your body, or you may find it difficult to fall asleep.

> **Review Video: The Importance of Sleep for Your Brain**
> Visit mometrix.com/academy and enter code: 319338

Along with sleep, other aspects of physical health are important in preparing for a test. Good nutrition is vital for good brain function. Sugary foods and drinks may give a burst of energy but this burst is followed by a crash, both physically and emotionally. Instead, fuel your body with protein and vitamin-rich foods.

Also, drink plenty of water. Dehydration can lead to headaches and exhaustion, especially if your brain is already under stress from the rigors of the test. Particularly if your test is a long one, drink water during the breaks. And if possible, take an energy-boosting snack to eat between sections.

> **Review Video: How Diet Can Affect your Mood**
> Visit mometrix.com/academy and enter code: 624317

Along with sleep and diet, a third important part of physical health is exercise. Maintaining a steady workout schedule is helpful, but even taking 5-minute study breaks to walk can help get your blood pumping faster and clear your head. Exercise also releases endorphins, which contribute to a positive feeling and can help combat test anxiety.

When you nurture your physical health, you are also contributing to your mental health. If your body is healthy, your mind is much more likely to be healthy as well. So take time to rest, nourish your body with healthy food and water, and get moving as much as possible. Taking these physical steps will make you stronger and more able to take the mental steps necessary to overcome test anxiety.

> **Review Video: How to Stay Healthy and Prevent Test Anxiety**
> Visit mometrix.com/academy and enter code: 877894

Mental Steps for Beating Test Anxiety

Working on the mental side of test anxiety can be more challenging, but as with the physical side, there are clear steps you can take to overcome it. As mentioned earlier, test anxiety often stems from lack of preparation, so the obvious solution is to prepare for the test. Effective studying may be the most important weapon you have for beating test anxiety, but you can and should employ several other mental tools to combat fear.

First, boost your confidence by reminding yourself of past success—tests or projects that you aced. If you're putting as much effort into preparing for this test as you did for those, there's no reason you should expect to fail here. Work hard to prepare; then trust your preparation.

Second, surround yourself with encouraging people. It can be helpful to find a study group, but be sure that the people you're around will encourage a positive attitude. If you spend time with others who are anxious or cynical, this will only contribute to your own anxiety. Look for others who are motivated to study hard from a desire to succeed, not from a fear of failure.

Third, reward yourself. A test is physically and mentally tiring, even without anxiety, and it can be helpful to have something to look forward to. Plan an activity following the test, regardless of the outcome, such as going to a movie or getting ice cream.

When you are taking the test, if you find yourself beginning to feel anxious, remind yourself that you know the material. Visualize successfully completing the test. Then take a few deep, relaxing breaths and return to it. Work through the questions carefully but with confidence, knowing that you are capable of succeeding.

Developing a healthy mental approach to test taking will also aid in other areas of life. Test anxiety affects more than just the actual test—it can be damaging to your mental health and even contribute to depression. It's important to beat test anxiety before it becomes a problem for more than testing.

> **Review Video: Test Anxiety and Depression**
> Visit mometrix.com/academy and enter code: 904704

Study Strategy

Being prepared for the test is necessary to combat anxiety, but what does being prepared look like? You may study for hours on end and still not feel prepared. What you need is a strategy for test prep. The next few pages outline our recommended steps to help you plan out and conquer the challenge of preparation.

Step 1: Scope Out the Test

Learn everything you can about the format (multiple choice, essay, etc.) and what will be on the test. Gather any study materials, course outlines, or sample exams that may be available. Not only will this help you to prepare, but knowing what to expect can help to alleviate test anxiety.

Step 2: Map Out the Material

Look through the textbook or study guide and make note of how many chapters or sections it has. Then divide these over the time you have. For example, if a book has 15 chapters and you have five days to study, you need to cover three chapters each day. Even better, if you have the time, leave an extra day at the end for overall review after you have gone through the material in depth.

If time is limited, you may need to prioritize the material. Look through it and make note of which sections you think you already have a good grasp on, and which need review. While you are studying, skim quickly through the familiar sections and take more time on the challenging parts. Write out your plan so you don't get lost as you go. Having a written plan also helps you feel more in control of the study, so anxiety is less likely to arise from feeling overwhelmed at the amount to cover. A sample plan may look like this:

- Day 1: Skim chapters 1–4, study chapter 5 (especially pages 31–33)
- Day 2: Study chapters 6–7, skim chapters 8–9
- Day 3: Skim chapter 10, study chapters 11–12 (especially pages 87–90)
- Day 4: Study chapters 13–15
- Day 5: Overall review (focus most on chapters 5, 6, and 12), take practice test

Step 3: Gather Your Tools

Decide what study method works best for you. Do you prefer to highlight in the book as you study and then go back over the highlighted portions? Or do you type out notes of the important information? Or is it helpful to make flashcards that you can carry with you? Assemble the pens, index cards, highlighters, post-it notes, and any other materials you may need so you won't be distracted by getting up to find things while you study.

If you're having a hard time retaining the information or organizing your notes, experiment with different methods. For example, try color-coding by subject with colored pens, highlighters, or post-it notes. If you learn better by hearing, try recording yourself reading your notes so you can listen while in the car, working out, or simply sitting at your desk. Ask a friend to quiz you from your flashcards, or try teaching someone the material to solidify it in your mind.

Step 4: Create Your Environment

It's important to avoid distractions while you study. This includes both the obvious distractions like visitors and the subtle distractions like an uncomfortable chair (or a too-comfortable couch that makes you want to fall asleep). Set up the best study environment possible: good lighting and a comfortable work area. If background music helps you focus, you may want to turn it on, but otherwise keep the room quiet. If you are using a computer to take notes, be sure you don't have any other windows open, especially applications like social media, games, or anything else that could distract you. Silence your phone and turn off notifications. Be sure to keep water close by so you stay hydrated while you study (but avoid unhealthy drinks and snacks).

Also, take into account the best time of day to study. Are you freshest first thing in the morning? Try to set aside some time then to work through the material. Is your mind clearer in the afternoon or evening? Schedule your study session then. Another method is to study at the same time of day that you will take the test, so that your brain gets used to working on the material at that time and will be ready to focus at test time.

Step 5: Study!

Once you have done all the study preparation, it's time to settle into the actual studying. Sit down, take a few moments to settle your mind so you can focus, and begin to follow your study plan. Don't give in to distractions or let yourself procrastinate. This is your time to prepare so you'll be ready to fearlessly approach the test. Make the most of the time and stay focused.

Of course, you don't want to burn out. If you study too long you may find that you're not retaining the information very well. Take regular study breaks. For example, taking five minutes out of every hour to walk briskly, breathing deeply and swinging your arms, can help your mind stay fresh.

As you get to the end of each chapter or section, it's a good idea to do a quick review. Remind yourself of what you learned and work on any difficult parts. When you feel that you've mastered the material, move on to the next part. At the end of your study session, briefly skim through your notes again.

But while review is helpful, cramming last minute is NOT. If at all possible, work ahead so that you won't need to fit all your study into the last day. Cramming overloads your brain with more information than it can process and retain, and your tired mind may struggle to recall even previously learned information when it is overwhelmed with last-minute study. Also, the urgent nature of cramming and the stress placed on your brain contribute to anxiety. You'll be more likely to go to the test feeling unprepared and having trouble thinking clearly.

So don't cram, and don't stay up late before the test, even just to review your notes at a leisurely pace. Your brain needs rest more than it needs to go over the information again. In fact, plan to finish your studies by noon or early afternoon the day before the test. Give your brain the rest of the day to relax or focus on other things, and get a good night's sleep. Then you will be fresh for the test and better able to recall what you've studied.

Step 6: Take a practice test

Many courses offer sample tests, either online or in the study materials. This is an excellent resource to check whether you have mastered the material, as well as to prepare for the test format and environment.

Check the test format ahead of time: the number of questions, the type (multiple choice, free response, etc.), and the time limit. Then create a plan for working through them. For example, if you have 30 minutes to take a 60-question test, your limit is 30 seconds per question. Spend less time on the questions you know well so that you can take more time on the difficult ones.

If you have time to take several practice tests, take the first one open book, with no time limit. Work through the questions at your own pace and make sure you fully understand them. Gradually work up to taking a test under test conditions: sit at a desk with all study materials put away and set a timer. Pace yourself to make sure you finish the test with time to spare and go back to check your answers if you have time.

After each test, check your answers. On the questions you missed, be sure you understand why you missed them. Did you misread the question (tests can use tricky wording)? Did you forget the information? Or was it something you hadn't learned? Go back and study any shaky areas that the practice tests reveal.

Taking these tests not only helps with your grade, but also aids in combating test anxiety. If you're already used to the test conditions, you're less likely to worry about it, and working through tests until you're scoring well gives you a confidence boost. Go through the practice tests until you feel comfortable, and then you can go into the test knowing that you're ready for it.

Test Tips

On test day, you should be confident, knowing that you've prepared well and are ready to answer the questions. But aside from preparation, there are several test day strategies you can employ to maximize your performance.

First, as stated before, get a good night's sleep the night before the test (and for several nights before that, if possible). Go into the test with a fresh, alert mind rather than staying up late to study.

Try not to change too much about your normal routine on the day of the test. It's important to eat a nutritious breakfast, but if you normally don't eat breakfast at all, consider eating just a protein bar. If you're a coffee drinker, go ahead and have your normal coffee. Just make sure you time it so that the caffeine doesn't wear off right in the middle of your test. Avoid sugary beverages, and drink enough water to stay hydrated but not so much that you need a restroom break 10 minutes into the test. If your test isn't first thing in the morning, consider going for a walk or doing a light workout before the test to get your blood flowing.

Allow yourself enough time to get ready, and leave for the test with plenty of time to spare so you won't have the anxiety of scrambling to arrive in time. Another reason to be early is to select a good seat. It's helpful to sit away from doors and windows, which can be distracting. Find a good seat, get out your supplies, and settle your mind before the test begins.

When the test begins, start by going over the instructions carefully, even if you already know what to expect. Make sure you avoid any careless mistakes by following the directions.

Then begin working through the questions, pacing yourself as you've practiced. If you're not sure on an answer, don't spend too much time on it, and don't let it shake your confidence. Either skip it and come back later, or eliminate as many wrong answers as possible and guess among the remaining ones. Don't dwell on these questions as you continue—put them out of your mind and focus on what lies ahead.

Be sure to read all of the answer choices, even if you're sure the first one is the right answer. Sometimes you'll find a better one if you keep reading. But don't second-guess yourself if you do immediately know the answer. Your gut instinct is usually right. Don't let test anxiety rob you of the information you know.

If you have time at the end of the test (and if the test format allows), go back and review your answers. Be cautious about changing any, since your first instinct tends to be correct, but make sure you didn't misread any of the questions or accidentally mark the wrong answer choice. Look over any you skipped and make an educated guess.

At the end, leave the test feeling confident. You've done your best, so don't waste time worrying about your performance or wishing you could change anything. Instead, celebrate the successful completion of this test. And finally, use this test to learn how to deal with anxiety even better next time.

> **Review Video: 5 Tips to Beat Test Anxiety**
> Visit mometrix.com/academy and enter code: 570656

Important Qualification

Not all anxiety is created equal. If your test anxiety is causing major issues in your life beyond the classroom or testing center, or if you are experiencing troubling physical symptoms related to your anxiety, it may be a sign of a serious physiological or psychological condition. If this sounds like your situation, we strongly encourage you to seek professional help.

Thank You

We at Mometrix would like to extend our heartfelt thanks to you, our friend and patron, for allowing us to play a part in your journey. It is a privilege to serve people from all walks of life who are unified in their commitment to building the best future they can for themselves.

The preparation you devote to these important testing milestones may be the most valuable educational opportunity you have for making a real difference in your life. We encourage you to put your heart into it—that feeling of succeeding, overcoming, and yes, conquering will be well worth the hours you've invested.

We want to hear your story, your struggles and your successes, and if you see any opportunities for us to improve our materials so we can help others even more effectively in the future, please share that with us as well. **The team at Mometrix would be absolutely thrilled to hear from you!** So please, send us an email (support@mometrix.com) and let's stay in touch.

If you'd like some additional help, check out these other resources we offer for your exam:

http://MometrixFlashcards.com/EMT

Additional Bonus Material

Due to our efforts to try to keep this book to a manageable length, we've created a link that will give you access to all of your additional bonus material.

Please visit **https://www.mometrix.com/bonus948/paramedic** to access the information.